Emerging and Re-Emerging Diseases—Novel Challenges in Today's World

Emerging and Re-Emerging Diseases—Novel Challenges in Today's World

Editor

João R. Mesquita

MDPI • Basel • Beijing • Wuhan • Barcelona • Belgrade • Manchester • Tokyo • Cluj • Tianjin

Editor
João R. Mesquita
Instituto de Ciências Biomédicas
Abel Salar (ICBAS)
Universidade do Porto
Porto
Portugal

Editorial Office
MDPI
St. Alban-Anlage 66
4052 Basel, Switzerland

This is a reprint of articles from the Special Issue published online in the open access journal *Animals* (ISSN 2076-2615) (available at: www.mdpi.com/journal/animals/special_issues/Emerging_Re-Emerging_Diseases_Novel_Challenges_Today_World).

For citation purposes, cite each article independently as indicated on the article page online and as indicated below:

LastName, A.A.; LastName, B.B.; LastName, C.C. Article Title. *Journal Name* **Year**, *Volume Number*, Page Range.

ISBN 978-3-0365-1897-8 (Hbk)
ISBN 978-3-0365-1896-1 (PDF)

Contents

About the Editor . . . . **vii**

Preface to "Emerging and Re-Emerging Diseases—Novel Challenges in Today's World" . . . . **ix**

João R. Mesquita
Emerging and Re-Emerging Diseases: Novel Challenges in Today's World or More of the Same?
Reprinted from: *Animals* **2021**, *11*, 2382, doi:10.3390/ani11082382 . . . . **1**

Jennah Green, Catherine Jakins, Eyob Asfaw, Nicholas Bruschi, Abbie Parker, Louise de Waal and Neil D'Cruze
African Lions and Zoonotic Diseases: Implications for Commercial Lion Farms in South Africa
Reprinted from: *Animals* **2020**, *10*, 1692, doi:10.3390/ani10091692 . . . . **5**

Saleh Al-Quraishy, Fathy Abdel-Ghaffar, Mohamed A. Dkhil and Rewaida Abdel-Gaber
Haemogregarines and Criteria for Identification
Reprinted from: *Animals* **2021**, *11*, 170, doi:10.3390/ani11010170 . . . . **21**

Danny Franciele da Silva Dias Moraes, João R. Mesquita, Valéria Dutra and Maria São José Nascimento
Systematic Review of Hepatitis E Virus in Brazil: A One-Health Approach of the Human-Animal-Environment Triad
Reprinted from: *Animals* **2021**, *11*, 2290, doi:10.3390/ani11082290 . . . . **47**

Abdelaziz Ghanemi, Mayumi Yoshioka and Jonny St-Amand
High-Fat Diet-Induced Trefoil Factor Family Member 2 (TFF2) to Counteract the Immune-Mediated Damage in Mice
Reprinted from: *Animals* **2021**, *11*, 258, doi:10.3390/ani11020258 . . . . **75**

Abdelaziz Ghanemi, Mayumi Yoshioka and Jonny St-Amand
Trefoil Factor Family Member 2 (TFF2) as an Inflammatory-Induced and Anti-Inflammatory Tissue Repair Factor
Reprinted from: *Animals* **2020**, *10*, 1646, doi:10.3390/ani10091646 . . . . **81**

Mohamed S. Ahmed, Reda E. Khalafalla, Ashraf Al-Brakati, Tokuma Yanai and Ehab Kotb Elmahallawy
Descriptive Pathological Study of Avian Schistosomes Infection in Whooper Swans (*Cygnus cygnus*) in Japan
Reprinted from: *Animals* **2020**, *10*, 2361, doi:10.3390/ani10122361 . . . . **87**

Diéssy Kipper, Laura M. Carroll, Andrea K. Mascitti, André F. Streck, André S. K. Fonseca, Nilo Ikuta and Vagner R. Lunge
Genomic Characterization of *Salmonella* Minnesota Clonal Lineages Associated with Poultry Production in Brazil
Reprinted from: *Animals* **2020**, *10*, 2043, doi:10.3390/ani10112043 . . . . **99**

Shaimaa Talat, Reham R. Abouelmaatti, Rafa Almeer, Mohamed M. Abdel-Daim and Wael K. Elfeil
Comparison of the Effectiveness of Two Different Vaccination Regimes for Avian Influenza H9N2 in Broiler Chicken
Reprinted from: *Animals* **2020**, *10*, 1875, doi:10.3390/ani10101875 . . . . **113**

Mohamed El-Tholoth, Michael G. Mauk, Yasser F. Elnaker, Samah M. Mosad, Amin Tahoun, Mohamed W. El-Sherif, Maha S. Lokman, Rami B. Kassab, Ahmed Abdelsadik, Ayman A. Saleh and Ehab Kotb Elmahallawy
Molecular Characterization and Developing a Point-of-Need Molecular Test for Diagnosis of Bovine Papillomavirus (BPV) Type 1 in Cattle from Egypt
Reprinted from: *Animals* **2020**, *10*, 1929, doi:10.3390/ani10101929 . . . . **125**

Zafer Yazici, Emre Ozan, Cuneyt Tamer, Bahadir Muftuoglu, Gerald Barry, Hanne Nur Kurucay, Ahmed Eisa Elhag, Abdurrahman Anil Cagirgan, Semra Gumusova and Harun Albayrak
Circulation of Indigenous Bovine Respiratory Syncytial Virus Strains in Turkish Cattle: The First Isolation and Molecular Characterization
Reprinted from: *Animals* **2020**, *10*, 1700, doi:10.3390/ani10091700 . . . . **139**

Patrícia F. Barradas, Clara Lima, Luís Cardoso, Irina Amorim, Fátima Gärtner and João R. Mesquita
Molecular Evidence of *Hemolivia mauritanica*, *Ehrlichia* spp. and the Endosymbiont *Candidatus* Midichloria Mitochondrii in *Hyalomma aegyptium* Infesting *Testudo graeca* Tortoises from Doha, Qatar
Reprinted from: *Animals* **2020**, *11*, 30, doi:10.3390/ani11010030 . . . . **149**

About the Editor

João R. Mesquita

João R. Mesquita (Mesquita JR) holds a bachelor in veterinary medicine and an MSc and a PhD in virology. He is a Diplomate of the European College of Veterinary Microbiology since 2019 and has been teaching since 2006, currently affiliated with Instituto de Ciências Biomédicas Abel Salazar, Universidade do Porto. His research interests are focused primarily on human and animal infectious diseases, particularly on zoonotic agents, with special emphasis on surveillance and epidemiological tools, as well with infection control. He is an author and co-author of several research papers and book chapters, as well as editor for several scientific journals. ORCID: 0000-0001-8769-8103.

Preface to "Emerging and Re-Emerging Diseases—Novel Challenges in Today's World"

It is known today that more than 61% of human pathogens are zoonotic, representing 75% of all emerging pathogens during the past decade, which is an increasing matter of concern, particularly in modern days where global warming aids is causing the introduction of exotic infectious agents or disease vectors into new regions. This book compiles studies that approach a myriad of zoonotic infectious diseases that broadly impact populations and the environment. This is a brief but in-depth collection that showcases the need to address health at the animal–human–environment interface, in a One Health perspective. The global perspective highlighted by the content of this Special Issue reinforces the need for joint and wide efforts by stakeholders. Acknowledgements are made to all authors who generated the data and provided meaningful contributions to this book, as well as to all colleagues who reviewed, read, and dispersed the information contained.

João R. Mesquita
Editor

animals

Editorial

Emerging and Re-Emerging Diseases: Novel Challenges in Today's World or More of the Same?

João R. Mesquita [1,2]

[1] Instituto de Ciências Biomédicas Abel Salar (ICBAS), Universidade do Porto, 4050-313 Porto, Portugal; jrmesquita@icbas.up.pt; Tel.: +351-220-428-000
[2] Epidemiology Research Unit (EPIUnit), Instituto de Saúde Pública da Universidade do Porto (ISPUP), 4050-313 Porto, Portugal

Abstract: More than 61% of all human pathogens are zoonotic, representing 75% of all emerging pathogens during the past decade. Albeit significant technological leaps in diagnostics development and disease surveillance, zoonotic emerging infectious diseases are evermore a matter of concern, particularly in modern days where global warming keeps providing ideal climatic conditions to the introduction of exotic infectious agents or disease vectors in new territories. Worryingly, the 2019 novel coronavirus epidemic acts as an extreme reminder of the role animal reservoirs play in public health, accounting for over 4,200,000 deaths worldwide until today. In this Special Issue, we approach a myriad of zoonotic infectious diseases and their complex mechanisms. This Special Issue is composed of three reviews on zoonotic diseases of African Lions, hemogregarine classification, and hepatitis E virus in Brazil, followed by one letter and one opinion piece that broadens the spectrum of disease emergence to mechanistic aspects of emerging non-communicable diseases. The Special Issue is completed by six research papers covering a wide array of emerging and re-emerging diseases of poultry, bovine, poultry and tortoises, of various nature such as parasitic, bacterial, and viral. This is a brief but assertive collection that showcases the need to address health at the animal–human–environment interface, in a One Health perspective.

check for updates

Citation: Mesquita, J.R. Emerging and Re-Emerging Diseases: Novel Challenges in Today's World or More of the Same?. *Animals* **2021**, *11*, 2382. https://doi.org/10.3390/ani11082382

Received: 4 August 2021
Accepted: 11 August 2021
Published: 12 August 2021

Publisher's Note: MDPI stays neutral with regard to jurisdictional claims in published maps and institutional affiliations.

1. Introduction

The notion of crossing the species barrier in infectious diseases derives from the relationship between infectious agents, such as viruses and bacteria, and their host species, which is restricted by genetic adaptations that develop through co-evolution [1]. Spillover of these agents is a reality that occurs frequently, potentially leading to the development of severe disease in the new hosts [1]. Pathogens cross the species barrier frequently that it is today known that over 61% of all human infectious diseases are of zoonotic origin, representing 75% of all emerging pathogens during the past 10 years [2]. Although substantial developments in medical/environmental surveillance and in diagnostic methods have been recently achieved, zoonotic emerging and re-emerging diseases are still a major global concern. In fact, such threats are expanding under global warming conditions, particularly in less developed regions. However, this has not started today. Emerging (and re-emerging) transmissible diseases have been impacting human populations since the Agricultural revolution, when hunter-gatherers settled and started crop cultivation and animal domestication, circa 12,000 years ago, reflecting man's first steps in nature's manipulation [3,4]. Since then, a vast number of animal and human diseases have circulated on the earth's surface [4], reaching to the current 2019 novel coronavirus epidemic as an extreme reminder of the role animal reservoirs play in public health [5], shedding SARS-CoV-2 to humans where it adapted and became transmissible by air [6] and surfaces [7].

This Special Issue of Animals: "Emerging and Re-Emerging Diseases—Novel Challenges in Today's World", presents a total of 11 manuscripts focusing on an important group of aspects related to diseases that are found to significantly imbalance ecosystems where humans/animals, pathogens, and the environment interact.

2. Reviews on Wildlife, Taxonomy, and Public Health

It first starts with three interesting reviews, the first on zoonotic diseases of African Lions, (*Panthera leo*) that are bred in captivity on commercial farms across South Africa and often have close contact with farm staff, tourists, and other industry workers, hence posing a potential risk of disease interchange between lions and humans [8]. The systematic review describes a total of 63 pathogenic organisms, with several known pathogens that can be transmitted from lions to other species, including humans. The second review [9] is focused on hemogregarines, apicomplexan blood parasites with an obligatory heteroxenous life cycle that are common blood parasites of fish, amphibians, lizards, snakes, turtles, tortoises, crocodilians, birds, and mammals. This work recognizes that proper classification for the hemogregarine complex is available and further develops on evolutionary relationships producing a reflection on the criteria of generic and unique diagnosis of these parasites. The last review proposes a systematic presentation of hepatitis E virus in humans, animals, and environment of Brazil, the fourth largest pig producer in the world [10]. The review shows that hepatitis E virus genotype 3 was the only retrieved genotype in humans, animals, and environment in Brazil. The South region of Brazil showed the highest human seroprevalence and also the highest density of pigs and related industry, suggesting a zoonotic link and allowing to infer that hepatitis E virus epidemiology in Brazil is similar to that of industrialized countries.

3. Letters and Opinions

These reviews are followed by one letter and one opinion piece that broadens the spectrum of disease emergence to mechanistic aspects of emerging non-communicable diseases by developing the topic of trefoil factor family member 2 (TFF2), discussing, particularly, the role of high-fat diet-induced TFF2 in counteracting immune-mediated damage [11] and as an inflammatory-induced and anti-inflammatory tissue repair factor [12].

4. A Wide Diversity of Original Research

The Special Issue is completed by six research papers covering a wide array of emerging and re-emerging diseases of poultry, bovine, poultry and tortoises, of various nature such as parasitic, bacterial, and viral. The first is a descriptive pathological study of avian schistosomes infection in Whooper Swans (*Cygnus cygnus*) from rescue/rehabilitation centers in Honshu, Japan, reporting that swans most likely died from obstructive phlebitis associated with *Allobilharzia visceralis* [13]. Additionally, more avian pathogens were assessed, initially bacteria, such as *Salmonella* Minnesota, with the genomic characterization of clonal lineages associated with poultry production in Brazil, demonstrating the dissemination of two distinct *S. Minnesota* lineages with high resistance to antibiotics and important virulence genetic clusters in Brazilian poultry farms [14]. A study on a viral pathogen of avian origin, specifically, avian influenza H9N2 in broiler chicken, compared the effectiveness of two different vaccination regimes, ultimately suggesting the use of a vaccine prepared from a recently circulating H9N2 that showed significantly higher protection than the other and was found to be more suitable for birds in the Middle East [15]. This Issue then presents a paper on bovine diseases, initially presenting a molecular approach on the characterization of bovine papillomavirus Type 1 (BPV-1) in cattle from Egypt. In addition, the development of a point-of-need molecular test for BPV-1 diagnosis is described, showing diagnostic utility comparable to PCR-based testing [16]. This article is followed by a study on the first isolation and molecular characterization of bovine respiratory syncytial virus strains in Turkish cattle, a disease with a huge economic burden on livestock industries of countries worldwide [17]. Lastly, the final work reports the molecular detection and characterization of tick-borne agents on *Hyalomma aegyptium* ticks from tortoises of a black market in Doha, Qatar. This study includes the detection of *Hemolivia mauritanica*, *Ehrlichia* spp., and *Candidatus* Midichloria Mitochondrii and highlights the dangers of the international trade of tortoises carrying ticks infected with pathogens of veterinary and medical importance [18].

5. Concluding Remarks

This is a brief but assertive collection that showcases the need to address health at the animal–human–environment interface, in a One Health approach. The global perspective highlighted by the content of this Special Issue reinforces the need of joint and wide efforts by stakeholders.

Funding: This work received no external funding.

Institutional Review Board Statement: Not applicable.

Informed Consent Statement: Not applicable.

Data Availability Statement: Not applicable.

Acknowledgments: I thank all authors who generated the data and contributed to this Special Issue and all our colleagues who reviewed, read, and dispersed the information contained within these studies.

Conflicts of Interest: The author declares no conflict of interest.

References

1. Wong, S.; Lau, S.K.P.; Woo, P.C.Y.; Yuen, K.-Y. Bats as a continuing source of emerging infections in humans. *Rev. Med. Virol.* **2007**, *17*, 67–91. [CrossRef] [PubMed]
2. Jones, K.; Patel, N.; Levy, M.; Storeygard, A.; Balk, D.; Gittleman, J.L.; Daszak, P. Global trends in emerging infectious diseases. *Nature* **2008**, *451*, 990–993. [CrossRef] [PubMed]
3. Dobson, A.P.; Carper, E.R. Infectious diseases and human population history. *BioScience* **1996**, *46*, 115–126. [CrossRef]
4. Morens, D.M.; Fauci, A.S. Emerging Pandemic Diseases: How We Got to COVID-19. *Cell* **2020**, *182*, 1077–1092, Correction in **2020**, *183*, 837. [CrossRef] [PubMed]
5. Da Silva, P.G.; Mesquita, J.R.; Nascimento, M.D.S.J.; Ferreira, V.A.M. Viral, host and environmental factors that favor anthropozoonotic spillover of coronaviruses: An opinionated review, focusing on SARS-CoV, MERS-CoV and SARS-CoV-2. *Sci. Total Environ.* **2021**, *750*, 141483. [CrossRef] [PubMed]
6. Da Silva, P.G.; Nascimento, M.S.J.; Soares, R.R.G.; Sousa, S.I.V.; Mesquita, J.R. Airborne spread of infectious SARS-CoV-2: Moving forward using lessons from SARS-CoV and MERS-CoV. *Sci. Total Environ.* **2021**, *764*, 142802. [CrossRef] [PubMed]
7. Gonçalves, J.; da Silva, P.G.; Reis, L.; Nascimento, M.S.J.; Koritnik, T.; Paragi, M.; Mesquita, J.R. Surface contamination with SARS-CoV-2: A systematic review. *Sci. Total Environ.* **2021**, *798*, 149231. [CrossRef] [PubMed]
8. Green, J.; Jakins, C.; Asfaw, E.; Bruschi, N.; Parker, A.; De Waal, L.; D'Cruze, N. African Lions and Zoonotic Diseases: Implications for Commercial Lion Farms in South Africa. *Animals* **2020**, *10*, 1692. [CrossRef] [PubMed]
9. Al-Quraishy, S.; Abdel-Ghaffar, F.; Dkhil, M.A.; Abdel-Gaber, R. Haemogregarines and Criteria for Identification. *Animals* **2021**, *11*, 170. [CrossRef] [PubMed]
10. Moraes, D.; Mesquita, J.; Dutra, V.; Nascimento, M. Systematic Review of Hepatitis E Virus in Brazil: A One-Health Approach of the Human-Animal-Environment Triad. *Animals* **2021**, *11*, 2290. [CrossRef]
11. Ghanemi, A.; Yoshioka, M.; St-Amand, J. High-Fat Diet-Induced Trefoil Factor Family Member 2 (TFF2) to Counteract the Immune-Mediated Damage in Mice. *Animals* **2021**, *11*, 258. [CrossRef] [PubMed]
12. Ghanemi, A.; Yoshioka, M.; St-Amand, J. Trefoil Factor Family Member 2 (TFF2) as an Inflammatory-Induced and Anti-Inflammatory Tissue Repair Factor. *Animals* **2020**, *10*, 1646. [CrossRef] [PubMed]
13. Ahmed, M.S.; Khalafalla, R.E.; Al-Brakati, A.; Yanai, T.; Elmahallawy, E.K. Descriptive Pathological Study of Avian Schistosomes Infection in Whooper Swans (*Cygnus cygnus*) in Japan. *Animals* **2020**, *10*, 2361. [CrossRef] [PubMed]
14. Kipper, D.; Carroll, L.M.; Mascitti, A.K.; Streck, A.F.; Fonseca, A.S.K.; Ikuta, N.; Lunge, V.R. Genomic Characterization of *Salmonella* Minnesota Clonal Lineages Associated with Poultry Production in Brazil. *Animals* **2020**, *10*, 2043. [CrossRef] [PubMed]
15. Talat, S.; Abouelmaatti, R.R.; Almeer, R.; Abdel-Daim, M.M.; Elfeil, W.K. Comparison of the Effectiveness of Two Different Vaccination Regimes for Avian Influenza H9N2 in Broiler Chicken. *Animals* **2020**, *10*, 1875. [CrossRef]
16. El-Tholoth, M.; Mauk, M.G.; Elnaker, Y.F.; Mosad, S.M.; Tahoun, A.; El-Sherif, M.W.; Lokman, M.S.; Kassab, R.B.; Abdelsadik, A.; Saleh, A.A.; et al. Molecular Characterization and Developing a Point-of-Need Molecular Test for Diagnosis of Bovine Papillomavirus (BPV) Type 1 in Cattle from Egypt. *Animals* **2020**, *10*, 1929. [CrossRef] [PubMed]
17. Yazici, Z.; Ozan, E.; Tamer, C.; Muftuoglu, B.; Barry, G.; Kurucay, H.N.; Elhag, A.E.; Cagirgan, A.A.; Gumusova, S.; Albayrak, H. Circulation of Indigenous Bovine Respiratory Syncytial Virus Strains in Turkish Cattle: The First Isolation and Molecular Characterization. *Animals* **2020**, *10*, 1700. [CrossRef]
18. Barradas, P.F.; Lima, C.; Cardoso, L.; Amorim, I.; Gärtner, F.; Mesquita, J.R. Molecular Evidence of *Hemolivia mauritanica*, *Ehrlichia* spp. and the Endosymbiont *Candidatus* Midichloria Mitochondrii in *Hyalomma aegyptium* Infesting *Testudo graeca* Tortoises from Doha, Qatar. *Animals* **2020**, *11*, 30. [CrossRef]

animals

MDPI

Review

African Lions and Zoonotic Diseases: Implications for Commercial Lion Farms in South Africa

Jennah Green [1], Catherine Jakins [2], Eyob Asfaw [1], Nicholas Bruschi [1], Abbie Parker [1], Louise de Waal [2] and Neil D'Cruze [1,*]

1 World Animal Protection 222 Gray's Inn Rd., London WC1X 8HB, UK; JennahGreen@worldanimalprotection.org (J.G.); EyobAsfaw@worldanimalprotection.org (E.A.); NicholasBruschi@worldanimalprotection.org (N.B.); AbbieParker@worldanimalprotection.org (A.P.)

2 Blood Lion NPC, P.O. Box 1548, Kloof 3640, South Africa; cathjakins@gmail.com (C.J.); louise@greengirlsinafrica.com (L.d.W.)

* Correspondence: NeilDCruze@worldanimalprotection.org

Received: 21 August 2020; Accepted: 17 September 2020; Published: 18 September 2020

check for updates

Simple Summary: In South Africa, thousands of African lions are bred on farms for commercial purposes, such as tourism, trophy hunting, and traditional medicine. Lions on farms often have direct contact with people, such as farm workers and tourists. Such close contact between wild animals and humans creates opportunities for the spread of zoonotic diseases (diseases that can be passed between animals and people). To help understand the health risks associated with lion farms, our study compiled a list of pathogens (bacteria, viruses, parasites, and fungi) known to affect African lions. We reviewed 148 scientific papers and identified a total of 63 pathogens recorded in both wild and captive lions, most of which were parasites (35, 56%), followed by viruses (17, 27%) and bacteria (11, 17%). This included pathogens that can be passed from lions to other animals and to humans. We also found a total of 83 diseases and clinical symptoms associated with these pathogens. Given that pathogens and their associated infectious diseases can cause harm to both animals and public health, we recommend that the lion farming industry in South Africa takes action to prevent and manage potential disease outbreaks.

Abstract: African lions (*Panthera leo*) are bred in captivity on commercial farms across South Africa and often have close contact with farm staff, tourists, and other industry workers. As transmission of zoonotic diseases occurs through close proximity between wildlife and humans, these commercial captive breeding operations pose a potential risk to thousands of captive lions and to public health. An understanding of pathogens known to affect lions is needed to effectively assess the risk of disease emergence and transmission within the industry. Here, we conduct a systematic search of the academic literature, identifying 148 peer-reviewed studies, to summarize the range of pathogens and parasites known to affect African lions. A total of 63 pathogenic organisms were recorded, belonging to 35 genera across 30 taxonomic families. Over half were parasites (35, 56%), followed by viruses (17, 27%) and bacteria (11, 17%). A number of novel pathogens representing unidentified and undescribed species were also reported. Among the pathogenic inventory are species that can be transmitted from lions to other species, including humans. In addition, 83 clinical symptoms and diseases associated with these pathogens were identified. Given the risks posed by infectious diseases, this research highlights the potential public health risks associated with the captive breeding industry. We recommend that relevant authorities take imminent action to help prevent and manage the risks posed by zoonotic pathogens on lion farms.

Keywords: zoonotic disease; *Panthera leo*; human health; biosecurity; wildlife farming; wildlife trade; disease transmission

1. Introduction

Zoonotic diseases are infectious diseases caused by pathogenic agents (including bacteria, parasites, fungi, viruses, and prions) that can be transmitted between vertebrate mammals and humans [1]. Outbreaks of zoonotic diseases can have widespread consequences for public health and are thought to cause two billion cases of human illness and over two million human deaths every year [2]. Disease outbreaks from wild animal sources periodically result in hundreds of billions of dollars of economic damage [3]. The most recent global health pandemic, coronavirus COVID-19, which was also thought to originate in a wild animal host [4], is likely to cost the global economy between 5–9 trillion USD [5].

The increasing rate of emerging infectious diseases is thought to be a result of human-induced changes in land use, extraction of natural resources, animal production systems, and the global wildlife trade [6,7]. Wildlife harbor a large and often unknown reservoir of infectious diseases [8] and zoonotic disease transmission to people occurs when wild animals are in close proximity with human activity [6]. Most recent global health pandemics [9], including COVID-19, are thought to have originated in wild animal hosts [4]. A range of solutions could be put in place to prevent future zoonotic epidemics (see Petrovan et al. [10]). However, it has been suggested that efforts to decrease contact between wild animals and humans could prove to be the most practical and cost-effective approach in reducing the global public health threat posed by zoonotic emerging infectious diseases [11].

Commercial use of wildlife, whether legal or illegal, puts humans in direct contact with a range of wild species [12]. Wildlife farms (herein referred to as facilities that breed non-domesticated species for commercial purposes) in particular can create opportunity for pathogen transmission between wild animals and their human caretakers because of regular or prolonged contact for husbandry purposes [13]. Furthermore, conditions often associated with wildlife farms, such as high concentrations of wild animals in the same enclosures, poor hygiene, and stress associated with captive conditions, can reduce resistance to pathogens and increase the risk for transmission of disease [14,15].

A diverse range of wild animal species are farmed around the world for a range of commercial purposes, for example as exotic pets (e.g., snake farms in West Africa [16]), traditional medicine (e.g., bear bile farms in China and South-East Asia [17]), leather (e.g., alligators farms in the USA [18]), or fur (e.g., mink and fox farms in Europe [19]). Cases of infectious disease emergence from pathogen transmission among farmed wildlife have been documented from across the taxonomic spectrum. For example, transmission of zoonotic tape worm *Armillifer armillatus* from snakes to a farm owner was reported in The Gambia [20], and rapid transmission of coronavirus COVID-19 occurred recently between mink and farm workers at a mink farm in the Netherlands [21].

African lions (*Panthera leo*) are bred and kept on commercial farms across South Africa. These lions are bred for a range of purposes that can involve direct contact with people, including interactive tourism experiences (e.g., paying international volunteers working with predators and day tourists involved in cub petting and walking activities), recreational hunting for 'trophies', and bone exports to Asia for use in traditional medicine products [22,23]. For example, lion bone and trophy exports require a number of 'middle-men' who are required to have direct contact with lions and/or handle their derivatives during transport, slaughter, and/or preparation. This relatively high level of direct contact between lions and people (or consumption of their parts and derivatives) provides ample opportunity for zoonotic exchange.

A review of diseases present among lions in the Kruger Park during the 1970s provides an important insight into the variety of infectious diseases that can affect populations in the wild (e.g., trichinosis, filariasis, sarcoptic mange, pentastomiasis, echinococcosis, taeniasis, hepatozoonosis, anthrax, and babesiosis), including some that are considered to be either directly or indirectly transmissible to humans [24]. Likewise, scientific studies have reported the transmission of zoonotic infectious diseases between humans and captive lions. For example, in 2015, a zoo-housed lion cub presented with 'dermatophytosis', a disease caused by infection with pathogenic fungi *Epidermophyton*,

Microsporum, or *Trichophyton*, was also contracted by a zookeeper caring for the lion as a result of continuous contact with the animal [25].

The number of lions bred on farms in South Africa has grown exponentially in the last two decades to a current captive population of up to 8500 individuals housed across more than 300 facilities [22]. The vast scale of these intensive breeding facilities further increases the number of people in close contact with lions and the opportunities for zoonotic disease transmission. Yet, to the authors' knowledge, despite its value for informing efforts to prevent, monitor, and manage any associated zoonotic disease outbreaks, no attempt has yet been made to compile a list of pathogenic organisms associated with African lions from recent scientific studies. Consequently, this review of the academic literature published in the last ten years provides an initial baseline of pathogenic organisms and discusses the potential animal and public health risks associated with the captive predator industry.

2. Materials and Methods

We conducted a systematic review of the scientific literature using the academic journal database Web of Science (Philadelphia, PA, USA). A total of 13 search terms relating to pathogenic health were searched on the database (Disease, Pathogen, Virus, Viral, Bacteria, Bacterial, Parasite, Parasitic, Fungus, Fungal, Zoonosis, Zoonotic, and Health). Each search term was employed with the Boolean operator 'AND', with the additional term *Panthera leo*. Searches were conducted for the time period 2009–2019, which returned a total of 252 results, comprising 152 individual academic papers. Of the 152 papers returned from the literature search, one could not be sourced due to institutional access and three were excluded because they were not published in English. The remaining 148 papers are included in the analysis.

Each paper was examined by one of six reviewers, who recorded any mention of 'bacteria', 'fungi', 'parasite', 'protozoa', or 'virus' in each article. All disorders, diseases, or conditions were recorded in relation to African and Asiatic lions, with a list of specific named pathogenic organisms compiled. The environment in which the lions were studied was recorded (wild or captive) with specific details on the type of captivity lions were housed in (commercial enterprises, zoos, private ownership, or mixed purposes). In addition, the papers were reviewed for information about disease transmission. The reviewers recorded where it was specified that pathogenic organisms were transmissible between African lions and other animal species, as well as between African lions and humans.

3. Results

A total of 63 different pathogenic organisms, known to affect lions, were reported (Table 1). Over half of the reported pathogenic organisms were parasites (35, 56%), including ticks (order Ixodida) (4, 6%), followed by viruses (17, 27%), and bacteria (11, 17%), with no pathogenic fungi reported. These 63 pathogenic organisms belong to 35 different genera across 30 different taxonomic families. Three novel pathogenic organisms representing unidentified and undescribed species were also reported.

The review also identified a total of 83 clinical symptoms and diseases associated with these pathogenic organisms (Table 2), highlighting the range of detrimental health risks that these pose to their feline hosts. With regards to information on the transmission of infectious disease, 38 (26%) of the scientific papers referred to transmission between lions and other species and three (2%) specifically referred to transmission between lions and humans.

Table 1. Pathogenic organisms (categorized into bacteria, parasites, and viruses) specified in the 148 papers in the dataset.

Pathogen Type	Family	Genus/Species	Source
Bacteria	Actinomycetaceae	*Actinomyces*	[26]
	Anaplasmataceae	*Ehrlichia canis*	[27]
	Bartonellaceae	*Bartonella koehlerae subsp. boulouisii; Bartonella henselae*	[28]
	Clostridiaceae	*Clostridia*	[26]
	Enterobacteriaceae	*Escherichia coli*	[26]
	Mycobacteriaceae	*Mycobacterium bovis*	[29–38]
	Mycoplasmataceae	*Mycoplasma haemominutum*	[39,40]
		Mycoplasma Hemoplasma spp.	[41]
	Rickettsiaceae	*Anaplasma phagocytophilum*	[27]
	Streptococcaceae	*Alpha-hemolytic streptococcus*	[26]
Viruses	Paramyxoviridae	*Morbillivirus* spp.	[42,43]
		Canine distemper virus	[32,37,42,44–59]
	Caliciviridae	*Feline calcivirus*	[44,47,51,56,60–62]
		Sapovirus Norovirus	[56]
	Herpesviridae	*Feline herpes virus*	[44,47,51,60,62]
	Retroviridae	*Feline immunodeficiency virus*	[32,38,47,51,52,57,60,62–71]
		Feline lentivirus	[72]
		Feline leukemia virus	[65,73,74]
		Feline panleukopenia virus	[44,51,61]
		Gammaretrovirus	[74]
	Parvoviridae	*feline panleukopenia virus*	[51]
		Parvovirus	[75]
	Coronaviridae	*Feline coronavirus*	[47,62]
	Picobirnaviridae	*Picobirnavirus*	[76]
	Reoviridae	*Mammalian orthoreovirus*	[77]
	Papillomaviridae	*Papillomavirus*	[78]
	Smacoviridae	*Smacovirus*	[79]
Parasites	Babesiidae	*Babesia canis*	[80,81]
		Babesia felis	[80,82]
		Babesia lengau	[80]
		Babesia leo	[27,80,82]
		Babesia. spp.	[32,51,82]
		Babesia vogeli	[27,80]
		Novel babesia (similar to lengau)	[80]
	Ixodidae	*Rhipicephalus simus; Rhipicephalus sulcatus; Rhipicephalus appendiculatus*	[51]
		Rhipicentor nuttalli	[51]
	Angiostrongylidae	*Aelurostrongylus abstrusus*	[83]
		Aelurostrongylus spp.	[83,84]
	Sarcocystidae	*Cystoisospora* spp.	[85]
		Cystoisospora felis like oocysts; Cystoisospora rivolta like oocysts	[86]
		Sarcocystis spp.	[84]
		Toxoplasma gondii	[87,88]
	Theileriidae	*Cytauxzoon manul*	[27]
		Theileria parva; Theileria sinensis	[27]
	Diphyllobothriidae	*Spirometra pretoriensis*	[89]
		Spirometra ranarum	[89,90]
		Spirometra theileri	[89–91]
		Spirometra spp.	[84,85,92]
	Trypanosomatidae	*Trypanosome b. rhodesiense; Trypanosome congolense; Trypanosome brucei s.l.*	[93]
	Taeniidae	*Taeniid cestodes*	[84]
		Taeniid spp.	[85]
	Toxocaridae	*Toxascaris leonine*	[94,95]
		Toxocara cati	[84]
	Trichinellidae	*Trichinella* spp.	[96]
	Hepatozoidae	*Hepatozoon canis; Hepatozoon felis*	[27,82]

Table 2. Associated diseases and clinical symptoms recorded in the 148 papers in the dataset.

Category	Terms from Source Papers
Diseases	Babesiosis [54]; bovine tuberculosis [29,30,32–34,37,47,52,62,64,71,97–99]; echinococcosis [52]; bilateral pulmonary disease [100]; encephalitis [42,43]; neurologic disease [43,50]; gingivitis [69]; gallbladder adenocarcinomas [26]; kidney disease [26]; biliary cystadenomas [26]; bacterial septicemia [26]; interstitial pneumonia [26,43]; necrotizing and neutrophilic hepatitis [26]; rabies [53]; pneumonia [94]
Clinical symptoms	Acute neurologic involvement [50]; anemia [32]; anisokaryosis [78]; anorexia [41,42,50]; ataxia [43,100]; bilateral submandibular swelling [100], cachexia [69]; congested lungs [26]; corneal opacity [100]; dehydration [26,32,69]; dehydration and hypertension due to kidney disease [101]; depletion of lymphoid organs [50]; depressed serum albumin [32]; profound depression or stupor [43]; dermal and/or mucocutaneous perioral masses [78]; diarrhea [94,95]; disorientation [43]; dyspnea [100]; elbow hygroma [33]; emaciation [33,35,100]; enlarged abdominal area [26]; facial and forelimb myoclonus (recurrent twitching) [43]; feline sarcoids [78]; fibropapilloma [78]; grand mal seizure [43]; hematologic derangements [64]; hyperglobulinemia [69]; immune depletion [70]; convulsions [102]; head tilt [102]; opisthotonos [102]; incoordination [102]; blindness [102]; hypoalbunemia [32]; monoytosis [32]; intraductular cholestasis [26]; ivermectin induced blindness [103]; lethargy [41]; leukopenia [75]; loss of coat condition [69]; lymphadenopathy [33,69]; lymphocytic depletion in lymph nodes and spleen [69]; lymphopenia [42]; hyperglobulinemia [32]; macroscopic abnormalities in the liver [26]; malnutrition [95]; mandibular swelling [33]; mange [33]; marked alopecia [100]; nasal discharge [42]; neutrophilic splenitis [26]; nodular polycystic lesion [26]; obstruction of the intestine [94]; papillomas [69]; peribiliary cysts [26]; polycystic liver [26]; pulmonary and bone lesions [35]; pyrexia [42]; severe seizures [104]; shoulder abscess [33]; tachypnoea [100]; vomiting [94,95]

Of the 109 papers that focused on African lions, 45 (41%) were based on data from captive lions, 61 (56%) from wild lions, and three (3%) from a mixture of both. Of the studies focusing on captive lions, only one collected data from a commercial breeding facility in South Africa. The study used samples from three deceased lions to analyze their evolutionary history and was unrelated to pathogens or disease. One further study focused on commercial facilities in South Africa but did not collect first-hand data and instead used literature sources to review the suitability of captive bred lions for reintroduction into the wild. The remainder of the captive data came from lions housed in zoos, wildlife sanctuaries, and reserves (34, 76%), in private ownership (5, 11%), or a combination of both (4, 9%).

4. Discussion

A systematic review of scientific literature confirmed that a range of 63 different pathogenic organisms are known to exist in both captive and wild free ranging lions (Tables 1 and 2). A number of novel pathogenic organisms, in some cases representing unidentified and undescribed species, were reported, including novel *Babesia* species and *Cystoisospora*-resembling oocysts.

There is a paucity of knowledge on disease susceptibility, transmission, epidemiology, and pathology in lions [100]. While the list of known pathogenic organisms will undoubtedly grow, this review provides an important baseline inventory. Given the conditions in which the lion farming industry currently operates, the considerable scale of trade in lions, and their susceptibility to such a wide range of multi-host pathogenic organisms, it is likely that farmed lions could play a central role in the emergence, amplification, and transmission of disease to both people and wild animal populations.

4.1. Significance for Lion Health

Some of the pathogenic organisms reported in this review are of significant health concern for captive and wild lions. For example, *Babesia* parasites, *Mycobacterium bovis* (a bacteria known for causing tuberculosis), canine distemper virus (CDV), canine parvovirus (CP), and feline panleukopenia virus (FPLV) (Table 1) are all highly contagious and cause significant morbidity and mortality in susceptible carnivore species. Infection with these pathogens is associated with a range of clinical symptoms, including but not limited to: emaciation, alopecia, diarrhea, seizures, recurrent twitching, and depression (Table 2) from which infected lions can suffer.

Some of these pathogenic organisms are particularly difficult to manage because infection of susceptible animals does not require direct physical contact. Infected lions shed pathogenic organisms in feces and other bodily secretions, e.g., aerosolized respiratory secretions [105,106] facilitating environmental contamination and rapid spread of disease. Furthermore, some of these organisms have longer incubation periods and can therefore lie undetected in the animals' systems until they reach hazardous levels. For example, tuberculosis onset is slow, in many cases with the majority of infected lions initially appearing healthy [100,107]. In a captive setting, this renders detection and prevention of spread of infections between individuals housed together very difficult.

In addition, some of these pathogenic organisms are likely to present a management challenge on commercial lion farms, as the onset of disease in lions often occurs suddenly after high stress situations, for example after repeated periods of pregnancy and lactation [100]. It has been suggested that intensive farming conditions and poor hygiene may be increasing the incidence of FPLV in captive carnivores, such as lions [108]. Disease transmission is promoted in immunocompromising conditions, and direct human–wildlife contact mixed with limited health and safety standards are all criteria for an emerging zoonosis hotspot [12].

Another challenge for captive facilities is that seemingly innocuous pathogens can cause harm when lions are 'co-infected' with multiple pathogens. For example, severe mortalities have occurred when individual lions were infected with both babesiosis and CDV, resulting in severe diseases like pneumonia and encephalitis, despite appearing healthy when infected with babesiosis alone [81]. This heightens the challenge of identifying infected individuals to manage diseases before transmission can occur.

4.2. *Significance for Human Health*

In addition to the potential significance for lion health, many of the pathogenic organisms reported in the reviewed scientific literature raise concerns for human health. For example, pathogenic strains of the Enterobacteriaceae *Escherichia coli* [26], the parasitic Sarcocystidae *Toxoplasma gondii* [14,87], and potentially, the parasitic Toxocaridae *Toxascaris leonine* [109] have a possible fecal–oral transmission route from lions to humans. For others, such as the Rickettsiaceae *Anaplasma phagocytophilum* [27], transmission via the bite of an infected arthropod tick is also possible.

Some pathogens possess the capacity to infect human tissue using keratin and therefore only require physical contact with the lion's fur; for example, *Microsporum gypseum*, the cause of dermatomycosis [110]. The adoption of prophylactic measures for sanitary maintenance for these animals and the professionals who maintain contact with them is paramount to reduce possible transmission of infection but is difficult to manage because of the asymptomatic nature of the pathogens in healthy lions [110]. Visitors to lion farms in South Africa have reported that basic hygiene protocols, for example hand sanitizing and stepping points to disinfect shoes between enclosures, are often absent for those intending to interact with the animals [111].

Lions have also been reported as hosts for diseases listed by the World Health Organization (WHO) as 'neglected tropical diseases (NTDs)' [112]. For example, human African trypanosomiasis caused by trypanosomes are multi-host parasites capable of infecting a wide range of wildlife species, including lions [93], that constitute a reservoir of infection for both people and domestic animals. *Echinococcosis*, a parasitic disease caused by tapeworms that reside in the intestines of carnivores, including lions [52], can cause serious morbidity and death in people. The prevalence of *Echinococcosis* is increasing in some African countries due to frequent contact between game animals (reservoir hosts), domestic animal hosts (such as dogs), and humans who are susceptible to transmission [113]. Neglecting these parasites can have severe socioeconomic consequences [113].

Captive carnivores can be predisposed to infections of *Toxoplasma*, a protozoan parasite with significant zoonotic potential [113]. Lions in particular have been identified as a susceptible host species [113]. Lions infected with *Toxoplasma* can transmit the parasites to people via blood and feces, causing severe pulmonary, cardiac, and brain inflammatory reactions (among others), sometimes with fatal outcomes [113]. Some *Toxoplasma* species have also been reported to cause abortion and fetal death; underestimating the impact of these parasites on humans could lead to a future epidemic where reduction in life expectancy, and increased child and maternal death, are rife [113].

Lions are also vulnerable to bovine tuberculosis (bTB), a disease caused by infection with the bacterial pathogen *M. bovis* [32,47]. Tuberculosis transmission at the wildlife–livestock–human interface is a growing concern worldwide, particularly in sub-Saharan Africa where infection is spreading [114]. Lions initially contracted bTB from infected buffalo carcasses [32], and although no direct spill-over from wildlife to humans (or vice-versa) has yet been documented [114], it is a growing concern, particularly in countries such as South Africa where there are a relatively high number of people living with HIV [115,116] and because HIV is the strongest known risk factor for TB [32]. Transmission of other pathogenic strains of tuberculosis from wild captive animals to humans has already been documented [117].

Epidemics caused by cats are possible (e.g., canine distemper in big cats) but are considered to be relatively rare [118]. While no evidence of lion-to-human transmission of feline coronavirus exists, isolation of pathogens with pandemic potential from any mammalian host is significant as it may provide conditions suitable for the virus to adapt to other mammalian hosts, enabling efficient mammal-to-human, and possibly also human-to-human, transmission, paving the way for a potentially devastating pandemic [119].

For example, it has recently been confirmed that big cats, including lions, can be infected with Sars-CoV-2 [120]. Some experts have publicly stated their belief that it is unlikely Sars-CoV-2 will naturally spread in a wild big cat population [118]. However, given the fact that the lions and tigers that tested positive for Sars-CoV-2 in the Bronx Zoo were likely to be infected by a zoo employee [121,122], there are on-going concerns that this virus could be passed from humans to big cats and vice versa in scenarios that involve captive individuals [118].

4.3. Significance for Lion Farming

The maintenance of wild species in captivity provides an opportunity for unnatural human-wildlife proximity, facilitating interspecies sharing of pathogenic organisms [123]. Lions are kept in captivity in zoos in many cases as part of conservation breeding programs [124], but also, and in far greater numbers, on commercial wildlife farms [125]. While published data detailing the scale of wildlife farming and lion farming in particular in South Africa are scant, the South African Minister of Environment, Forestry and Fisheries stated in July 2019 in response to a Parliamentary question that the captive lion population in South Africa amounted to 7979 lions housed across 366 facilities.

Scientific papers that focus on the welfare conditions on commercial lion farms prevalent across South Africa are currently lacking. However, the living conditions and environments provided are frequently reported as low welfare, involving large numbers of lions, often in poor physical condition and in over-crowded spaces [126,127] (Figure 1). High concentrations of wild animals in the same enclosures can increase the risk for transmission of disease to and from wild animals due to reduced resistance to pathogens from factors associated with captivity, such as poor hygiene, poor diet, or stress [14,128]. Furthermore, cub separation from their mothers and the provision of alternative milk formulas (a practice reported at some lion farms [111]] can lead to nutritional deficiencies [129], which weakens immune systems and leaves animals more susceptible to pathogens [130].

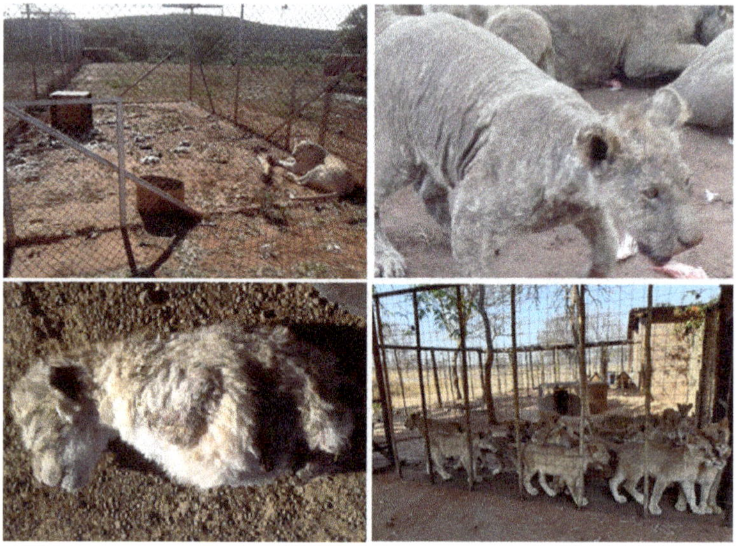

Figure 1. Environments provided for lions at commercial captive breeding facilities in South Africa are frequently reported as low welfare, involving large numbers of lions, often in poor physical condition and in over-crowded spaces. (**Top left**) Lioness housed in an enclosure with fecal matter and decaying carcasses. (**Top right**) Lions with little to no fur left as a result of severe and untreated mange. (**Bottom left**) Lion cub born with severe deformities, likely due to inbreeding. (**Bottom right**) Lions housed in overcrowded conditions. Images copyright Blood Lions.

A key part of this industry is "ecotourism", where people are provided with the opportunity to come into close and unnatural proximity with lions via cub "petting" and "walking with" interactions or international volunteers paying to hand-rear lion cubs. The process of preparation of carcasses for human consumption also presents a considerable risk for transmission of disease to and from wild animals [131], a risk that is amplified in situations where slaughter and preparation take place at unregulated slaughterhouses, unbound by official hygiene standards [132]. Furthermore, the regulatory body that governs the international export of lion bones (The Convention of International Trade of Endangered Species, 'CITES') dictates quotas based on conservation science [133] and is not specifically aimed at preventing zoonotic disease introduction, despite the major role wildlife trade has as a transmission pathway for pathogenic organisms [12].

It is also important to note that any pathogenic organisms present in the captive lion population may pose a threat to the conservation of wild populations, particularly in scenarios where lion farms are located close to a wild lion habitat and where lion farm staff and visitors are actively engaged in other activities (e.g., conservation-focused field research, hunting, and photo tourism) that bring them into close proximity to free-ranging lions. For example, wild racoon dogs (*Nyctereutes procyonoides*) are thought to have transmitted CDV to a group of zoo-housed tigers in Japan [42] and records of transmission of intestinal nematodes between captive felids and local feral cats have been reported in Brazil [134]. Multi-host pathogenic organisms may pose a particular threat in scenarios where lion farm activity overlaps with areas inhabited by other free-ranging carnivore species (both wild and domesticated).

4.4. Mitigating Animal and Public Health Risks

Remedial measures, such as improved animal welfare standards, veterinary interventions, and biosecurity protocols can partially mitigate the risk of zoonosis at captive lion breeding facilities [135]. However, due to the potential of asymptomatic pathogens affecting lions [110], biosecurity would require sophisticated disease surveillance, which could prove challenging [136,137]. Even with comprehensive surveillance, identification of emerging pathogens is still a challenge that poses significant animal and public health risks [12]. There is currently no publicly available information detailing the biosecurity protocols and regulatory standards within the lion breeding industry and, from our initial review of the literature, an apparent lack of national norms and standards for the health of the lions housed on commercial farms.

Alternatively, a phased reduction in the scale of, or end to, the commercial captive breeding of lions for non-conservation purposes in South Africa could help to remove the animal and public health risks associated with this industry. However, efforts focused on improving animal husbandry, reducing consumer demand for lions (and their derivatives), increased enforcement effort, and the provision of economic incentives for farm staff would need to be considered to prevent any unintended consequences on lion welfare, conservation, and local livelihoods.

4.5. Limitations

We acknowledge that restricting our search to a ten-year time period and to one academic database will limit the number of relevant articles in our review. In addition, we recognize that additional onsite research is required to determine the incidence and prevalence of particular pathogenic organisms (in both captive and wild lion populations) and to help identify which infectious diseases are more likely to affect them under certain conditions. However, it was not our intention to provide a comprehensive overview of all pathogens affecting African lions or to provide specific statistics on their occurrence. Rather, the aim of our study was to create a baseline inventory of key pathogens and associated diseases and to describe the potential associated health concerns for both lions and people. Although our review may omit some relevant pathogens, we hope to demonstrate that, by only scratching the surface of this field, we identify a previously neglected area of consideration that will stimulate increased attention in future.

5. Conclusions

There are many socio-cultural, political, economic, and conservation factors that create a complex and nuanced debate around the commercial captive lion breeding industry in South Africa [133]. However, all economic, ethical, and environmental considerations aside, the data presented here indicate that the industry poses a potential risk to wild animal and public health. This initial literature review reveals a long and varied list of pathogenic organisms known to affect African lions, some of which can be transmitted to people. Given the range of pathogens identified, the growth of the industry over the last couple of decades, and the increasing number of people who have direct contact with live lions and/or their parts and derivatives, we recommend that a closer examination of the current policies and practices associated with commercial lion farming is required, particularly under a biosecurity lens. Furthermore, to properly safeguard lion and public health, it is paramount that the recommendations of any such examinations should be acted on with clear time-bound objectives relating to both implementation and enforcement.

Author Contributions: Conceptualization, N.D., J.G. and L.d.W.; methodology, N.D. and J.G.; formal analysis, J.G.; investigation, N.D., J.G., C.J., L.d.W., E.A., A.P. and N.B.; resources, N.D., J.G., C.J., L.d.W., E.A., A.P. and N.B.; data curation, J.G.; writing—original draft preparation, J.G. and N.D.; writing—review and editing, J.G., N.D., L.d.W., C.J.; visualization, J.G.; supervision, N.D. and L.d.W.; project administration, J.G. All authors have read and agreed to the published version of the manuscript.

Funding: This research received no external funding.

Acknowledgments: We would like to thank Gilbert Sape, Edith Kabesiime, Patrick Muinde, and Paul Giess for providing helpful comments and feedback on an earlier version of this manuscript.

Conflicts of Interest: The authors declare no conflict of interest.

References

1. Can, Ö.E.; D'Cruze, N.; Macdonald, D.W. Dealing in deadly pathogens: Taking stock of the legal trade in live wildlife and potential risks to human health. *Glob. Ecol. Conserv.* **2019**, *17*, e00515. [CrossRef] [PubMed]
2. Grace, D.; Gilbert, J.; Randolph, T.; Kang'ethe, E. The multiple burdens of zoonotic disease and an ecohealth approach to their assessment. *Trop. Anim. Health Prod.* **2012**, *44*, 67–73. [CrossRef]
3. Fukushima, C.S.; Mammola, S.; Cardoso, P. Global wildlife trade permeates the Tree of Life. *Biol. Conserv.* **2020**, *247*, 108503. [CrossRef]
4. Zhang, T.; Wu, Q.; Zhang, Z. Probable pangolin origin of SARS-CoV-2 associated with the COVID-19 outbreak. *Curr. Biol.* **2020**, *30*, 1346–1351.e2. [CrossRef] [PubMed]
5. Chapman, B. Coronavirus could Deliver $8.8 Trillion Hit to Global Economy without Government Intervention, Bank Says. *Independent* **2020**. Available online: https://www.independent.co.uk/news/business/news/coronavirus-global-economy-impact-gdp-covid-19-a9516806.html (accessed on 28 August 2020).
6. Karesh, W.B.; Dobson, A.; Lloyd-Smith, J.O.; Lubroth, J.; Dixon, M.A.; Bennett, M.; Aldrich, S.; Harrington, T.; Formenty, P.; Loh, E.H.; et al. Ecology of zoonoses: Natural and unnatural histories. *Lancet* **2012**, *380*, 1936–1945. [CrossRef]
7. Smith, K.M.; Zambrana-Torrelio, C.; White, A.; Asmussen, M.; Machalaba, C.; Kennedy, S.; Lopez, K.; Wolf, T.M.; Daszak, P.; Travis, D.A. Summarizing US wildlife trade with an eye toward assessing the risk of infectious disease introduction. *EcoHealth* **2017**, *14*, 29–39. [CrossRef]
8. Levinson, J.; Bogich, T.L.; Olival, K.J.; Epstein, J.H.; Johnson, C.K.; Karesh, W.; Daszak, P. Targeting Surveillance for Zoonotic Virus Discovery. *Emerg. Infect. Dis.* **2013**, *19*, 743–747. [CrossRef] [PubMed]
9. Morse, S.S.; Mazet, J.A.; Woolhouse, M.; Parrish, C.R.; Carroll, D.; Karesh, W.B.; Zambrana-Torrelio, C.; Lipkin, W.I.; Daszak, P. Prediction and prevention of the next pandemic zoonosis. *Lancet* **2012**, *380*, 1956–1965. [CrossRef]
10. Petrovan, V.; Murgia, M.V.; Wu, P.; Lowe, A.D.; Jia, W.; Rowland, R.R. Epitope mapping of African swine fever virus (ASFV) structural protein, p54. *Virus Res.* **2020**, *279*, 197871. [CrossRef]
11. Karesh, W.B.; Cook, R.A.; Bennett, E.L.; Newcomb, J. Wildlife trade and global disease emergence. *Emerg. Infect. Dis.* **2005**, *11*, 1000. [CrossRef]
12. Watsa, M.; Group, W.D.S.F. Rigorous wildlife disease surveillance. *Science* **2020**, *369*, 145–147. [CrossRef] [PubMed]
13. Kimman, T.; Hoek, M.; de Jong, M.C. Assessing and controlling health risks from animal husbandry. *NJAS Wagening J. Life Sci.* **2013**, *66*, 7–14. [CrossRef]
14. Mukarati, N.L.; Vassilev, G.D.; Tagwireyi, W.M.; Tavengwa, M. Occurrence, prevalence and intensity of internal parasite infections of African lions (Panthera leo) in enclosures at a recreation park in Zimbabwe. *J. Zoo Wildl. Med.* **2013**, *44*, 686–693. [CrossRef] [PubMed]
15. Whitehouse-Tedd, K.M.; Lefebvre, S.L.; Janssens, G.P. Dietary factors associated with faecal consistency and other indicators of gastrointestinal health in the captive cheetah (Acinonyx jubatus). *PLoS ONE* **2015**, *10*, e0120903. [CrossRef]
16. Auliya, M.; Hofmann, S.; Segniagbeto, G.H.; Assou, D.; Ronfot, D.; Astrin, J.J.; Forat, S.; Ketoh, G.K.K.; D'Cruze, N. The first genetic assessment of wild and farmed ball pythons (Reptilia, Serpentes, Pythonidae) in southern Togo. *Nat. Conserv.* **2020**, *38*, 37. [CrossRef]
17. Dutton, A.J.; Hepburn, C.; Macdonald, D.W. A stated preference investigation into the Chinese demand for farmed vs. wild bear bile. *PLoS ONE* **2011**, *6*, e21243. [CrossRef]
18. Moyle, B. Conservation that's more than skin-deep: Alligator farming. *Biodivers. Conserv.* **2013**, *22*, 1663–1677. [CrossRef]
19. Wong, T.C.; Ng, R.; Cai, L.M. Sustainability in the Fur Industry. In *Sustainability in Luxury Fashion Business*; Springer: New York City, NY, USA, 2018; pp. 133–152.
20. Tappe, D.; Meyer, M.; Oesterlein, A.; Jaye, A.; Frosch, M.; Schoen, C.; Pantchev, N. Transmission of Armillifer armillatus ova at snake farm, The Gambia, West Africa. *Emerg. Infect. Dis.* **2011**, *17*, 251–254. [CrossRef]
21. Enserink, M. Coronavirus rips through Dutch mink farms, triggering culls. *Science* **2020**, *368*, 1169. [CrossRef]
22. Hutchinson, A.; Roberts, D.L. Differentiating captive and wild African lion (Panthera leo) populations in South Africa, using stable carbon and nitrogen isotope analysis. *Biodivers. Conserv.* **2020**, 1–19. [CrossRef]
23. Outhwaite, W. *The Legal and Illegal Trade in African Lions*; TRAFFIC: Cambridge, UK, 2018.

24. Young, E. Some important parasitic and other diseases of lion, Panthera leo, in the Kruger National Park. *J. S. Afr. Vet. Assoc.* **1975**, *46*, 181–183. [PubMed]
25. Kim, K.T.; Lee, S.H.; mi Kwak, D. Dermatophytosis on an African lion and transmission to human. 대한수의학회 학술대회발표집 **2015**, 543.
26. Caliendo, V.; Bull, A.C.; Stidworthy, M.F. Congenital biliary tract malformation resembling biliary cystadenoma in a captive juvenile African lion (Panthera leo). *J. Zoo Wildl. Med.* **2012**, *43*, 922–926. [CrossRef] [PubMed]
27. Kelly, P.; Marabini, L.; Dutlow, K.; Zhang, J.; Loftis, A.; Wang, C. Molecular detection of tick-borne pathogens in captive wild felids, Zimbabwe. *Parasites Vvectors* **2014**, *7*, 514. [CrossRef] [PubMed]
28. Molia, S.; Kasten, R.W.; Stuckey, M.J.; Boulouis, H.-J.; Allen, J.; Borgo, G.M.; Koehler, J.E.; Chang, C.C.; Chomel, B.B. Isolation of Bartonella henselae, Bartonella koehlerae subsp. koehlerae, Bartonella koehlerae subsp. bothieri and a new subspecies of B. koehlerae from free-ranging lions (Panthera leo) from South Africa, cheetahs (Acinonyx jubatus) from Namibia and captive cheetahs from California. *Epidemiol. Infect.* **2016**, *144*, 3237–3243. [PubMed]
29. Brüns, A.C.; Tanner, M.; Williams, M.C.; Botha, L.; O'Brien, A.; Fosgate, G.T.; Van Helden, P.D.; Clarke, J.; Michel, A.L. Diagnosis and implications of Mycobacterium bovis infection in banded mongooses (Mungos mungo) in the Kruger National Park, South Africa. *J. Wildl. Dis.* **2017**, *53*, 19–29. [CrossRef]
30. Cross, P.C.; Heisey, D.M.; Bowers, J.A.; Hay, C.T.; Wolhuter, J.; Buss, P.; Hofmeyr, M.; Michel, A.L.; Bengis, R.G.; Bird, T.L.F. Disease, predation and demography: Assessing the impacts of bovine tuberculosis on African buffalo by monitoring at individual and population levels. *J. Appl. Ecol.* **2009**, *46*, 467–475. [CrossRef]
31. Kosmala, M.; Miller, P.; Ferreira, S.; Funston, P.; Keet, D.; Packer, C. Estimating wildlife disease dynamics in complex systems using an Approximate Bayesian Computation framework. *Ecol. Appl.* **2016**, *26*, 295–308. [CrossRef]
32. Maas, M.; Keet, D.F.; Rutten, V.P.; Heesterbeek, J.A.P.; Nielen, M. Assessing the impact of feline immunodeficiency virus and bovine tuberculosis co-infection in African lions. *Proc. R. Soc. B Biol. Sci.* **2012**, *279*, 4206–4214. [CrossRef]
33. Miller, M.; Buss, P.; Hofmeyr, J.; Olea-Popelka, F.; Parsons, S.; van Helden, P. Antemortem diagnosis of Mycobacterium bovis infection in free-ranging African lions (Panthera leo) and implications for transmission. *J. Wildl. Dis.* **2015**, *51*, 493–497. [CrossRef]
34. Miller, M.; Joubert, J.; Mathebula, N.; De Klerk-Lorist, L.-M.; Lyashchenko, K.P.; Bengis, R.; van Helden, P.; Hofmeyr, M.; Olea-Popelka, F.; Greenwald, R. Detection of antibodies to tuberculosis antigens in free-ranging lions (Panthera leo) infected with Mycobacterium bovis in Kruger National Park, South Africa. *J. Zoo Wildl. Med.* **2012**, *43*, 317–323. [CrossRef] [PubMed]
35. Miller, M.A.; Buss, P.; Sylvester, T.T.; Lyashchenko, K.P.; deKlerk-Lorist, L.-M.; Bengis, R.; Hofmeyr, M.; Hofmeyr, J.; Mathebula, N.; Hausler, G. Mycobacterium bovis in free-ranging lions (panthera leo)—Evaluation of serological and tuberculin skin tests for detection of infection and disease. *J. Zoo Wildl. Med.* **2019**, *50*, 7–15. [PubMed]
36. Newkirk, K.M.; Beard, L.K.; Sun, X.; Ramsay, E.C. Investigation of enrofloxacin-associated retinal toxicity in nondomestic felids. *J. Zoo Wildl. Med.* **2017**, *48*, 518–520. [CrossRef] [PubMed]
37. Olivier, T.T.; Viljoen, I.M.; Hofmeyr, J.; Hausler, G.A.; Goosen, W.J.; Tordiffe, A.S.W.; Buss, P.; Loxton, A.G.; Warren, R.M.; Miller, M.A. Development of a Gene Expression Assay for the Diagnosis of M ycobacterium bovis Infection in African Lions (P anthera leo). *Transbound. Emerg. Dis.* **2017**, *64*, 774–781. [CrossRef] [PubMed]
38. Sylvester, T.T.; Martin, L.E.R.; Buss, P.; Loxton, A.G.; Hausler, G.A.; Rossouw, L.; van Helden, P.; Parsons, S.D.C.; Olea-Popelka, F.; Miller, M.A. Prevalence and risk factors for Mycobacterium bovis infection in African lions (Panthera leo) in the Kruger National Park. *J. Wildl. Dis.* **2017**, *53*, 372–376. [CrossRef] [PubMed]
39. de Sousa, K.C.M.; Herrera, H.M.; Secato, C.T.; do Vale Oliveira, A.; Santos, F.M.; Rocha, F.L.; Barreto, W.T.G.; Macedo, G.C.; de Andrade Pinto, P.C.E.; Machado, R.Z. Occurrence and molecular characterization of hemoplasmas in domestic dogs and wild mammals in a Brazilian wetland. *Acta Trop.* **2017**, *171*, 172–181. [CrossRef]

40. Ribeiro, C.M.; de Matos, A.C.; Richini-Pereira, V.B.; Lucheis, S.B.; Azzolini, F.; Sipp, J.P.; Lima, P.P.; Katagiri, S.; Vidotto, O. Occurrence and phylogenetic analysis of 'Candidatus Mycoplasma haemominutum'in wild felines from Paraná, Brazil. *Semin. Ciências Agrárias* **2017**, *38*, 2837–2844. [CrossRef]
41. Krengel, A.; Meli, M.L.; Cattori, V.; Wachter, B.; Willi, B.; Thalwitzer, S.; Melzheimer, J.; Hofer, H.; Lutz, H.; Hofmann-Lehmann, R. First evidence of hemoplasma infection in free-ranging Namibian cheetahs (Acinonyx jubatus). *Vet. Microbiol.* **2013**, *162*, 972–976. [CrossRef]
42. Nagao, Y.; Nishio, Y.; Shiomoda, H.; Tamaru, S.; Shimojima, M.; Goto, M.; Une, Y.; Sato, A.; Ikebe, Y.; Maeda, K. An outbreak of canine distemper virus in tigers (Panthera tigris): Possible transmission from wild animals to zoo animals. *J. Vet. Med. Sci.* **2011**, 1112250745. [CrossRef]
43. Roelke-Parker, M.E.; Munson, L.; Packer, C.; Kock, R.; Cleaveland, S.; Carpenter, M.; O'Brien, S.J.; Pospischil, A.; Hofmann-Lehmann, R.; Lutz, H. A canine distemper virus epidemic in Serengeti lions (Panthera leo). *Nature* **1996**, *379*, 441–445. [CrossRef]
44. Alexander, K.A.; McNutt, J.W.; Briggs, M.B.; Standers, P.E.; Funston, P.; Hemson, G.; Keet, D.; Van Vuuren, M. Multi-host pathogens and carnivore management in southern Africa. *Comp. Immunol. Microbiol. Infect. Dis.* **2010**, *33*, 249–265. [CrossRef] [PubMed]
45. Broekhuis, F.; Cushman, S.A.; Elliot, N.B. Identification of human–carnivore conflict hotspots to prioritize mitigation efforts. *Ecol. Evol.* **2017**, *7*, 10630–10639. [CrossRef] [PubMed]
46. Caillaud, D.; Craft, M.E.; Meyers, L.A. Epidemiological effects of group size variation in social species. *J. R. Soc. Interface* **2013**, *10*, 20130206. [CrossRef] [PubMed]
47. Hunter, L.T.; White, P.; Henschel, P.; Frank, L.; Burton, C.; Loveridge, A.; Balme, G.; Breitenmoser, C.; Breitenmoser, U. Walking with lions: Why there is no role for captive-origin lions Panthera leo in species restoration. *Oryx* **2013**, *47*, 19–24. [CrossRef]
48. Jackson, C.R.; Masenga, E.H.; Mjingo, E.E.; Davies, A.B.; Fossøy, F.; Fyumagwa, R.D.; Røskaft, E.; May, R.F. No evidence of handling-induced mortality in Serengeti's African wild dog population. *Ecol. Evol.* **2019**, *9*, 1110–1118. [CrossRef]
49. Jhala, Y.V.; Banerjee, K.; Chakrabarti, S.; Basu, P.; Singh, K.; Dave, C.; Gogoi, K. Asiatic lion: Ecology, economics and politics of conservation. *Front. Ecol. Evol.* **2019**, *7*, 312. [CrossRef]
50. Konjević, D.; Sabočanec, R.; Grabarević, Ž.; Zurbriggen, A.; Bata, I.; Beck, A.; Kurilj, A.G.; Cvitković, D. Canine distemper in Siberian tiger cubs from Zagreb ZOO: Case report. *Acta Vet. Brno* **2011**, *80*, 47–50. [CrossRef]
51. McDermid, K.R.; Snyman, A.; Verreynne, F.J.; Carroll, J.P.; Penzhorn, B.L.; Yabsley, M.J. Surveillance for viral and parasitic pathogens in a vulnerable African Lion (Panthera Leo) population in the Northern Tuli Game Reserve, Botswana. *J. Wildl. Dis.* **2017**, *53*, 54–61. [CrossRef]
52. Miller, S.M.; Bissett, C.; Burger, A.; Courtenay, B.; Dickerson, T.; Druce, D.J.; Ferreira, S.; Funston, P.J.; Hofmeyr, D.; Kilian, P.J. Management of reintroduced lions in small, fenced reserves in South Africa: An assessment and guidelines. *Afr. J. Wildl. Res.* **2013**, *43*, 138–154. [CrossRef]
53. Norton, B.B.; Tunseth, D.; Holder, K.; Briggs, M.; Hayek, L.-A.; Murray, S. Causes of morbidity in captive African lions (Panthera leo) in North America, 2001–2016. *Zoo Biol.* **2018**, *37*, 354–359. [CrossRef]
54. Oates, L.; Rees, P.A. The historical ecology of the large mammal populations of N gorongoro C rater, T anzania, east A frica. *Mammal Rev.* **2013**, *43*, 124–141. [CrossRef]
55. O'brien, S.J.; Troyer, J.L.; Brown, M.A.; Johnson, W.E.; Antunes, A.; Roelke, M.E.; Pecon-Slattery, J. Emerging viruses in the Felidae: Shifting paradigms. *Viruses* **2012**, *4*, 236–257. [CrossRef] [PubMed]
56. Olarte-Castillo, X.A.; Hofer, H.; Goller, K.V.; Martella, V.; Moehlman, P.D.; East, M.L. Divergent sapovirus strains and infection prevalence in wild carnivores in the Serengeti ecosystem: A long-term study. *PLoS ONE* **2016**, *11*, e0163548. [CrossRef] [PubMed]
57. Packer, C. The African lion: A long history of interdisciplinary research. *Front. Ecol. Evol.* **2019**, *7*, 259. [CrossRef]
58. Rafiqi, S.I.; Kumar, S.; Reena, K.K.; Garg, R.; Ram, H.; Karikalan, M.; Mahendran, K.; Pawde, A.M.; Sharma, A.K.; BANERJEE10, P. Molecu-lar characterization of Hepatozoon sp. and Babesia sp. isolated from endangered asiatic lion (Panthera leo persica). *Indian J. Anim. Sci.* **2018**, *88*, 662–666.
59. Watts, H.E.; Holekamp, K.E. Ecological determinants of survival and reproduction in the spotted hyena. *J. Mammal.* **2009**, *90*, 461–471. [CrossRef]

60. Chaber, A.-L.; Cozzi, G.; Broekhuis, F.; Hartley, R.W.; McNutt, J. Serosurvey for selected viral pathogens among sympatric species of the African large predator guild in northern Botswana. *J. Wildl. Dis.* **2017**, *53*, 170–175. [CrossRef]
61. Risi, E.; Agoulon, A.; Allaire, F.; Le Dréan-Quénec'hdu, S.; Martin, V.; Mahl, P. Antibody response to vaccines for rhinotracheitis, caliciviral disease, panleukopenia, feline leukemia, and rabies in tigers (Panthera tigris) and lions (Panthera leo). *J. Zoo Wildl. Med.* **2012**, *43*, 248–255. [CrossRef]
62. Trinkel, M.; Cooper, D.; Packer, C.; Slotow, R. Inbreeding depression increases susceptibility to bovine tuberculosis in lions: An experimental test using an inbred–outbred contrast through translocation. *J. Wildl. Dis.* **2011**, *47*, 494–500. [CrossRef]
63. Adams, H.; Van Vuuren, M.; Kania, S.; Bosman, A.-M.; Keet, D.; New, J.; Kennedy, M. Sensitivity and specificity of a nested polymerase chain reaction for detection of lentivirus infection in lions (Panthera leo). *J. Zoo Wildl. Med.* **2010**, *41*, 608–615. [CrossRef]
64. Broughton, H.M.; Govender, D.; Shikwambana, P.; Chappell, P.; Jolles, A. Bridging gaps between zoo and wildlife medicine: Establishing reference intervals for free-ranging african lions (panthera leo). *J. Zoo Wildl. Med.* **2017**, *48*, 298–311. [CrossRef] [PubMed]
65. Filoni, C.; Helfer-Hungerbuehler, A.K.; Catão-Dias, J.L.; Marques, M.C.; Torres, L.N.; Reinacher, M.; Hofmann-Lehmann, R. Putative progressive and abortive feline leukemia virus infection outcomes in captive jaguarundis (Puma yagouaroundi). *Virol. J.* **2017**, *14*, 226. [CrossRef] [PubMed]
66. Fountain-Jones, N.M.; Packer, C.; Troyer, J.L.; VanderWaal, K.; Robinson, S.; Jacquot, M.; Craft, M.E. Linking social and spatial networks to viral community phylogenetics reveals subtype-specific transmission dynamics in African lions. *J. Anim. Ecol.* **2017**, *86*, 1469–1482. [CrossRef] [PubMed]
67. Hayward, J.J.; Rodrigo, A.G. Molecular epidemiology of feline immunodeficiency virus in the domestic cat (Felis catus). *Vet. Immunol. Immunopathol.* **2010**, *134*, 68–74. [CrossRef]
68. Kerr, T.J.; Matthee, S.; Govender, D.; Tromp, G.; Engelbrecht, S.; Matthee, C.A. Viruses as indicators of contemporary host dispersal and phylogeography: An example of feline immunodeficiency virus (FIVP le) in free-ranging African lion (Panthera leo). *J. Evol. Biol.* **2018**, *31*, 1529–1543. [CrossRef]
69. Roelke, M.E.; Brown, M.A.; Troyer, J.L.; Winterbach, H.; Winterbach, C.; Hemson, G.; Smith, D.; Johnson, R.C.; Pecon-Slattery, J.; Roca, A.L. Pathological manifestations of feline immunodeficiency virus (FIV) infection in wild African lions. *Virology* **2009**, *390*, 1–12. [CrossRef]
70. Troyer, J.L.; Roelke, M.E.; Jespersen, J.M.; Baggett, N.; Buckley-Beason, V.; MacNulty, D.; Craft, M.; Packer, C.; Pecon-Slattery, J.; O'Brien, S.J. FIV diversity: FIVPle subtype composition may influence disease outcome in African lions. *Vet. Immunol. Immunopathol.* **2011**, *143*, 338–346. [CrossRef]
71. Van Hooft, P.; Keet, D.F.; Brebner, D.K.; Bastos, A.D. Genetic insights into dispersal distance and disperser fitness of African lions (Panthera leo) from the latitudinal extremes of the Kruger National Park, South Africa. *BMC Genet.* **2018**, *19*, 21. [CrossRef]
72. Meoli, R.; Eleni, C.; Cavicchio, P.; Tonnicchia, M.C.; Biancani, B.; Galosi, L.; Rossi, G. B-cell chronic lymphocytic leukaemia in an African lion (Panthera leo). *Veterinární Med.* **2018**, *63*, 433–437. [CrossRef]
73. Harrison, T.M.; McKnight, C.A.; Sikarskie, J.G.; Kitchell, B.E.; Garner, M.M.; Raymond, J.T.; Fitzgerald, S.D.; Valli, V.E.; Agnew, D.; Kiupel, M. Malignant lymphoma in African lions (Panthera leo). *Vet. Pathol.* **2010**, *47*, 952–957. [CrossRef]
74. Mourier, T.; Mollerup, S.; Vinner, L.; Hansen, T.A.; Kjartansdóttir, K.R.; Frøslev, T.G.; Boutrup, T.S.; Nielsen, L.P.; Willerslev, E.; Hansen, A.J. Characterizing novel endogenous retroviruses from genetic variation inferred from short sequence reads. *Sci. Rep.* **2015**, *5*, 15644. [CrossRef]
75. Duarte, M.D.; Barros, S.C.; Henriques, M.; Fernandes, T.L.; Bernardino, R.; Monteiro, M.; Fevereiro, M. Fatal infection with feline panleukopenia virus in two captive wild carnivores (Panthera tigris and Panthera leo). *J. Zoo Wildl. Med.* **2009**, *40*, 354–359. [CrossRef]
76. Gillman, L.; Sánchez, A.M.; Arbiza, J. Picobirnavirus in captive animals from Uruguay: Identification of new hosts. *Intervirology* **2013**, *56*, 46–49. [CrossRef] [PubMed]
77. Ahasan, M.S.; Subramaniam, K.; Sayler, K.A.; Loeb, J.C.; Popov, V.L.; Lednicky, J.A.; Wisely, S.M.; Krauer, J.M.C.; Waltzek, T.B. Molecular characterization of a novel reassortment Mammalian orthoreovirus type 2 isolated from a Florida white-tailed deer fawn. *Virus Res.* **2019**, *270*, 197642. [CrossRef] [PubMed]
78. Orbell, G.M.B.; Young, S.; Munday, J.S. Cutaneous sarcoids in captive African lions associated with feline sarcoid-associated papillomavirus infection. *Vet. Pathol.* **2011**, *48*, 1176–1179. [CrossRef]

79. Kraberger, S.; Serieys, L.; Fountain-Jones, N.; Packer, C.; Riley, S.; Varsani, A. Novel smacoviruses identified in the faeces of two wild felids: North American bobcat and African lion. *Arch. Virol.* **2019**, *164*, 2395–2399. [CrossRef] [PubMed]
80. Chhibber-Goel, J.; Joshi, S.; Sharma, A. Aminoacyl tRNA synthetases as potential drug targets of the Panthera pathogen Babesia. *Parasites Vectors* **2019**, *12*, 482. [CrossRef]
81. Githaka, N.; Konnai, S.; Kariuki, E.; Kanduma, E.; Murata, S.; Ohashi, K. Molecular detection and characterization of potentially new Babesia and Theileria species/variants in wild felids from Kenya. *Acta Trop.* **2012**, *124*, 71–78. [CrossRef] [PubMed]
82. Williams, B.M.; Berentsen, A.; Shock, B.C.; Teixiera, M.; Dunbar, M.R.; Becker, M.S.; Yabsley, M.J. Prevalence and diversity of Babesia, Hepatozoon, Ehrlichia, and Bartonella in wild and domestic carnivores from Zambia, Africa. *Parasitol. Res.* **2014**, *113*, 911–918. [CrossRef]
83. Di Cesare, A.; Laiacona, F.; Iorio, R.; Marangi, M.; Menegotto, A. Aelurostrongylus abstrusus in wild felids of South Africa. *Parasitol. Res.* **2016**, *115*, 3731–3735. [CrossRef]
84. Berentsen, A.R.; Becker, M.S.; Stockdale-Walden, H.; Matandiko, W.; McRobb, R.; Dunbar, M.R. Survey of gastrointestinal parasite infection in African lion (Panthera leo), African wild dog (Lycaon pictus) and spotted hyaena (Crocuta crocuta) in the Luangwa Valley, Zambia. *Afr. Zool.* **2012**, *47*, 363–368. [CrossRef]
85. Seltmann, A.; Webster, F.; Ferreira, S.C.M.; Czirják, G.Á.; Wachter, B. Age-specific gastrointestinal parasite shedding in free-ranging cheetahs (Acinonyx jubatus) on Namibian farmland. *Parasitol. Res.* **2019**, *118*, 851–859. [CrossRef]
86. Dubey, J.P. A review of Cystoisospora felis and C. rivolta-induced coccidiosis in cats. *Vet. Parasitol.* **2018**, *263*, 34–48. [CrossRef] [PubMed]
87. Alvarado-Esquivel, C.; Gayosso-Dominguez, E.A.; Villena, I.; Dubey, J.P. Seroprevalence of Toxoplasma gondii infection in captive mammals in three zoos in Mexico City, Mexico. *J. Zoo Wildl. Med.* **2013**, 803–806. [CrossRef] [PubMed]
88. Ferreira, S.C.M.; Torelli, F.; Klein, S.; Fyumagwa, R.; Karesh, W.B.; Hofer, H.; Seeber, F.; East, M.L. Evidence of high exposure to Toxoplasma gondii in free-ranging and captive African carnivores. *Int. J. Parasitol. Parasites Wildl.* **2019**, *8*, 111–117. [CrossRef] [PubMed]
89. Eom, K.S.; Park, H.; Lee, D.; Choe, S.; Kang, Y.; Bia, M.M.; Lee, S.-H.; Keyyu, J.; Fyumagwa, R.; Jeon, H.-K. Molecular and morphologic identification of Spirometra ranarum found in the stool of African lion, Panthera leo in the Serengeti plain of Tanzania. *Korean J. Parasitol.* **2018**, *56*, 379. [CrossRef]
90. Eom, K.S.; Park, H.; Lee, D.; Choe, S.; Kang, Y.; Bia, M.M.; Ndosi, B.A.; Nath, T.C.; Eamudomkarn, C.; Keyyu, J. Identity of Spirometra theileri from a Leopard (Panthera pardus) and Spotted Hyena (Crocuta crocuta) in Tanzania. *Korean J. Parasitol.* **2019**, *57*, 639–645. [CrossRef] [PubMed]
91. Jeon, H.-K.; Kim, K.-H.; Sohn, W.-M.; Eom, K.S. Differential Diagnosis of Human Sparganosis Using Multiplex PCR. *Korean J. Parasitol.* **2018**, *56*, 295. [CrossRef]
92. Eberhard, M.L.; Thiele, E.A.; Yembo, G.E.; Yibi, M.S.; Cama, V.A.; Ruiz-Tiben, E. Thirty-Seven Human Cases of Sparganosis from Ethiopia and South Sudan Caused by Spirometra Spp. *Am. J. Trop. Med. Hyg.* **2015**, *93*, 350–355. [CrossRef]
93. Anderson, N.E.; Mubanga, J.; Fevre, E.M.; Picozzi, K.; Eisler, M.C.; Thomas, R.; Welburn, S.C. Characterisation of the wildlife reservoir community for human and animal trypanosomiasis in the Luangwa Valley, Zambia. *PLoS Negl. Trop. Dis.* **2011**, *5*. [CrossRef]
94. Sheng, Z.-H.; Chang, Q.-C.; Tian, S.-Q.; Lou, Y.; Zheng, X.; Zhao, Q.; Wang, C.-R. Characterization of Toxascaris leonina and Tococara canis from cougar (Panthera leo) and common wolf (Canis lupus) by nuclear ribosomal DNA sequences of internal transcribed spacers. *Afr. J. Microbiol. Res.* **2012**, *6*, 3545–3549.
95. Xue, L.-M.; Chai, J.-B.; Guo, Y.-N.; Zhang, L.-P.; Li, L. Further studies on Toxascaris leonina (Linstow, 1902) (Ascaridida: Ascarididae) from Felis lynx (Linnaeus) and Panthera leo (Linnaeus) (Carnivora: Felidae). *Acta Parasitol.* **2015**, *60*, 146–153. [CrossRef]
96. Marucci, G.; La Grange, L.J.; La Rosa, G.; Pozio, E. Trichinella nelsoni and Trichinella T8 mixed infection in a lion (Panthera leo) of the Kruger National Park (South Africa). *Vet. Parasitol.* **2009**, *159*, 225–228. [CrossRef] [PubMed]
97. Maruping-Mzileni, N.T.; Funston, P.J.; Ferreira, S.M. State-shifts of lion prey selection in the Kruger National Park. *Wildl. Res.* **2017**, *44*, 28–39. [CrossRef]

98. Groom, R.J.; Funston, P.J.; Mandisodza, R. Surveys of lions Panthera leo in protected areas in Zimbabwe yield disturbing results: What is driving the population collapse? *Oryx* **2014**, *48*, 385–393. [CrossRef]
99. Roos, E.O.; Olea-Popelka, F.; Buss, P.; Hausler, G.A.; Warren, R.; Van Helden, P.D.; Parsons, S.D.; de Klerk-Lorist, L.-M.; Miller, M.A. Measuring antigen-specific responses in Mycobacterium bovis-infected warthogs (Phacochoerus africanus) using the intradermal tuberculin test. *BMC Vet. Res.* **2018**, *14*, 1–7. [CrossRef]
100. Viljoen, I.M.; Van Helden, P.D.; Millar, R.P. Mycobacterium bovis infection in the lion (Panthera leo): Current knowledge, conundrums and research challenges. *Vet. Microbiol.* **2015**, *177*, 252–260. [CrossRef]
101. McCain, S.; Allender, M.C.; Schumacher, J.; Ramsay, E. The effects of a probiotic on blood urea nitrogen and creatinine concentrations in large felids. *J. Zoo Wildl. Med.* **2011**, *42*, 426–429. [CrossRef]
102. Gross-Tsubery, R.; Chai, O.; Shilo, Y.; Miara, L.; Horowitz, I.H.; Shmueli, A.; Aizenberg, I.; Hoffman, C.; Reifen, R.A.M.; Shamir, M.H. Computed tomographic analysis of calvarial hyperostosis in captive lions. *Vet. Radiol. Ultrasound* **2010**, *51*, 34–38. [CrossRef]
103. Saqib, M.; Abbas, G.; Mughal, M.N. Successful management of ivermectin-induced blindness in an African lion (Panthera leo) by intravenous administration of a lipid emulsion. *BMC Vet. Res.* **2015**, *11*, 287. [CrossRef]
104. Loots, A.K.; Cardoso-Vermaak, E.; Venter, E.H.; Mitchell, E.; Kotzé, A.; Dalton, D.L. The role of toll-like receptor polymorphisms in susceptibility to canine distemper virus. *Mamm. Biol.* **2018**, *88*, 94–99. [CrossRef]
105. Deem, S.L.; Spelman, L.H.; Yates, R.A.; Montali, R.J. Canine distemper in terrestrial carnivores: A review. *J. Zoo Wildl. Med.* **2000**, *31*, 441–451. [PubMed]
106. Steinel, A.; Parrish, C.R.; Bloom, M.E.; Truyen, U. Parvovirus infections in wild carnivores. *J. Wildl. Dis.* **2001**, *37*, 594–607. [CrossRef] [PubMed]
107. Keet, D.F.; Michel, A.L.; Bengis, R.G.; Becker, P.; Van Dyk, D.S.; Van Vuuren, M.; Rutten, V.; Penzhorn, B.L. Intradermal tuberculin testing of wild African lions (Panthera leo) naturally exposed to infection with Mycobacterium bovis. *Vet. Microbiol.* **2010**, *144*, 384–391. [CrossRef]
108. Lane, E.P.; Brettschneider, H.; Caldwell, P.; Oosthuizen, A.; Dalton, D.L.; du Plessis, L.; Steyl, J.; Kotze, A. Feline panleukopaenia virus in captive non-domestic felids in South Africa. *Onderstepoort J. Vet. Res.* **2016**, *83*, 1–8. [CrossRef]
109. Moudgil, A.D.; Singla, L.D.; Singh, M.P. An issue of Public Health concern due to emerging drug resistance against Toxascaris leonina (Linstow, 1909) in Asiatic lions (Panthera leo persica). *Int. J. Infect. Dis.* **2016**, *45*, 105. [CrossRef]
110. Bentubo, H.D.L.; Fedullo, J.D.L.; Corrêa, S.H.R.; Teixeira, R.H.F.; Coutinho, S.D. Isolation of Microsporum gypseum from the haircoat of health wild felids kept in captivity in Brazil. *Braz. J. Microbiol.* **2006**, *37*, 148–152. [CrossRef]
111. *Anonymous Personal Comms*; 2019.
112. *World Health Organisation Neglected Tropical Diseases*; World Health Organisation: Geneva, Switzerland, 2020.
113. Odeniran, P.O.; Ademola, I.O. Zoonotic parasites of wildlife in Africa: A review. *Afr. J. Wildl. Res.* **2016**, *46*, 1–13. [CrossRef]
114. De Garine-Wichatitsky, M.; Caron, A.; Kock, R.; Tschopp, R.; Munyeme, M.; Hofmeyr, M.; Michel, A. A review of bovine tuberculosis at the wildlife–livestock–human interface in sub-Saharan Africa. *Epidemiol. Infect.* **2013**, *141*, 1342–1356. [CrossRef]
115. Probst, C.; Parry, C.D.; Rehm, J. Socio-economic differences in HIV/AIDS mortality in South Africa. *Trop. Med. Int. Health* **2016**, *21*, 846–855. [CrossRef]
116. Tadokera, R.; Bekker, L.-G.; Kreiswirth, B.N.; Mathema, B.; Middelkoop, K. TB transmission is associated with prolonged stay in a low socio-economic, high burdened TB and HIV community in Cape Town, South Africa. *BMC Infect. Dis.* **2020**, *20*, 120. [CrossRef] [PubMed]
117. Kiers, A.; Klarenbeek, A.; Mendelts, B.; Van Soolingen, D.; Koëter, G. Transmission of Mycobacterium pinnipedii to humans in a zoo with marine mammals. *Int. J. Tuberc. Lung Dis.* **2008**, *12*, 1469–1473. [PubMed]
118. IUCN SSC Cat Specialist Group 2020. Available online: https://www.facebook.com/IUCN-SSC-Cat-Specialist-Group-1478766355730648/ (accessed on 29 August 2020).
119. Peiris, J.M.; De Jong, M.D.; Guan, Y. Avian influenza virus (H5N1): A threat to human health. *Clin. Microbiol. Rev.* **2007**, *20*, 243–267. [CrossRef] [PubMed]
120. Opriessnig, T.; Huang, Y. Update on possible animal sources for COVID-19 in humans. *Xenotransplantation* **2020**, *27*. [CrossRef]

121. Goldstein, J.D. Bronx Zoo Tiger is Sick with Coronavirus. *The New York Times*. 2020. Available online: https://www.nytimes.com/2020/04/06/science/tiger-cats-coronavirus.html (accessed on 13 August 2020).
122. Steenhuisen, F.J.; Lorimer, J.; Street, P. Didiza's Attempt to Legalise the Consumption of Wild Animals Is Unfathomable. Available online: https://www.da.org.za/2020/05/didizas-attempt-to-legalise-the-consumption-of-wild-animals-is-unfathomable. (accessed on 25 August 2020).
123. Daszak, P.; Cunningham, A.A.; Hyatt, A.D. Anthropogenic environmental change and the emergence of infectious diseases in wildlife. *Acta Trop.* **2001**, *78*, 103–116. [CrossRef]
124. Association of Zoos and Aquiariums African Lion Breeding Program Receives Award from Association of Zoos & Aquariums. *News Releases*. 2018. Available online: https://www.aza.org/aza-news-releases/posts/african-lion-breeding-program-receives-award-from-association-of-zoos--aquariums (accessed on 18 August 2020).
125. Williams, V.L.; Michael, J. Born captive: A survey of the lion breeding, keeping and hunting industries in South Africa. *PLoS ONE* **2019**, *14*, e0217409. [CrossRef]
126. Fobar, R. More than 100 Neglected Lions Found in a South African Breeding Facility. *National Geographic*. 2019. Available online: https://www.nationalgeographic.co.uk/animals/2019/05/more-100-neglected-lions-discovered-south-africa-breeding-facility (accessed on 12 August 2020).
127. Katz, B. 108 Neglected Lions Found on South African Breeding Farm. *Smithsonian Magazine*. 2019. Available online: https://www.smithsonianmag.com/smart-news/108-neglected-lions-found-south-african-breeding-farm-180972146/ (accessed on 20 August 2020).
128. Humphrey, T. Are happy chickens safer chickens? Poultry welfare and disease susceptibility. *Br. Poult. Sci.* **2006**, *47*, 379–391. [CrossRef]
129. Saragusty, J.; Shavit-Meyrav, A.; Yamaguchi, N.; Nadler, R.; Bdolah-Abram, T.; Gibeon, L.; Hildebrandt, T.B.; Shamir, M.H. Comparative skull analysis suggests species-specific captivity-related malformation in lions (Panthera leo). *PLoS ONE* **2014**, *9*, e94527. [CrossRef]
130. Beck, M.A.; Levander, O.A. Host nutritional status and its effect on a viral pathogen. *J. Infect. Dis.* **2000**, *182*, S93–S96. [CrossRef]
131. Woo, P.C.; Lau, S.K.; Yuen, K. Infectious diseases emerging from Chinese wet-markets: Zoonotic origins of severe respiratory viral infections. *Curr. Opin. Infect. Dis.* **2006**, *19*, 401–407. [CrossRef]
132. Wildlife Conservation Society. *Commercial Wildlife Farms in Vietnam: A Problem or Solution for Conservation?* Wildlife Conservation Society: Hanoi, Vietnam, 2008.
133. Coals, P.; Burnham, D.; Loveridge, A.; Macdonald, D.W.; Sas-Rolfes, M.T.; Williams, V.L.; Vucetich, J.A. The Ethics of Human-Animal Relationships and Public Discourse: A Case Study of Lions Bred for Their Bones. *Animals* **2019**, *9*, 52. [CrossRef] [PubMed]
134. Rendón-Franco, E.; Romero-Callejas, E.; Villanueva-García, C.; Osorio-Sarabia, D.; Muñoz-García, C.I. Cross transmission of gastrointestinal nematodes between captive neotropical felids and feral cats. *J. Zoo Wildl. Med.* **2013**, *44*, 936–940. [CrossRef]
135. Saegerman, C.; Dal Pozzo, F.; Humblet, M.-F. Reducing hazards for humans from animals: Emerging and re-emerging zoonoses. *Ital. J. Public Health* **2012**, *9*. [CrossRef]
136. Halliday, J.; Daborn, C.; Auty, H.; Mtema, Z.; Lembo, T.; de Bronsvoort, B.M.C.; Handel, I.; Knobel, D.; Hampson, K.; Cleaveland, S. Bringing together emerging and endemic zoonoses surveillance: Shared challenges and a common solution. *Philos. Trans. R. Soc. B Biol. Sci.* **2012**, *367*, 2872–2880. [CrossRef] [PubMed]
137. Halliday, J.E.B.; Hampson, K.; Hanley, N.; Lembo, T.; Sharp, J.P.; Haydon, D.T.; Cleaveland, S. Driving improvements in emerging disease surveillance through locally relevant capacity strengthening. *Science* **2017**, *357*, 146–148. [CrossRef]

animals

MDPI

Review

Haemogregarines and Criteria for Identification

Saleh Al-Quraishy [1], Fathy Abdel-Ghaffar [2], Mohamed A. Dkhil [1,3] and Rewaida Abdel-Gaber [1,2,*]

1 Department of Zoology, College of Science, King Saud University, Riyadh 11451, Saudi Arabia; guraishi@yahoo.com (S.A.-Q.); mohameddkhil@yahoo.com (M.A.D.)
2 Zoology Department, Faculty of Science, Cairo University, Cairo 12613, Egypt; fathyghaffar@yahoo.com
3 Department of Zoology and Entomology, Faculty of Science, Helwan University, Cairo 11795, Egypt
* Correspondence: rabdelgaber.c@ksu.edu.sa

Simple Summary: Taxonomic classification of haemogregarines belonging to Apicomplexa can become difficult when the information about the life cycle stages is not available. Using a self-reporting, we record different haemogregarine species infecting various animal categories and exploring the most systematic features for each life cycle stage. The keystone in the classification of any species of haemogregarines is related to the sporogonic cycle more than other stages of schizogony and gamogony. Molecular approaches are excellent tools that enabled the identification of apicomplexan parasites by clarifying their evolutionary relationships.

Abstract: Apicomplexa is a phylum that includes all parasitic protozoa sharing unique ultrastructural features. Haemogregarines are sophisticated apicomplexan blood parasites with an obligatory heteroxenous life cycle and haplohomophasic alternation of generations. Haemogregarines are common blood parasites of fish, amphibians, lizards, snakes, turtles, tortoises, crocodilians, birds, and mammals. Haemogregarine ultrastructure has been so far examined only for stages from the vertebrate host. PCR-based assays and the sequencing of the *18S rRNA* gene are helpful methods to further characterize this parasite group. The proper classification for the haemogregarine complex is available with the criteria of generic and unique diagnosis of these parasites.

Keywords: haemogregarines; gamogony; sporogony; schizongony; molecular analysis

check for updates

Citation: Al-Quraishy, S.; Abdel-Ghaffar, F.; Dkhil, M.A.; Abdel-Gaber, R. Haemogregarines and Criteria for Identification. *Animals* **2021**, *11*, 170. https://doi.org/10.3390/ani11010170

Received: 27 November 2020
Accepted: 7 January 2021
Published: 12 January 2021

1. Introduction

Phylum Apicomplexa was described by Levine [1] to include parasitic protozoa sharing unique ultrastructural features known as the "apical complex" (Figure 1). Haemogregarines (Figure 2) are ubiquitous adeleorine apicomplexan protists inhabiting the blood cells of a variety of ectothermic and some endothermic vertebrates [2–4]. They have also an obligatory heteroxenous life cycle (Figure 3), where asexual multiplication occurs in the vertebrate host; while sexual reproduction occurs in the hematophagous invertebrate vector [5]. This family contains four genera, according to Levine [6]: *Haemogregarina* Danilewsky [7], *Karyolysus* Labbé [8], *Hepatozoon* Miller [9], and *Cyrilia* Lainson [10]. Barta [11] conducted a phylogenetic analysis of representative genera in phylum Apicomplexa using biological and morphological features to infer evolutionary relationships in this phylum among the widely recognized groups. The data showed that the biologically diverse Haemogregarinidae family should be divided into at least three families (as suggested by Mohammed and Mansour [12]), were family Haemogregarinidae, containing the genera *Haemogregarina* and *Cyrilia*; family Karyolysidae Wenyon [13], of the genus *Karyolysus*; and family Hepatozoidae Wenyon [13], of the genus *Hepatozoon*, since the four genera currently in the family do not constitute a monophyletic group. The picture is further complicated by evidence from a study by Petit et al. [14] of a new Brazilian toad haemogregarine parasite *Haemolivia stellata*.

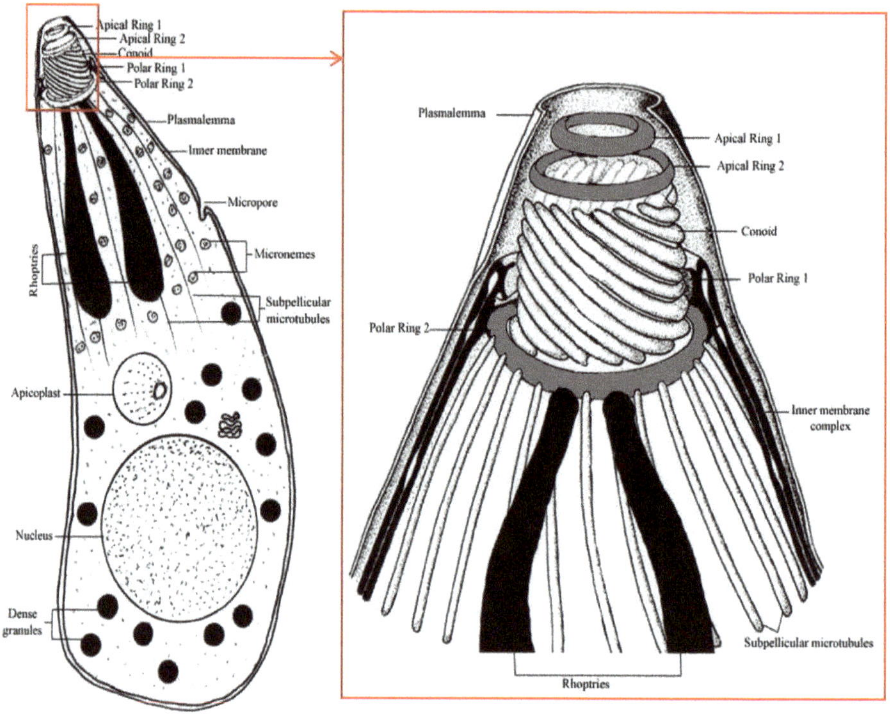

Figure 1. The general structure for the apical complex for Apicomplexa.

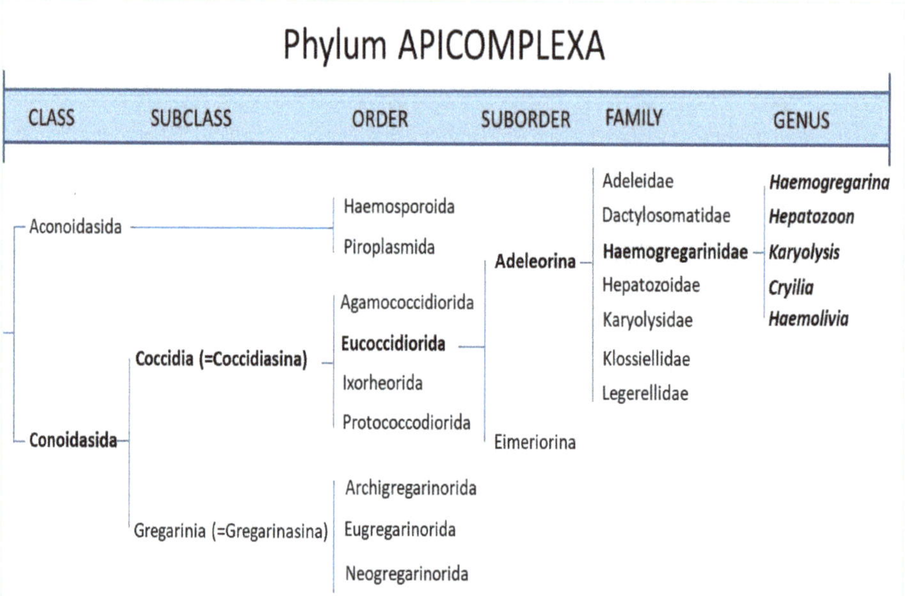

Figure 2. Haemogregarines as a part of phylum Apicomplexa.

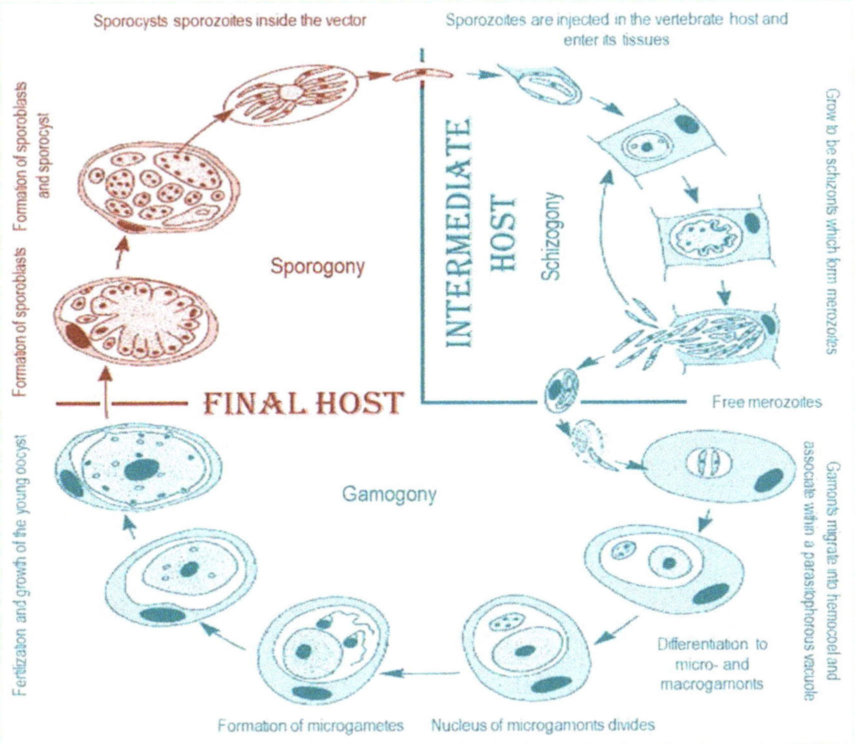

Figure 3. The life cycle of the apicomplexan parasites.

It undergoes sporogonic development in its tick host's gut wall and has a complex life cycle that resembles *Karyolysus* species much more than *Hepatozoon*, *Haemogregarina*, and *Cyrilia* species. Haemogregarines can be morphologically classified based on the developmental details of sporogonic phases of the parasite in the vector, which provide the main characters for classification, the morphology of gametocytes in the red blood cells, and an evaluation of the stages of development [15,16]. Although useful, this methodology is not sufficient for a taxonomic diagnosis [17,18] also the classical systematics has been problematic because of the variability to which morphological details are subjected [19]. Therefore, the use of molecular methods from blood or tissue samples [20–22], with appropriate molecular phylogeny study, became an essential adjunct to existing morphological and biological characters for use in the inference of evolutionary history relationships among haemoprotozoan parasites [23–25]. Molecular data has been carried out based using PCR assays targeting the nuclear 18s ribosomal RNA gene, which have been extensively applied to characterize hemoparasites DNA more fully in the absence of complete life cycles [26–32].

In the present critical review of the haemogregarines complex, the proper classification, the criteria of generic and unique diagnosis, and the cosmopolitan distribution of haemogregarines among the vertebrate and invertebrate hosts are examined because of their relevant characteristic and taxonomic revisions.

2. Materials and Methods

This review included all related published scientific articles from January 1901 to December 2020. This article was conducted by searching the electronic databases NCBI, ScienceDirect, Saudi digital library, and GenBank database, to check scientific articles and

M.Sc./Ph.D. Thesis related to the research topic of this review. Studies published in the English language were only included and otherwise are excluded.

Relevant studies were reviewed through numerous steps. In the first step, target published articles were identified by using general related terms related to the morphological features, such as "Haemogregarines" and "Apicomplex". The second step involved screening the resulting articles by using highly specific keywords of the generic features for stages in the life cycle of haemogregarines species, including "Merogony", "Gamogony", "Sporogony", "Infective stages", "Motile stage", "Infection sites", and "sporozoites". The last step of the review focused on selected studies involving the use of molecular analysis for accurate taxonomic identification by using highly specific keywords, including "PCR", "Genetic markers", "Variable regions", "*18S rRNA*", and "Phylogenetic analysis".

The obtained data were presented in tables and figures and were: Table 1 representing the characteristic features for the haemogregarines genera, Tables 2–6 showing haemogregarines species, the vertebrate host, site of the merogonic stage, the invertebrate vectors, site of gamogony and sporogonic stages, geographical locality for hosts, and the authors for publishing data, Table 7 with the primer sets used for the amplification and sequencing for the appropriate gene of *18S rRNA* for haemogregarines, and Table 8 representing all the sequenced and deposited haemogregarines in the GenBank database until now.

3. Results and Discussion

In this review, the different stages of the apicomplexan life cycle were used to identify haemogregarines. However, in most cases, their assignment to one or another genus cannot be considered more than provisional. Accordingly, about 82 haemogregarines in 155 research articles were identified previously. Osimani [33] stated that the differences between the haemogregarines relied more on the host's identity than the parasite's characteristics. Mohammed and Mansour [12] reported that haemogregarines gamonts morphology does not provide generic identification with a reliable key. However, Telford et al. [34], and Herbert et al. [35] stated that the determination of generic haemogregarines should not be based exclusively on the gamonts' form, the type of parasitized host cells, and their effect on the host and site merogony in host cells. While the most characteristic feature for the basic identification via the sporogonic stage.

The reviewed species belonged to the four genera within Hemogregarinidae (Table 1). Following the parsimony analysis in the phylogenetic study of the representative genera in phylum Apicomplexa performed by Siddall and Desser [36] primarily based on ultrastructural observations, it was concluded that the variations between the different haemogregarines genera are mainly reflected by the sporogony features. Besides, Dvořáková et al. [37] added that the host specificity, together with the haemogregarine's careful morphological and biological analysis, is a sound criterion for accurate identification. These species are common in different animals as fish (Table 2), amphibians (Table 3), reptiles (Tables 4–7), birds (Table 8), and mammals (Table 9).

Table 1. Characters of different groups of haemogregarines used in the parsimony analysis carried out by Barta [19] and Siddall and Desser [36].

Comparable Features	*Karyolysis*	*Haemogregarina*	*Cryilia*	*Hepatozoon*	*Haemolivia*
Conoid present	In all non-gametes	In all non-gametes	In all non-gametes	In all non-gametes	In all non-gametes
Crystalloid bodies +/-	?	+	?	+	+ (fragmented)
Merogeny +/-	+ Intra-cellular	+ Intra-cellular	+ Intra-cellular	+ Intra-cellular	+ Intra-cellular
Micropores +/-	+	+	+	+	+
Mitochondria.	Cristate	Cristate	Cristate	Cristate	Cristate
Mitosis	Centriolar	Centriolar	?	Centriolar	Centriolar
Amylopectin granules +/-	+	-	-	+	+
Polar ring complex +/-	+	+	+	+	+
Gametogenesis	Extra-cellular	Extra-cellular	Extra-cellular	Extra-cellular	Intra-cellular
No. of microgametes/each microgamont	2	4	4	4	2–4
Gamonts	Anisogamous	Anisogamous	Anisogamous	Anisogamous	Anisogamous
Syzygy	+	+	+	+	+
Zygote	Non-motile	Non-motile	Non-motile	Non-motile	Non-motile
Sporogony	Extra-cellular	Extra-cellular	Extra-cellular	Extra-cellular	Intra-cellular
Persistent cysts +/-	-	-	-	+	+
No. of flagella/microgametes	1	1	Absent	1	?
Arrangement of flagella in microgametes	Terminal	Terminal	?	Terminal	Terminal
No. of sporozoites/oocyst	20–30	8	>20	4–16	10–25

Note: (+) presence, (-) absence, (?) not detected.

Table 2. Haemogregarines of fish.

Species of Haemogregarines	The Vertebrate Host	Site of Merogony	Invertebrate Vector	Site of Gamogony and Sporogony	Locality	Authors
Cyrilia gomesi	*Synbranchus marmoratus*	Leucocytes	*Haementeria lutzi*	Stomach	Sao Paulo, Brazil	Nakamoto et al. [38]
Haemogregarina bigemina	*Lipophrys folis* and *Coryphoblrnnius galerita*	Blood cells	*Gnathia maxillaris*	Hindgut	Portugal Atlantic west coast	Davies et al. [39]
Haemogregarina vltavensis	*Perca fluviatilis*	Intra-erythrocytic gamonts are only described	–	–	Czechoslovakia	Lom et al. [40]
Haemogregarina leptocotti	*Leptocottus armatus*	Blood cells	–	–	California USA	Hill and Hendrickson [41]
Haemogregarina roelofsi	*Sebastes melanops*	Blood cells	–	–	California USA	Hill and Hendrickson [41]
Haemogregarina bigemina	*Clinus superciliosus* and *Clinus cottoides*	Intra-erythrocytic	*Gnathia africana*	–	South Africa	Davies and Smit [42]
Haemogregarine sp.	*Scomber scombrus* L.	Leucocytes	–	–	Northwest and Northeast Atlantic ocean	Maclean and Davies [43]
Haemogregarina curvata	*Clinus cottoides*, *Parablennius cornutus*	Intra-erythrocytic	*Zeylanicobdella arugamensis*	Host gut tissue	South Africa	Hayes et al. [44]
Haemogregarina balistapi	*Rhinecanthus aculeatus*	Intra-erythrocytic	*Gnathia aureamaculosa*	Host gut tissue	Great Barrier Reef, Australia	Curtis et al. [45]
Cyrilia sp.	*Potamotrygon wallacei*	Intra-erythrocytic	–	–	Rio Negri	Oliveira et al. [46]
Haemogregarina daviesensis	*Lepidosiren paradoxa*	Intra-erythrocytic	–	–	Eastern Amazon region	Esteves-Silva et al. [47]

Table 3. Haemogregarines of amphibians.

Species of Haemogregarines	The Vertebrate Host	Site of Merogony	Invertebrate Vector	Site of Gamogony and Sporogony	Locality	Authors
Pseudohaemogregarina nutti	*Rana nutti*	Erythrocytes and liver	–	–	Germany	Awerenzew [48]
Haemogregarina theileri	*Rana angloensis*	Erythrocytes and liver	–	–	Njoro, Kenya	Ball [49]
Haemolivia stellate	Brazilian toads	Liver	Ticks	Gut wall	Brazil	Petit et al. [14]
Haemogregarina nucleobisecans	*Bufo himalayanus*	Erythrocytes and liver	–	–	India	Ray [50]
Hepatozoon sipedon	*Nerodia sipedon* and *Rana pipiens*	Various internal organs	*Culex pipiens* and *Culex territans*	Hemocoel	Ontario, Canada	Smith et al. [51]
Hepatozoon catesbianae	*Rana catesbeiana*	Erythrocytes and liver	*Culex territans*	Malpighian tubules	Ontario, Canada	Desser et al. [52]
Hepatozoon caimani	*Rana catesbeiana*	Intra-erythrocytic	*Culex fatigans*	Extra-erythrocytic gametocytes	State of Mato Grosso	Lainson et al. [53]
Hepatozoon theileri	*Amietia quecketti*	Intra-erythrocytic gamonts are only described	–	–	South Africa	Conradie et al. [54]
Hepatozoon involucrum	*Hyperolius marmoratus*	Intra-erythrocytic	–	–	KwaZulu-Natal, South Africa	Netherlands et al. [55]
Hepatozoon tenuis	*Afrixalus fornasinii*	Intra-erythrocytic	–	–	KwaZulu-Natal, South Africa	Netherlands et al. [55]
Hepatozoon thori	*Hyperolius marmoratus*	Intra-erythrocytic	–	–	KwaZulu-Natal, South Africa	Netherlands et al. [55]

Table 4. Haemogregarines of lizards.

Species of Haemogregarines	The Vertebrate Host	Site of Merogony	Invertebrate Vector	Site of Gamogony and Sporogony	Locality	Authors
Hepatozoon mesnili	*Gecko verticillatus*	Endothelial cells of all host organs	*Culex fatigans* and *Aedes albopictus*	Stomach	Saigon	Robin [56]
Haemogregarina triatomae	*Tupinambis teguixin*	Liver and lung	*Triatoma subrovaria*	Intestine	South America	Osimani [33]
Hepatozoon argantis	*Agama mossambica*	Liver	*Argas brumpti*	Gut and homocoelomic cavity	East Africa, Mossambic	Garnham [57]
Hepatozoon sauromali	*Sauromalus* sp.	Liver	*Ophionyssus* sp.	Hemocoel	–	Lewis and Wagner [58]
Haemogregarina sp.	*Tarentola annularis*	Lung	–	–	Sudan	Elwasila [59]
Hepatozoon lygosomarum	*Leiolopisma nigriplantare*	Liver and spleen	*Ophionissus saurarum*	Wall of the gut caeca	Canterbury, New Zealand	Allison and Desser [60]
Haemogregarina waltairensis	*Calotes versicolor*	Peripheral blood, liver, lung, and bone marrow	–	–	India	Saratchandra [61]
Hepatozoon gracilis	*Mabuya quinquetaeniata*	Liver	*Culex pipienis molesus*	Hemocoel	Giza, Egypt	Bashtar et al. [62]
Haemogregarina sp.	*Podarcis bocagei* and *Podarcis carbonelli*	Intra-erythrocytic	–	–	NW Portugal	Roca and Galdón [63]
Haemogregarina ramadani	*Acanthodactylus boskianus*	Intra-erythrocytic	–	–	Giza, Egypt	Abdel-Baki and Al-Quraishy [64]
Hepatozoon sp.	*Podarcis vaucheri*	Intra-erythrocytic	–	–	Oukaimeden	Moreira et al. [65]
Haemogregarina sp.	*Tarentola annularis*	Intra-erythrocytic	–	–	Qena, Egypt	Rabie and Hussein [66]
Karyolysus lacazei *Karyolysus* sp. *Karyolysus latus*	*Lacerta agilis* *Zootoca vivipara* *Podarcis muralis*	Intra-erythrocytic	*Ophionyssus saurarum* and *Ixodes ricinus*		Poland, Slovakia	Haklová-Kočíková et al. [18]
Karyolysus paradoxa	*Varanus albigularis*, *Varanus niloticus*	Intra-erythrocytic	–	–	Ndumo Game Reserve, South Africa	Cook et al. [31]
Haemogregarina daviesensis	*Lepidosiren paradoxa*	Intra-erythrocytic	–	–	Eastern Amazon region	Esteves-Silva et al. [47]
Haemogregarina sp.	*Scincus scincus*	Intra-erythrocytic	–	–	South Sinai, Egypt	Abou Shafeey et al. [67]
Karyolysus lacazei	*Lacerta schreiberi*	Intra-erythrocytic	*Ixodes ricinus*	–	Czech Republic	Zechmeisterová et al. [68]

Table 5. Haemogregarines of snakes.

Species of Haemogregarines	The Vertebrate Host	Site of Merogony	Invertebrate Vector	Site of Gamogony and Sporogony	Locality	Authors
Hepatozoon rarefaciens	*Drymachon corais*	Lung	*Culex tarsalis, Anopheles albintarus, Aedes sierrensis*	Hemocoel	California, USA	Ball and Oda [69]
Haemogregarnia matruhensis	*Psammophis schokari*	Intra-erythrocytic	–	–	Egypt	Ramadan [70]
Hepatozoon fusifex	*Boa constrictor*	Lung	*Culex tarsalis*	Hemocoel	USA	Ball et al. [71]
Hepatozoon aegypti	*Spalerosophis diadema*	Lung	*Culex pipiens molestus*	Hemocoel	Egypt	Bashtar et al. [72]
Hepatozoon mocassini	*Agkistrodon piscivorus leucostoma*	Liver parenchyma cells	*Aedes aegypti*	Hemocoel	Louisiana, USA	Lowichik et al. [73]
Hepatozoon seurati	*Cerastes cerastes*	Liver, lung, and spleen	*Culex pipiens molestus*	Hemocoel	Aswan, Egypt	Abdel-Ghaffar et al. [74]
Hepatozoon mehlhorni	*Echis carinatus*	Liver, lung, and spleen	*Culex pipiens molestus*	Hemocoel	Siwah and Baharia Oasis, Egypt	Bashtar et al. [75]
Hepatozoon matruhensis	*Psammophis schokari*	Liver and lung	*Culex pipiens molestus*	Hemocoel	Faiyum, Ismailia, Egypt	Bashtar et al. [76]
Hepatozoon ghaffari	*Cerastes vipera*	Liver, lung, and spleen	*Culex pipiens molestus*	Hemocoel	Aswan, Egypt	Shazly et al. [77]
Hepatozoon sipedon	*Nerodia sipedon* and *Rana pipiens*	Liver and internal organs	*Culex pipiens*, and *Culex territans*	Hemocoel	Ontario, Canada	Smith et al. [51]
Haemogregarnia garnhami	*Psammophis schokari*	Intra-erythrocytic	–	–	Egypt	Saoud et al. [78]
Hepatozoon ayorgbor	*Python regius*	Intra-erythrocytic	–	–	Ghana	Sloboda et al. [79]
Haemogregarnia sp.	*Cerastes cerastes gasperetti*	Intra-erythrocytic	–	–	Jizan, Saudi Arabia	Al-Farraj [80]
Hepatozoon garnhami	*Psammophis schokari*	Intra-erythrocytic	–	–	Riyadh, Saudi Arabia	Abdel-Baki et al. [29]
Hepatozoon sp.	*Zamenis longissimus*	Intra-erythrocytic	–	–	Iran	Sajjadi and Javanbakht [81]
Hepatozoon aegypti	*Spalerosophis diadema*	Intra-erythrocytic	–	–	Riyadh, Saudi Arabia	Abdel-Haleem et al. [82]

Table 6. Haemogregarines of turtles and tortoises.

Species of Haemogregarines	The Vertebrate Host	Site of Merogony	Invertebrate Vector	Site of Gamogony and Sporogony	Locality	Authors
Hemogregarina nicoriae	*Nicoria trijuga*	Circulating blood and lung	*Ozobranchus shipleyi*	Intestinal epithelium	Ceylon	Robertson [83]
Haemogregarina balli	*Chelydra serpentine serpentina*	Lacunar endothelial cells, liver, lung, and spleen	*Placobdella ornata*	Gastric and intestinal caeca	Ontario, Canada	Siddall and Desser [84]
Hepatozoon mauritanicum	*Testudo graeca*	Endothelial cells of all host organs as liver, lung, spleen . . . etc	*Hyalomma aegyptium*	The intestinal epithelium of the tick	–	Michel [85]
Haemogregarina pseudomydis	*Pseudemys scripta elegans*	Leucocytes and Erythrocytes	*Placobdella parasitica*	The intestinal epithelium of the leech	Louisiana, USA	Acholonu [86]
Haemogregarina gangetica (=*H. simondi*)	*Trionyx gangeticus*	Erythrocytes and lung	–	–	India	Misra [87]
Haemogregarina ganapatii	*Lissemys punctata granosa*	Peripheral blood and Liver and lung	–	–	India	Saratchandra [61]
Haemogregarina sinensis	*Trionyx sinensis*	Erythrocytes and Kupffer's cells of the liver	*Mooreotorix cotylifer*	Gastric and intestinal caeca of the leech	China	Chai and Chen [88]
Haemogregarina sp.	*Emys orbicularis*	Intra-erythrocytic	*Placobdella costata*	–	Romania	Mihalca et al. [89]
Haemolivia mauritanica	*Testudo graeca*	Intra-erythrocytic	*Hyalomna aegyptium*	Gut cells	Israel	Paperna [90]
Haemolivia mauritanica	Tortoises	Intra-erythrocytic	*Hyalomma aegyptium*	–	Western Palaearctic realm	Široký et al. [91]
Haemogregarina macrochelysi	*Macrochelys temminckii*	Intra-erythrocytic	*Leech*	–	Georgia and Florida	Telford et al. [92]
Haemogregarina stepanowi	*Emys orbicularis, Mauremys caspica, M. rivulata, M. leprosa*	Intra-erythrocytic	–	–	Western Palaearctic	Dvořáková et al. [23]
Haemogregarina sp.	*Lissemys punctata* and *Geoclemys hamiltonii*	Intra-erythrocytic	–	–	West Bengal, India	Hossen et al. [4]
Haemolivia mauritanica	*Testudo graeca* and *Testudo marginata*	Intra-erythrocytic		–	North African	Harris et al. [93]

Table 6. *Cont.*

Species of Haemogregarines	The Vertebrate Host	Site of Merogony	Invertebrate Vector	Site of Gamogony and Sporogony	Locality	Authors
Haemogregarina sp.	*Rhinoclemmys funera* and *Kinosternon leucostomum*	Intra-erythrocytic	–	–	Costa Rica	Rossow et al. [94]
Haemogregarina sp.	*Podocnemis unifilis*	Intra-erythrocytic	–	–	Brazilian Amazonia	Soares et al. [95]
Haemogregarina sundarbanensis	*Lissemys punctata*	Intra-erythrocytic	–	–	West Bengal, India	Molla et al. [96]
Haemogregarina stepanowi	*Emys orbicularis*	Intra-erythrocytic	–	–	Belgrade Zoo	Jòzsef et al. [24]
Haemogregarina sp.	*Podocnemis expansa*	Intra-erythrocytic	–	–	Araguaia River Basin, Brazil	Picelli et al. [97]
Haemogregarina sacaliae *Haemogregarina pellegrini*	*Cuora galbinifrons, Leucocephalon yuwonoi, Malayemys subtrijuga, Platysternon megacephalum,*	Intra-erythrocytic	–	–	Southeast Asia	Dvořáková et al. [37]
Haemogregarina fitzsimonsi *Haemogregarina parvula*	Land tortorise, *Stigmochelys pardalis*	Intra-erythrocytic	–	–	South African	Cook et al. [31]
Haemogregarina stepanowi	*Emys trinacris*	Intra-erythrocytic	–	–	Sicily	Arizza et al. [98]
Haemogregarina sp.	*Mauremys caspica*	Intra-erythrocytic	–	–	Iran	Rakhshandehroo et al. [99]
Haemogregarina sp.	*Macrochelys temminckii*	Intra-erythrocytic	–	–	Caldwell Zoo, Texas	Alhaboubi et al. [100]
Haemogregarina sp.	*Mesoclemmys vanderhaegei*	Intra-erythrocytic	–	–	Brazil	Goes et al. [101]
Haemogregarina podocnemis	*Podocnemis Unifilis*	Intra-erythrocytic	–	–	Brazil	Úngari et al. [102]

Table 7. Haemogregarines of crocodilians.

Species of Haemogregarines	The Vertebrate Host	Site of Merogony	Invertebrate Vector	Site of Gamogony and Sporogony	Locality	Authors
Haemogregarina crocodilinorum	*Alligator mississippiensis*	Intra-erythrocytic	*Placobdella multilineata*	Intestinal epithelial cells of the leech	Southern USA includes Arkansas, Carolina, and Florida	Börner [103]
Haemogregarina caimani (= *Hepatozoon caimani*)	*Caiman latirostris*	Intra-erythrocytic	*Culex dolosus*	Hemocoel	Brazil	Pessôa and de Biasi [104]
Haemogregarina pettiti (=*Hepatozoon pettiti Hoare 1932)*	*Crocodilus niloticus*	Erythrocytes and liver	*Glossina palpalis*	Intestine	Uganda, Senegal, West Africa	Hoare [105]
Hepatozoon sp.	*Caiman c. yacare*	Intra-erythrocytic	*Phaeotabanus fervens*	Intestine	Pantanal	Viana and Marques [106]
Hepatozoon caimani	*Caiman yacare*	Intra-erythrocytic	–	–	Pantanal region, Brazil	Viana et al. [107]

Table 8. Haemogregarines of birds.

Species of Haemogregarines	The Vertebrate Host	Site of Merogony	Invertebrate Vector	Site of Gamogony and Sporogony	Locality	Authors
Hepatozoon atticorae	*Hirundo spilodera*	Intra-erythrocytic	*Ornithodoros peringueyi* and *Xenopsylia trispinis*	Hemolymph	South Africa, South America, Jamaica, Europea	Bennett et al. [108]
Hepatozoon prionopis	*Prionops plumatus*	Intra-erythrocytic	–	–	Transvaal, South Africa	Bennett and Earle [109]
Hepatozoon lanis	*Lanius collaris*	Intra-erythrocytic	–	–	South Africa	Bennett et al. [108]
Hepatozoon malacotinus	*Dryoscopus cubla*	Intra-erythrocytic	–	–	South Africa	Bennett et al. [108]
Hepatozoon numidis	*Numida meleagris*	Intra-erythrocytic	–	–	South Africa	Bennett et al. [108]
Hepatozoon pittae	*Pitta arcuate*	Intra-erythrocytic	–	–	Sabah	Bennett et al. [108]
Hepatozoon estrildus	*Lonchura cucullata*	Intra-erythrocytic	–	–	Zambia	Bennett et al. [108]
Hepatozoon sylvae	*Parisoma subcaeruleum*	Intra-erythrocytic	–	–	South Africa	Bennett et al. [108]
Hepatozoon zosteropis	*Zosterops pallida*	Intra-erythrocytic	–	–	South Africa	Bennett et al. [108]
Hepatozoon passeris	*Sporopipes squamifrons*	Intra-erythrocytic	–	–	Botswana, South Africa	Bennett et al. [108]

Table 9. Haemogregarines of mammals.

Species of Haemogregarines	The Vertebrate Host	Site of Merogony	Invertebrate Vector	Site of Gamogony and Sporogony	Locality	Authors
Hepatozoon perniciosum	Laboratory white rats	The liver	*Echinolaelaps echidninus*	Stomach	Washington, USA	Miller [9]
Hepatozoon griseisciuri	*Sciurus carolinensis*	Bone marrow, liver, lung, and spleen (with intra-leucocytic gametocytes)	*Euhaemogamasus ambulans, Echinolaelaps echidninus* and *Haemogamasus reidi*	Stomach	Washington, Marland, Georgia, USA	Desser [110]
Hepatozoon erhardovae	*Clethrionomys glareolus*	Lung	*Xenopsylla cheopis, Ctenophthalmus agyrtes, C. assimilis* and *Nosopsyllus fasciatus*	Stomach and fat-body cells	Munich, Germany	Göbel and Krampitz [111]
Hepatozoon sylvatici	*Apodemus sylvaticus* and *Apodemus flavicollis*	Bone marrow and liver	*Laelaps agilis*	Stomach	Austria	Frank [112]
Hepatozoon sp.	Dogs	Intra-erythrocytic	–	–	Brazil	Forlano et al. [113]
Hepatozoon canis	Dogs	Intra-erythrocytic	–	–	Italy	Otranto et al. [114]
Hepatozoon felis	Cats	Intra-erythrocytic	–	–	India	Baneth et al. [115]
Hepatozoon canis	Dogs	Intra-erythrocytic	*Rhipicephalus sanguineus*	–	Mato Grosso do Sul, Brazil	Ramos et al. [116]
Hepatozoon canis	Dogs	Intra-erythrocytic	–	–	Central-western Brazil	Paiz et al. [117]
Hepatozoon sp.	*Cerdocyon thous, Nasua nasua, Leopardus pardalis, Canis familiaris, Thrichomys fosteri, Oecomys mamorae, Clyomys laticeps, Thylamys macrurus, Monodelphis domestics*	Intra-erythrocytic	*Amblyomma sculptum, A. parvum, A. tigrinum, Rhipicephalus microplus, R. sanguineus, A. auricularium*	–	Brazil	De Sousa et al. [118]
Hepatozoon felis	*Panthera leo*	–	*Rhipicephalus sanguineus*	–	Thailand	Bhusri et al. [119]
Hepatozoon canis	Dogs	Intra-erythrocytic	–	–	Czech Republic	Mitkova et al. [120]
Hepatozoon felis	Dogs	Intra-erythrocytic	–	–	Northeastern Iran	Barati and Razmi [121]
Hepatozoon sp.	Cats	Intra-erythrocytic	–	–	Turkey	Tuna et al. [122]
Hepatozoon canis	Dogs	Intra-erythrocytic	–	–	United Kingdom	Attipa et al. [123]
Hepatozoon felis	*Felis silvestris, Caracal caracal, Panthera pardus, P. leo, Leptailurus serval*	Muscle and Liver	–	–	Limpopo and Mpumalanga	Harris et al. [124]
Hepatozoon luiperdjie	*Panthera pardus*	Leukocytes	–	–	Limpopo Province, South Africa	Van As et al. [125]
Hepatozoon canis	*Dogs*	Intra-erythrocytic	–	–	Manila, Philippines	Baticados et al. [126]

In the schizogony (merogony) stage, haemogregarines are characterized by their considerable ability to invade and develop within different organs and cell types inside the vertebrate host (Tables 2–9). Bray [127] proposed that haemogregarines with schizonts in the liver should be placed in the genus *Hepatozoon*. In contrast, those species that precede schizogony in other organs should belong to another genus as *Haemogregarina* or *Karyolysus*. However, only in the lung of the river turtle, *Trionyx gangeticus* infected with *Haemogregarina gangetica*, was described by Misra [87]. In addition to the usual location of merogonic development in the liver, lung, and spleen, Ball et al. [71] have found certain merogonic stages in the highly infected snakes' brain and heart. Siddall and Desser [84] described merogonic stages in the lacunar endothelial cells of the circulatory system of the leech and its proboscis, besides the liver, lung, and spleen in the turtle. Yanai et al. [128] also described nodular lesions containing schizonts and merozoites of *Hepatozoon* sp. of the heart's martens, perisplenic, and perirenal adipose tissues, the diaphragm, mesentery, and tongue. Úngari et al. [102] reported that the genus *Haemogregarina* underwent schizogony in the circulating blood cells as in turtles and fish, and the genus *Hepatozoon* underwent schizogony in the liver. Additionally, there are two morphologically different meronts were the micro- and macromeronts. The presence of these two forms of meronts was mentioned to be a fundamental feature of the whole haemogregarine [74,129,130].

Gametocytes are usually the only stages of the parasite detected by scientists. Their morphology, unfortunately, does not provide a reliable clue to the generic differentiation. Together with other relevant data, their morphological characteristics offer a reliable basis for specific identification [35,67]. The haemogregarines gametocytes appeared as sausage-shaped and generally lie singly within erythrocytes (Tables 2–9), but sometimes free in extracellular space, which is consistent with Telford et al. [34], Sloboda et al. [79] as the presence of free extracellular gametocytes. They are also observed in the leucocytes of fish (Table 2), birds (Table 8), and mammals (Table 9).

The shape, size, and structure of infected blood-corpuscles often undergo considerable changes. Hypertrophy may result directly from the gametocyte's added intraerythrocytic volume or represent an erythrocyte adaptation to the gametocyte's presence [53,82,131,132]. An entirely different cell response occurred when the gametocytes of *Hemogregarina* sp. invaded erythrocytes of *Rana berlandieri*. The erythrocytes undergo hypertrophy, and the plasmalemma of the infected erythrocyte demonstrated numerous microvilli-like outgrowings. Hussein [133] also described the hypertrophy of *Karyolysus*-infected erythrocytes. Most haemogregarine gametocytes do not invade the host cell's nucleus but instead move it to the opposite side or the other host cell's other pole. This is contrary to the effect of the genus *Karyolysus* on the infected erythrocytes. *Karyolysus* has a karyolytic impact on the host cell's nucleus and is therefore identified *Karyolysus* Reichenow [134].

Little work had been done to identify the actual arthropod vectors of haemogregarines, as the transmission by inoculation of blood was rarely successful. In general, the invertebrate vectors of haemogregarines were the most challenging problem facing this group's research progress [49]. The haemogregarines displayed a wide distribution of vertebrate host infections, and a large number of invertebrate vectors (Tables 2–9). In all haemogregarines, fertilization is of Adelea type; both micro- and macrogamonts lie in syzygy within the same parasitophorous vacuole. Syzygy can stimulate the production of the associated gamonts in haemogregarines, since only the parasites found in pairs were mostly differentiated, which is consistent with Davies and Smit [42]. Regarding the number of microgametes produced by each microgamont, the members of the suborder Adeleidea were characterized by the production of only a few (four or less) microgametes [135]. Simultaneously, the formation of multiple microgametes has been identified in most haemogregarines species [52]. However, there are some suggestions that multiple microgamete formation does not occur in the entire genus *Hepatozoon* [111]. Regarding the number of flagella in microgametes in haemogregarines, contradictions were recorded. While monoflagellated microgametes have been described for haemogregarines species [74], biflagellated microgametes were also recorded for other haemogregarines [52]. On the other hand, Michel [85] reported non-flagellated microgametes in *Hepatozoon mauritanicum*.

Fertilization follows, leading to the formation of a zygote that becomes an oocyst. The oocyst is surrounded by a flexible membrane rather than a wall, and it produces sporozoites that may undergo further merogony. Sporogony is elucidated for just a few known haemogregarines species, the vast majority of which is supposed to investigate this aspect of their life-cycle, as reported by Forlano et al. [113]. There is also another potential criterion for distinguishing between *Hepatozoon* and *Haemogregarina* based on the presence or absence of oocysts containing sporocysts in the invertebrate vector, which is consistent with Levine [6]. When the developing mite reaches the nymphal stage, the sporozoites attain their maturity. The sporozoites eventually get the nymph's stomach and pass out with their faeces, which are considered infection sources of the vertebrate host (lizard). The morphological characteristics of the gamonts and meronts found in the blood cells sometimes provide inadequate information for differential diagnoses [37], meaning that assigning species of haemogregarines to one of these genera must be based on the characteristics of its sporogony in the invertebrate vectors [6,64]. However, data on invertebrate vectors and sporogony are missing for the majority of species [23].

Until now, the current taxonomy of haemogregarines is facing a great challenge due to the high variation in gamont morphology, low host specificity, unknown invertebrate hosts in many cases, and fewer details of sporogony. Therefore, molecular approaches are now available to distinguish populations of morphologically identical but genetically different parasites, including DNA and polymerase chain reaction (PCR) based approaches [22,136–141]. Some studies based on PCR-based assays as the reference diagnostic test for epidemiological studies, which given their greater sensitivity, particularly for testing different hosts with intermittent levels of parasitemia via a low infection rate by gamonts, as Otranto et al. [114], Haklová-Kočíková et al. [18], Jòzsef et al. [24], Ramos et al. [116], and Mitkova et al. [120]. Notably, all the molecular evidence comes from the complete and partial sequences of the small subunit (SSU) ribosomal DNA (rDNA) 18S gene is a sufficient phylogenetic marker to approximate ordinal level relationships and those within orders [68,98,119,142–145]. Previous molecular studies of Harris et al. [22] and Barta et al. [19] demonstrated that the haemogregarine species are clustered in sister clades with interspecies linked more with the host geographic distribution, rather than host species. There are universal primer sets that were able to molecularly characterize haemogregarines, as mentioned in Table 10. However, many species with sequences deposited in the GenBank database are not identified correctly at the generic level. Table 11 expressed only haemogregarines identified at the species level and others identified at the generic level are excluded.

Table 10. Primer sets used in the phylogenetic analysis of haemogregarines by *18S rRNA* gene.

Primer Set	Primer Sequence	Reference
4558F 2733R	5′- GCT AAT ACA TGA GCA AAA TCT CAA -3′ 5′- CGG AAT TAA CCA GAC AAA T -3′	Mathew et al. [146]
2867F 2868R	5′- AAC CTG GTT GAT CCT GCC AG -3′ 5′- TGA TCC TTC TGC AGG TTC ACC TAC -3′	Mathew et al. [146]
HEMO1 HEMO2	5′ - TAT TGG TTT TAA GAA CTA ATT TTA TGA TTG - 3′ 5′ - CTT CTC CTT CCT TTA AGT GAT AAG GTT CAC - 3′	Perkins and Keller [147]
HepF HepR	5′- ATA-CAT-GAG-CAA-AAT-CTC-AAC -3′ 5′- CTT-ATT-ATT-CCA-TGC-TGC-AG -3′	Inokuma et al. [148]
HepF300 HepR900	5′- GTTTCTGACCTATCAGCTTTCGAC -3′ 5′- CAAATCTAAGAATTTCACCTCTGAC -3′	Ujvari et al. [20]

Table 10. *Cont.*

Primer Set	Primer Sequence	Reference
HEP-1	5′- CGC GAA ATT ACC CAA TT -3′	Criado-Fornelio et al. [149]
HEP-2	5′- CAG ACC GGT TAC TTT YAG CAG -3′	
Piroplasmid-F	5′- CCA GCA GCC GCG GTA ATT -3′	Tabar et al. [150]
Piroplasmid-R	5′- CTT TCG CAG TAG TTY GTC TTT AAC AAA TCT -3′	
EF	5′-GAA ACT GCG AAT GGC TCA TT-3′	Kvičerová et al. [26]
ER	5′-CTT GCG CCT ACT AGG CAT TC-3′	
Hep-001F	5′- CCT GGC TAT ACA TGA GCA AAA TCT CAA CTT -3′	Kledmanee et al. [151]
Hep-737R	5′- CCA ACT GTC CCT ATC AAT CAT TAA AGC -3′	
BTH-1F	5′- CCT GAG AAA CGG CTA CCA CAT CT -3′	Zintl et al. [152]
BTH-1R	5′- TTG CGA CCA TAC TCC CCC CA -3′	
GF2	5′- GTC TTG TAA TTG GAA TGA TGG -3′	Hodžić et al. [153]
GR2	5′- CCA AAG ACT TTG ATT TCT CTC -3′	
Haemog11_F	5′- ATT GGA GGG CAA GTC TGG TG -3′	Rakhshandehroo et al. [99]
Haemog11_R	5′- GCG TTA GAC ACG CAA AGT CT -3′	
HemoFN	5′- CCG TGG TAA TTC TAG AGC TAA TAC ATG AGC -3′	Alhaboubi et al. [100]
HemoRN	5′- GAT AAG GTT TAC GAA ACT TTC TAT ATT TA -3′	

Table 11. List of sequences for haemogregarines from GenBank database based on the *18S rRNA* gene.

Parasites	Hosts	Accession Number in GenBank
Haemogregarina podocnemis	*Podocnemis unifilis*	MF476203.1 - MF476205.1
Haemogregarina pellegrini	*Platysternon megacephalum*	KM887509.1
	Malayemys subtrijuga	KM887508.1
Haemogregarina sacaliae	*Sacalia quadriocellata*	KM887507.1
	Emys orbicularis	MT345287.1
Haemogregarina stepanowi	*Mauremys leprosa*	MT345284.1 - MT345286.1, KX691418.1, KX691417.1
	Emys orbicularis	KT749877.1, KF257928.1
	Mauremys leprosa	KF257929.1
	Mauremys rivlata	KF257927.1
	Mauremys caspica	KF257926.1, KF992697.1
Haemogregarina bigemina	*Lipophrys pholis*	MK393799.1 - MK393801.1
Haemogregarina balli	*Chelydra serpentine*	HQ224959.1
Hepatozoon fitzsimonsi	*Kinixys zombensis*	KR069084.1
	Chersina angulate	KJ702453.1
Hepatozoon ursi	*Ursus thibetanus japonicus*	EU041718.1, AB586028.1, LC431855.1 - LC431853.1
	Melursus ursinus	HQ829437.1 - HQ829429.1
Hepatozoon seychellensis	*Gradisonia alternans*	KF246566.1, KF246565.1,
	Apodemus sylvaticus	KT274177.1, KT274178.1
Hepatozoon ayorgbor	*Ctenophthalmus agyrtes*	KJ634066.1
	Python regius	EF157822.1
	Rhombomys opimus	MW342705.1
Hepatozoon musa	*Crotalus durissus*	MF497763.1 - MF497767.1
	Philodryas natterei	KX880079.1
Hepatozoon involucrum	*Hyperolius marmoratus*	MG041591.1 - MG041594.1
	Ursus arctos	MN150506.1 - MN150504.1
Hepatozoon clamatae	*Rana pipiens*	MN310689.1
Hepatozoon catesbianae	*Rana clamitans*	MN244529.1, MN244528.1, AF040972.1,
Hepatozoon aegypti	*Spalerosophis diadema*	MH198742.1
Hepatozoon martis	*Martes foina*	MG136688.1, MG136687.1
Hepatozoon procyonis	*Nasua nasua*	MF685386.1 - MF685409.1
Hepatozoon griseisciuri	*Scinurus carolinensis*	MK452389.1, MK452388.1, MK452253.1, MK452252.1,

Table 11. *Cont.*

Parasites	Hosts	Accession Number in GenBank
Hepatozoon sciuri	*Scinus vulgaris*	MN104636.1 - MN104640.1,
Hepatozoon americanum	*Canis familiaris*	AF206668.1, KU729739.1
Hepatozoon ingwe	*Panthera pardus pardus*	MN793001.1, MN793000.1
Hepatozoon theileri	*Amietia queckettii* *Amietia delalandii*	KP119773.1, KX512804.1, KJ599676.1, MG041605.1
Hepatozoon caimani	*Caiman crocodilus yacare* *Caiman crocodilus*	MF322538.1, MF322539.1 MF435046.1 - MF435049.1
Hepatozoon silvestris	*Felis silvestris silvestris*	KX757032.1
	Felis catus	MH078194.1, KY649445.1
Hepatozoon tenuis	*Afrixalus fornasini*	MG041595.1 - MG041599.1
Hepatozoon thori	*Hyperolius argus*	MG041600.1 - MG041603.1
Hepatozoon ixoxo	*Amietophrynus maculatus*	KP119772.1
Hepatozoon luiperdjie	*Panthera pardus pardus*	MN793002.1 - MN793004.1,
Hepatozoon cuestensis	*Crotalus durissus*	MF497769.1, MF497770.1
Hepatozoon sipedon	*Snakes*	AF110249.1 - AF110241.1
Hepatozoon erhardovae	*Megabothris turbidus*	KJ608372.1
Hepatozoon domerguei	*Furcifer* sp.	KM234649.1 - KM234646.1
Hepatozoon tuatarae	*Sphenodon punctatus*	GU385473.1 - GU385470.1
Hepatozoon cf. *ophisauri*	*Rhombomys opimus*	MW256822.1
Hepatozoon colubri	–	MN723844.1
Hepatozoon canis	*Amblyomma cajennense*	KT215377.1 - KT215353.1
	Amblyomma sculptum	KP167594.1
	Tapir tapir	MT458172.1
	Haemaphysalis longicornis	MT107092.1 - MT107097.1, MT107087.1 - MT107089.1, LC169075.1
	Haemaphysalis concinna	KC509532.1 - KC509527.1
	Rhipicephalus sanguineus	MH595911.1 - MH595892.1, MG807347.1, KY056823.1, MG241229.1, KT587790.1, KT587789.1, KY196999.1, KY197000.1 - KY197002.1, JQ867389.1, MN207197.1
	Rhipicephalus microplus	HQ605710.1
	Rhipicephalus decoloratus	MN294724.1
	Canis lupus familiaris	MH615003.1, EU289222.1, DQ071888.1, MK910141.1 - MK910144.1, MK757793.1 - MK757815.1, MN791089.1, MN791088.1, MN393913.1, MN393910.1, MK645971.1 - MK645946.1, MK214285.1 - MK214282.1, MG254613.1 - MG254622.1, MK091084.1 - MK091092.1, KY940658.1, MG772658.1, MG254573.1 - MG254611.1, KY021176.1 - KY021184.1, MG496257.1, MG496273.1, MG062866.1, MG076961.1, MG209580.1 - MG209594.1, KX588232.1, KU729737.1, KU729738.1, KY026191.1, KY026192.1, KX880502.1 - KX880506.1, KX761384.1, KU232309.1, KU232310.1, KT736298.1, LC012839.1 - LC012821.1, LC053450.1, JX976545.1, JN584478.1 - JN584475.1, JF459994.1, GQ176285.1, EU571737.1, EF650846.1, MW019643.1 - MW019630.1, MT909554.1, MT081051.1, MT081050.1, MT821184.1, MT499356.1 - MT499354.1, MT754266.1, LC556379.1, MT433126.1 - MT433121.1
	Lycalopex vetulus	AY150067.2, MT458173.1
	Kinixys species	MT704950.1
	Lycalopex gymnocercus	KX816958.1
	Didelphis albiventris	KY392884.1, KY392885.1
	Canis aureus	KF322145.1, KC886721.1, KC886729.1 - KC886733.1, KJ868814.1, KJ572977.1 - KJ572975.1, KJ634654.1, JX466886.1 - JX466880.1,

Table 11. *Cont.*

Parasites	Hosts	Accession Number in GenBank
	Felis catus	KY469446.1, MN689671.1 - MN689661.1
	Vulpes vulpes	KF322141.1-KF322144.1, KC886720.1 - KC886728.1, MK757741.1 - MK757792.1, MN103520.1, MN103519.1, MH699884.1 - MH699892.1, MG077084.1 - MG077087.1, KY693670.1, KJ868819.1 - KJ868815.1, KU893118.1 - KU893127.1, KM096414.1 - KM096411.1, KJ572979.1, KJ572978.1, EU165370.1, GU376458.1 - GU376446.1, DQ869309.1, AY731062.1, MW295531.1, MN463026.1 - MN463021.1
	Ixodes ricinus	KU597235.1 - KU597242.1, KC584780.1
	Hydrochoerus hydrochaeris	KY965141.1 - KY965144.1
	Cuon alpinus	HQ829448.1 - HQ829438.1, MK144332.1
	Dermacentor reticulatus	KC584777.1 - KC584773.1
	Pseudalopex gymnocercus	AY471615.1, AY461376.1, AY461375.1
	Panthera leo	MT814748.1
	Panthera tigris	MT232064.1 - MT232062.1
	Camelus dromedrius	MN989311.1
Hepatozoon apri	*Sus scrofa leucomystax*	LC314791.1
	Amietophrynus gutturalis	KP119771.1
	Amietophrynus garmani	KP119770.1,
	Sclerophrys maculata	KX512803.1
	Sclerophrys pusilla	MG041604.1
Hepatozoon cf. *felis*	*Felis catus*	MK301457.1 - MK301462.1, MK724001.1, MG386482.1 - MG386484.1, KY649442.1 - KY649444.1, AY628681.1, AY620232.1
	Felis silvestris silvestris	KX757033.1, MT210593.1 - MT210598.1,
	Puma concolor	MT458171.1
	Eira barbara	MT458170.1
	Lycalopex gymnocercus	HQ020489.1
	Leopardus pardalis	KY684005.1
	Asiatic lion	KX017290.1
	Prionailurus bengalensis	AB771577.1 - AB771501.1, GQ377218.1 - GQ377216.1
	Prionailurus iriomotensis	AB636287.1 - AB636285.1
	Panthera onca	KU232302.1 - KU232308.1
	Panthera tigris	MT645336.1, MT634695.1
	Rhipicephalus sanguineus	JQ867388.1
	Eurasian lynx	MN905025.1, MN905023.1, MN905027.1
Haemolivia parvula	*Kinixys zombensis*	KR069083.1, KR069082.1
Haemolivia stellata	*Amblyomma dissimile*	MH196477.1 - MH196482.1, MH196475
	Amblyomma rotundatum	KP881349.1
Haemolivia mariae	*Egernia stokesii*	KF992712.1, KF992711.1
	Tiliqua rugosa	JN211118.1, HQ224961.1
Haemolivia mauritanica	*Hyalomma aegyptium*	MH618775.1, MN463032.1, MN463031.1, MW092781.1 - MW092776.1, MK918611.1 - MK918608.1, MH497199.1 - MH497190.1, MH975037.1, MH975031.1, MH975026.1, MH975025.1,
	Hyalomma sp.	MF383512. - MF383506.1,
Haemolivia mauritanica	*Canis lupus familiaris*	KP719092.1
	Testudo marginata	KF992710.1, KF992699.1
	Testudo graeca	KF992709.1 - KF992698.1, MH975039.1 - MH975032.1, MH975030.1 - MH975027.1, MH975024.1 - MH975021.1,
Karyolysus paradoxa	*Varanus albigularis*	KX011039.1, KX011040.1
Karyolysus cf. *lacazei*	*Ixodes ricinus*	MK497254.1

4. Conclusions

Few haemogregarine characteristics provide a reliable basis for the related parasite to recognized genera. Details of the sporogonic cycle seem to be the only reliable criterion as they are the "Key-stone" in the classification system. Morphological characteristics of the gametocytes do not help in this respect. Features of the schizogonic stages, when these are known, are not much better as criteria of generic value. Molecular phylogenetic studies using the appropriate genetic markers are helpful tools for the accurate taxonomic identification for haemogregarines. Further studies are recommended to include other nuclear and mitochondrial genes to provide more information about the genetic variability among haemogregarines.

Author Contributions: Conceptualization, S.A.-Q., F.A.-G. and M.A.D.; methodology, F.A.-G. and R.A.-G.; validation, M.A.D.; formal analysis, R.A.-G. and M.A.D.; investigation, S.A.-Q. and F.A.-G.; resources, R.A.-G. and M.A.D.; data curation, R.A.-G. and M.A.D.; writing—original draft preparation, S.A.-Q., F.A.-G., R.A.-G. and M.A.D.; writing—review and editing, S.A.-Q., F.A.-G., R.A.-G. and M.A.D.; visualization, R.A.-G. and M.A.D.; supervision, S.A.-Q., F.A.-G. and M.A.D. All authors have read and agreed to the published version of the manuscript.

Funding: This research was funded by the Deanship for Research and Innovation, "Ministry of Education" in Saudi Arabia, grant number IFKSURP-131.

Institutional Review Board Statement: Not applicable.

Informed Consent Statement: Not applicable.

Data Availability Statement: All data generated or analysed during this study are included in this published article.

Acknowledgments: The authors extend their appreciation to the Deanship for Research and Innovation, "Ministry of Education" in Saudi Arabia for funding this research work through the project number IFKSURP-131".

Conflicts of Interest: The authors declare no conflict of interest.

References

1. Levine, N.D. Taxonomy of the Sporozoa. *J. Parasitol.* **1970**, *56*, 208–209.
2. Davies, A.J.; Johnston, M.R.L. The biology of some intraerythrocytic parasites of fishes, amphibian and reptiles. *Adv. Parasitol.* **2000**, *45*, 1–107. [PubMed]
3. Adl, S.M.; Simpson, A.G.B.; Lane, C.E.; Lukeš, J.; Bass, D.; Bowser, S.S.; Brown, M.W.; Burki, F.; Dunthorn, M.; Hampl, V.; et al. The revised classification of eukaryotes. *J. Eukaryot. Microbiol.* **2012**, *59*, 429–514. [CrossRef] [PubMed]
4. Hossen, M.S.; Bandyopadhyay, P.K.; Gürelli, G. On the occurrence of a Haemogregarinae (Apicomplexa) parasite from freshwater turtles of South 24 Parganas, West Bengal, India. *Tutkiye Parazitol. Derg.* **2013**, *37*, 118–122. [CrossRef] [PubMed]
5. Telford, S.R. *Hemoparasites of the Reptilia: Color Atlas and Text*; CRC Press, Taylor and Francis Group: Boca Raton, FL, USA, 2009.
6. Levine, N.D. Some corrections in Haemogregarine (Apicomplexa: Protozoa) Nomenclature. *J. Protozool.* **1982**, *29*, 601–603. [CrossRef] [PubMed]
7. Danilewsky, B. Die Hematozoen der Kaltblüter. *Arch. Mikr. Anat.* **1885**, *24*, 588–598. [CrossRef]
8. Labbé, A. Recherches zoologiques et biologiques sur les parasites endoglobulaires du sang des Vertébrés. *Arch. Zool. Exp. Gen.* **1894**, *2*, 55–258.
9. Miller, W.W. *Hepatozoon perniciosum* n. g. n. sp., a haemogregarines pathogenic for white rats: With a brief description of the sexual cycle in the intermediate host a mite (*Laelaps echidninus* Berlese). *Hyg. Lab. Bull. (Washington)* **1908**, *46*, 51–123.
10. Lainson, R. On *Cyrilia gomesi* (Neiva and Pinto, 1926) gen. nov. (Haemogregarinidae) and *Trypanosoma bourouli* Neiva and Pinto. In the fish *Synbranchus marmoratus*: Simultaneous transmission by the leech *Haementeria lutzi*. In *Parasitological Topics*; Special Publication; Canning, E.U., Ed.; Society of Protozoologists, Inc.: Lawrence, KS, USA, 1981; Volume 1, pp. 150–158.
11. Barta, J.R. Phylogenetic analysis of the Class Sporozoa (Phylum Apicomplexa Levine 1970): Evidence for the independent evaluation of heteroxenous life cycles. *J. Parasitol.* **1989**, *75*, 195–206. [CrossRef]
12. Mohammed, A.H.H.; Mansour, N.S. The haemogregarines complex (an analytical systematic review). *Bull. Fac. Pharm. Cairo Univ. (BFPC)* **1959**, *35*, 39–52.
13. Wenyon, C.M. *Protozoology*; Bailliere, Tindall and Cox: London, UK, 1926; Volume 2.
14. Petit, G.; Landau, I.; Baccam, D.; Lainson, R. Description et cycle biologique *d'Hemolivia stellate* n. g., n. sp., hémogregarine de crapauds Brésiliens. [Desription and life cycle of *Hemolivia stellate* n.g., n. sp., a haemogregarines of Brazilian toads]. *Ann. Parasitol. Hum. Comp.* **1990**, *65*, 3–15. [CrossRef]

15. Široký, P.; Kamler, M.; Modrý, D. Long-term occurrence of *Hemolivia* cf. *mauritanica* (Apicomplexa: Adeleina: Haemogregarinidae) in the captive *Testudo marginata* (Reptilia: Testudinidae): Evidence for cyclic merogony? *J. Parasitol.* **2004**, *90*, 1391–1393.
16. Jacobson, E.R. Parasites and parasitic diseases of reptiles. In *Infectious Diseases and Pathology of Reptiles: Color Atlas and Text*; Jacobson, E.R., Ed.; CRC Press, Taylor & Francis Group: Boca Raton, FL, USA, 2007; pp. 579–580.
17. Pineda-Catalan, O.; Perkins, S.L.; Peirce, M.A.; Engstrand, R.; Garcia-Davila, C.; Pinedo-Vasquez, M.; Aguirre, A.A. Revision of hemoproteid genera and description and redescription of two species of chelonian hemoproteid parasites. *J. Parasitol.* **2013**, *99*, 1089–1098. [CrossRef] [PubMed]
18. Haklová-Kočíková, B.; Hižňanová, A.; Majláth, I.; Račka, K.; Harris, D.G.; Földvári, G. Molecular characterization of *Karyolysus*– a neglected but common parasite infecting some European lizards. *Parasite. Vector.* **2014**, *7*, 555. [CrossRef] [PubMed]
19. Barta, J.R.; Ogedengbe, J.D.; Martin, D.S.; Smith, T.G. Phylogenetic position of the adeleorinid coccidia (Myzozoa, Apicomplexa, Coccidia, Eucoccidiorida, Adeleorina) inferred using 18S rDNA sequences. *J. Eukaryot. Microbiol.* **2012**, *59*, 171–180. [CrossRef]
20. Ujvari, B.; Madsen, T.; Olsson, M. High prevalence of *Hepatozoon* spp. (Apicomplexa, Hepatozoidae) infection in water pythons (*Liasis fuscus*) from tropical Australia. *J. Parasitol.* **2004**, *90*, 670–672. [CrossRef]
21. Johnson, A.J.; Origgi, F.C.; Wellehan, J.F.X., Jr. Molecular diagnostics. In *Infectious Diseases and Pathology of Reptiles: Color Atlas and Text*; Jacobson, E.R., Ed.; CRC Press, Taylor & Francis Group: Boca Raton, FL, USA, 2007; pp. 351–380.
22. Harris, D.J.; Maia, J.P.M.C.; Perera, A. Molecular characterization of *Hepatozoon* species in reptiles from the Seychelles. *J. Parasitol.* **2011**, *97*, 106–110. [CrossRef]
23. Dvořáková, N.; Kvičerova, J.; Papousek, I.; Javanbakht, H.; Tiar, G.; Kami, H.G. Haemogregarines from western Palaearctic freshwater turtles (genera *Emys*, *Mauremys*) are conspecifi c with *Haemogregarina stepanowi* Danilewsky, 1885. *Parasitology* **2014**, *141*, 522–530.
24. Jòzsef, Ö.; Darko, M.; Milos, V.; Bojan, G.; Jevrosima, S.; Dejan, K.; Sanja, A.-K. Cytological and molecular identification of *Haemogregarina stepanowi* in blood samples of the European pond turtle (*Emys orbicularis*) from quarantine at Belgrade Zoo. *Acta Vet.-Beograd* **2015**, *65*, 443–453.
25. O'Donoghue, P. Haemoprotozoa: Making biological sense of molecular. *Int. J. Parasitol. Parasites Wildl.* **2017**, *6*, 241–256.
26. Kvičerová, J.; Hypša, V.; Pakandl, M. Phylogenetic relationships among *Eimeria* spp. (Apicomplexa, Eimeriidae) infecting rabbits: Evolutionary significance of biological and morphological features. *Parasitology* **2008**, *135*, 443–452. [CrossRef] [PubMed]
27. Kubo, M.; Jeong, A.; Kim, S.I.; Kim, Y.J.; Lee, H.; Kimura, J.; Agatsuma, T.; Sakai, H.; Yanai, T. The first report of *Hepatozoon* species infection in leopard cats (*Prionailurus bengalensis*) in Korea. *J. Parasitol.* **2010**, *96*, 437–439. [CrossRef] [PubMed]
28. Pawar, R.M.; Poornachandar, A.; Srinivas, P.; Rao, K.R.; Lakshmikantan, U.; Shivaji, S. Molecular characterization of *Hepatozoon* spp. infection in endangered Indian wild felids and canids. *Vet. Parasitol.* **2012**, *186*, 475–479. [CrossRef] [PubMed]
29. Abdel-Baki, A.S.; Al-Quraishy, S.; Zhang, J.Y. Redescription of *Haemogregarina garnhami* (Apicomplexa: Adeleorina) from the blood of Psammophis schokari (Serpentes: Colubridae) as *Hepatozoon garnhami* n. comb. based on molecular, morphometric and morphologic characters. *Acta Parasitol.* **2014**, *59*, 294–300. [CrossRef] [PubMed]
30. Cook, C.A.; Lawton, S.P.; Davies, A.J.; Smit, N.J. Reassignment of the land tortoise haemogregarine *Haemogregarina fitzimonsi* Dias 1953 (Adeleorina: Haemogregarinidae) to the genus *Hepatozoon* Miller 1908 (Adeleorina: Hepatozoidae) based on parasite morphology, life cycle and phylogenetic analysis of 18S rDNA sequence fragments. *Parasitology* **2014**, *141*, 1611–1620.
31. Cook, C.A.; Netherlands, E.C.; Smit, N.J. Redescription, molecular characterisation and taxonomic re-evaluation of a unique African monitor lizard haemogregarine *Karyolysus paradoxa* (Dias, 1954) n. comb. (Karyolysidae). *Parasit. Vectors.* **2016**, *9*, 347. [CrossRef]
32. Cook, C.A.; Netherlands, E.C.; Van As, J.; Smit, N.J. Two new species of *Hepatozoon* (Apicomplexa: Hepatozoidae) parasitizing species of *Philothamnus* (Ophidia: Colubridae) from South Africa. *Folia Parasitol.* **2018**, *65*, 004. [CrossRef]
33. Osimani, J.J. *Haemogregarina triatomae* n. sp. from a South American lizard, *Tupinambis teguixin* transmitted by the Reduviid *Triatoma rebrovaria*. *J. Parasite.* **1942**, *28*, 147–154. [CrossRef]
34. Telford, S.R., Jr.; Ernst, J.A.; Clark, A.M.; Butler, J.F. *Hepatozoon sauritus*: A polytopic haemogregarine of three genera and four species of snakes in North Florida, with specific identity verified from genome analysis. *J. Parasitol.* **2004**, *90*, 352–358. [CrossRef]
35. Herbert, J.D.K.; Godfrey, S.; Bull, C.M.; Menz, I. Developmental stages and molecular phylogeny of *Hepatozoon tuatarae*, a parasite infecting the New Zealand tuatara, *Sphenodon punctatus* and the tick, *Amblyomma sphenodonti*. *Int. J. Parasitol.* **2010**, *40*, 1311–1315. [CrossRef]
36. Siddall, M.E.; Desser, S.S. Merogonic development of *Haemogregarina balli* (Apicomplexa: Adeleina: Haemogregarinidae) in the leech *Placobdella ornate* (Glossiphoniidae), its transmission to a chelonian intermediate host and phylogenetic implications. *J. Parasitol.* **1991**, *77*, 426–436. [CrossRef]
37. Dvořáková, N.; Kvičerová, J.; Hostovský, M.; Široký, P. Haemogregarines of freshwater turtles from Southeast Asia with a description of *Haemogregarina sacaliae* sp. n. and a redescription of *Haemogregarina pellegrini* Laveran and Pettit, 1910. *Parasitology* **2015**, *142*, 816–826.
38. Nakamoto, W.; Silva, A.J.; Machado, P.E.; Padovani, C.R.; Januario, S.A.; De Abreu, M.E. Leukocytes and *Cyrilia gomesi* (blood parasite) in *Synbranchus marmoratus* Bloch, 1975 (Pisces, Synbranchidae) from the Biriqui region of Sao Paulo (Brazil). *Rev. Bras. Biol.* **1991**, *51*, 755–761.
39. Davies, A.J.; Eiras, J.C.; Austin, R.T.E. Investigations into the transmission of *Haemogregarina bigemina* Laveran and Mesnil, 1901 (Apicomplexa: Adeleorina) between intertidal fishes in Portugal. *J. Fish. Dis.* **1994**, *17*, 283–289. [CrossRef]

40. Lom, J.; Tomas, K.; Dykova, I. *Haemogregarina vltavensis*, new species from perch (*Perca fluviatilis*) in Czechoslovakia. *Syst. Parasitol.* **1989**, *13*, 193–196. [CrossRef]
41. Hill, J.P.; Hendrickson, G.L. Haematozoa of fishes in Humboldt Bay, California. *J. Wildl. Dis.* **1991**, *27*, 701–705. [CrossRef]
42. Davies, A.J.; Smit, N.J. The life cycle of *Haemogregarina bigemina* (Adeleina: Haemogregarinidae) in South African hosts. *Folia Parasit.* **2001**, *48*, 169–177. [CrossRef]
43. MacLean, S.A.; Davies, A.J. Prevalence and development of intraleucocytic haemogregarines from northwest and northeast Atlantic mackerel, *Scomber scombrus* L. *J. Fish. Dis.* **1990**, *13*, 59–68. [CrossRef]
44. Hayes, P.M.; Smit, N.J.; Seddon, A.M.; Wertheim, D.F.; Davies, A.J. A new fish haemogregarine from South Africa and its suspected dual transmission with trypanosomes by a marine leech. *Folia Parasit.* **2006**, *53*, 241–248. [CrossRef]
45. Curtis, L.M.; Grutter, A.S.; Smit, N.J.; Davies, A.J. *Gnathia aureamaculosa*, a likely definitive host of *Haemogregarina balistapi* and potential vector for *Haemogregarina bigemina* between fishes of the Great Barrier Reef, Australia. *Int. J. Parasitol.* **2013**, *43*, 361–370. [CrossRef]
46. Oliveira, A.; Araújo, M.L.G.; Pantoja-Lima, J.; Aride, P.; Tavares-Dias, M.; Brinn, R.P.; Marcon, J.L. Cyrilia sp. (Apicomplexa: Haemogregarinidae) in the Amazonian freshwater stingray *Potamotrygon wallacei* (cururu stingray) in different hydrological phases of the Rio Negro. *Rev. Bras. Biol.* **2016**, *77*, 1–6. [CrossRef] [PubMed]
47. Esteves-Silva, P.H.; da Silva, M.R.L.; O'Dwyer, L.H.; Tavares-Dias, M.; Viana, L.A. *Haemogregarina daviesensis* sp. nov. (Apicomplexa: Haemogregarinidae) from South American lungfish *Lepidosiren paradoxa* (Sarcopterygii: Lepidosirenidae) in the eastern Amazon region. *Parasitol. Res.* **2019**, *118*, 2773–2779. [CrossRef] [PubMed]
48. Awerenzew, S. Parasiten aus dem Blute von Rana nuti. *Arch. Protistenk.* **1941**, *95*, 15–21.
49. Ball, G.H. Some blood sporozoans from East African reptiles. *J. Protozool.* **1967**, *14*, 198–210. [CrossRef]
50. Ray, R. Studies on the anuran blood parasites of sub-Himalayan West Bengal, India. *J. Beng. Nat. Hist. Soc.* **1992**, *11*, 4–8.
51. Smith, T.G.; Desser, S.S.; Martin, D.S. The development of *Hepatozoon sipedon* n. sp. (Apicomplexa: Adeleina: Hepatozoidae) in its natural host, the northern water snake (*Nerodia sipedon sipedon*), its culicine vectors (*Culex pipiens* and *Culex territans*) and its intermediate host, the northern leopard frog (*Rana pipiens*). *Parasitol. Res.* **1994**, *80*, 559–568.
52. Desser, S.S.; Hong, H.; Martin, D.S. The life history, ultrastructure and experimental transmission of *Hepatozoon catesbiana* n. comb., an apicomplexan parasite of the bullfrog, *Rana catesbeiana* and the mosquito, *Culex territans* in Algonquin Park, Ontario. *J. Parasitol.* **1995**, *81*, 212–222. [CrossRef]
53. Lainson, R.; Paperna, I.; Naiff, R.D. Development of *Hepatozoon caimani* (Carini, 1909) Pessôa, de Biasi & de Souza, 1972 in the Caiman c. Crocodilus, the frog *Rana catesbeiana* and the mosquito *Culex fatigans*. *Mem. Inst. Oswaldo. Cruz.* **2003**, *98*, 103–113.
54. Conradie, R.; Cook, C.A.; Preez, L.H.; Jordaan, A.; Netherlands, E.C. Ultrastructural comparison of *Hepatozoon ixoxo* and *Hepatozoon theileri* (Adeleorina: Hepatozoidae), parasitising South African anurans. *J. Eukaryot. Microbiol.* **2017**, *64*, 193–203. [CrossRef]
55. Netherlands, E.C.; Cook, C.A.; Du Preez, L.H.; Vanhove, M.P.M.; Brendonck, L.; Smit, N.J. Monophyly of the species of *Hepatozoon* (Adeleorina: Hepatozoidae) parasitizing (African) anurans, with the description of three new species from hyperoliid frogs in South Africa. *Parasitology* **2018**, *145*, 1039–1050. [CrossRef]
56. Robin, L.A. Cycle évolutif d'un Hepatozoon de *Greko verticillatus*. *Ann. Inst. Pasteur.* **1936**, *56*, 376–394.
57. Garnham, P.C.C.C. A haemogregarines in *Argas brumpti*. *Riv. Parasitol.* **1954**, *15*, 425–435.
58. Lewis, J.E.; Wagner, E.D. *Hepatozoon sauromali* sp. n., a haemogregarines from the Chuckwalla (*Sauromalus* spp.) with notes on the life history. *J. Parasitol.* **1964**, *50*, 11–14. [CrossRef]
59. Elwasila, M. *Haemogregarina* sp. (Apicomplexa: Adeleorina) from the gecko *Tarentola annularis* in the Sudan: Fine structure and life-cycle trials. *Parasitol. Res.* **1989**, *75*, 444–448. [CrossRef]
60. Allison, B.; Desser, S.S. Developmental stages of *Hepatozoon lygosomarum* (Dore 1919) comb. N. (Protozoa, Haemogregarinidae), a parasite of a new Zealand skink, *Leiolopisma nigriplamtare*. *J. Parasitol.* **1981**, *67*, 852–858. [CrossRef]
61. Saratchandra, B. Two new haemogregarines, Haemogregarina waltairensis n. sp. from Calotes versicolor (Daudin) and H. ganapatii n. sp. from Lissemys punctata granosa (Shoepff). *Proc. Indian Acad. Sci. (Anim. Sci.)* **1981**, *90*, 365–371. [CrossRef]
62. Bashtar, A.-R.; Abdel-Ghaffar, F.; Shazly, M.A. Developmental stages of *Hepatozoon gracilis* (Wenyon, 1909) comb. Nov., a parasite of the Egyptian Skink, *Mabuya quinquetaeniata*. *Parasitol. Res.* **1987**, *73*, 507–514. [CrossRef]
63. Roca, V.; Galdón, M.A. Haemogregarine blood parasites in the lizards *Podarcis bocagei* (Seoane) and *P. carbonelli* (Pérez-Mellado) (Sauria: Lacertidae) from NW Portugal. *Syst. Parasitol.* **2010**, *75*, 75–79. [CrossRef]
64. Abdel-Baki, A.S.; Al-Quraishy, S. Morphological characteristics of a new species of *Haemogregarina* Danilewsky, 1885 (Apicomplexa: Adeleorina) in naturally infected *Acanthodactylus boskianus* (Daudin) (Sauria: Lacertidae) in Egypt. *Syst. Parasitol.* **2012**, *82*, 65–69. [CrossRef]
65. Moreira, I.D.; Harris, D.J.; Rosado, D.; Tavares, I.; Maia, J.P.; Salvi, D.; Perera, A. Consequences of haemogregarine infection on the escape distance in the lacertid lizard, *Podarcis vaucheri*. *Acta Herpetol.* **2014**, *9*, 119–123.
66. Rabie, S.A.H.; Hussein, A.-N.A. A description of *Haemogregarina* species naturally infecting white-spotted gecko (*Tarentola annularis*) in Qena, Egypt. *J. Egypt Soc. Parasitol.* **2014**, *44*, 351–358. [CrossRef] [PubMed]
67. Abou Shafeey, H.; Mohamadain, H.S.; Abdel-Gaber, R.; Emara, N.M. Haemogregarines infecting reptiles in Egypt: 1- Blood and Merogenic stages of *Haemogregarine* sp. infecting the skink *Scincus scincus*. *Egypt J. Exp. Biol. (Zool.)* **2019**, *15*, 127–133.

68. Zechmeisterová, K.; De Bellocq, J.G.; Široký, P. Diversity of *Karyolysus* and *Schellackia* from the Iberian lizard *Lacerta schreiberi* with sequence data from engorged ticks. *Parasitology* **2019**, *146*, 1690–1698. [CrossRef] [PubMed]
69. Ball, G.H.; Oda, S.N. Sexual stages in the life history of the haemogregarines *Hepatozoon rarefaciens* (Sambon and Seligmann 1907). *J. Protozool.* **1971**, *18*, 697–700. [CrossRef]
70. Ramadan, N.F. Morphological, experimental and taxonomic studies on protozoan blood parasite of Egyptian reptiles. Ph.D. Thesis, Ain Shams University, Cairo, Egypt, 1974; 220p.
71. Ball, G.H.; Chao, J.; Telford, S.R. *Hepatozoon fusifex* sp. n. a haemogregarine from the Boa constrictor producing marked morphological changes in the infected erythrocytes. *J. Parasitol.* **1969**, *55*, 800–813. [CrossRef]
72. Bashtar, A.R.; Boules, R.; Mehlhorn, H. *Hepatozoon aegypti* nov. sp. 1- Life cycle. *Z. Parasitenkd.* **1984**, *70*, 29–41. [CrossRef]
73. Lowichik, A.; Lanners, H.N.; Lowrie, R.C.; Meiners, N.E. Gametogenesis and sporogony of *Hepatozoon mocassinin* (Apicomplexa: Adeleina: Hepatozoidae) in an experimental mosquito host, *Aedes aegypti*. *J. Eukaryot. Microbiol.* **1993**, *40*, 287–297. [CrossRef] [PubMed]
74. Abdel-Ghaffar, F.A.; Bashtar, A.R.; Shazly, M.A. Life cycle of *Hepatozoon seurati* comb. Nov. 1- Gamogony and sporogony inside the vector, *Culex pipiens molestus*. *J. Egypt Ger. Soc. Zool.* **1991**, *3*, 211–226.
75. Bashtar, A.R.; Abdel-Ghaffar, F.A.; Shazly, M.A. Life cycle of *Hepatozoon mehlhorni* sp. nov. in the viper Echis carinatus and the mosquito *Culex pipiens*. *Parasitol. Res.* **1991**, *77*, 402–410. [CrossRef]
76. Bashtar, A.R.; Shazly, M.A.; Ahmed, A.K.; Fayed, H.M. Life cycle of *Hepatozoon matruhensis* comb. nov. 1- Blood stages and merogony inside the snake *Psammophis schokari*. *J. Egypt Ger. Soc. Zool.* **1994**, *14*, 117–131.
77. Shazly, M.A.; Ahmed, A.K.; Bashtar, A.R.; Fayed, H.M. Life cycle of *Hepatozoon matruhensis* comb. nov. 2. Gamogony and sporogony inside the vector *Culex pipiens molestus*. *J. Egypt Ger. Soc. Zool.* **1994**, *14*, 323–340.
78. Saoud, M.; Ramadan, N.; Mohammed, S.; Fawzi, S. On two new haemogregarines (Protozoa: Apicomplexa) from Colubrid and Elapidae snakes in Egypt. *Qatar Univ. Sci. J.* **1996**, *16*, 127–139.
79. Sloboda, M.; Kamler, M.; Bulantová, J.; Votýpka, J.; Modrý, D. A new species of *Hepatozoon* (Apicomplexa: Adeleorina) from *Python regius* (Serpentes:Pythonidae) and its experimental transmission by a mosquito vector. *J. Parasitol.* **2007**, *93*, 1189–1198. [CrossRef]
80. Al-Farraj, S. Light and electron microscopic study on a haemogregarine species infecting the viper *Cerastes cerastes gasperitti* from Saudi Arabia. *Pak. J. Biol. Sci.* **2008**, *11*, 1414–1421. [CrossRef]
81. Sajjadi, S.S.; Javanbakht, H. Study of blood parasites of the three snake species in Iran: *Natrix natrix*, *Natrix tessellate* and *Zamenis longissimus* (Colubridae). *J. Genet. Resour.* **2017**, *3*, 1–6.
82. Abdel-Haleem, H.M.; Mansour, L.; Holal, M.; Qasem, M.A.; Al-Quraishy, S.; Abdel-Baki, A.S. Molecular characterisation of *Hepatozoon aegypti* Bashtar, Boulos & Mehlhorn, 1984 parasitising the blood of *Spalerosophis diadema* (Serpentes: Colubridae). *Parasitol. Res.* **2018**, *117*, 3119–3125. [PubMed]
83. Robertson, M. Studies on Ceylon haematozoa. II- Notes on the life cycle of *Haemogregarina nicoriae*. *Q. J. Microsc. Sci.* **1910**, *55*, 741–762.
84. Siddall, M.E.; Desser, S.S. Ultrastructure of gametogenesis and sporogony of Haemogregarina (sensu lato) myoxoxephali (Apicomplexa: Adeleina) in the Marine Leech *Malmianta scorpii*. *J. Protozool.* **1992**, *39*, 545–554. [CrossRef]
85. Michel, J.C. *Hepatozoon mauritanicum* (Et. Et Ed. Sergent, 1904) n. comb., parasite de Testudo graeca: Redescription de la sporogone chez *Hyalomma aegyptium* et de la schizogonie tissularie d'apres le material d'E. Brump. *Ann. Parasitol. Hum. Comp.* **1973**, *48*, 11–21. [CrossRef]
86. Acholonu, A.D. *Haemogregarina pseudemydis* n sp (Apicomplexa: Haemogregarinidae) and *Pirhemocyton chelonarum* n. sp. in turtles from Louisiana. *J. Protozool.* **1947**, *21*, 659–664. [CrossRef]
87. Misra, K.K. Erythrocytic Schizogony in Haemogregarina gangetica of a River Turtle, Trionyx gangeticus Cuvier. *Proc. Zool. Soc. (Calcutta)* **1981**, *32*, 141–143.
88. Chai, J.Y.; Chen, C.H. Six new species of Haemogregarina from chinese turtles. *Acta Hydrobiol. Sin.* **1990**, *14*, 129–137.
89. Mihalca, A.D.; Achelăriţei, D.; Popescu, P. Haemoparasites of the genus Haemogregarina in a population of european pond turtles (*Emys orbicularis*) from Drăgăşani, Vâlcea county, Romania. *Rev. Sci. Parasitol.* **2002**, *3*, 22–27.
90. Paperna, I. *Hemolivia mauritanica* (Haemogregarindae: Apicomplex) infection in the tortoise *Testudo graeca* in the Near East with data on sporogonous development in the tick vector *Hyalomna aegyptium*. *Parasite* **2006**, *13*, 267–273. [CrossRef]
91. Široký, P.; Mikulíček, P.; Jandzik, D.; Kami, H.; Mihalca, A.; Rouag, R.; Kamler, M.; Schneider, C.; Zaruba, M.; Modrý, D. Co-distribution pattern of a haemogregarine *Hemolivia mauritanica* (Apicomplexa: Haemogregarinidae) and its vector *Hyalomma aegyptium* (Metastigmata: Ixodidae). *J. Parasitol.* **2009**, *95*, 728–733.
92. Telford, S.R., Jr.; Norton, T.M.; Moler, P.E.; Jensen, J.B. A new *Haemogregarina* species of the alligator snapping turtle, *Macrochelys temminckii* (Testudines: Chelydridae), in Georgia and Florida that produces macromeronts in circulating erythrocytes. *J. Parasitol.* **2009**, *95*, 208–214. [CrossRef]
93. Harris, D.J.; Graciá, E.; Jorge, F.; Maia, J.P.M.C.; Perera, A.; Carretero, M.A.; Giménez, A. Molecular detection of *Hemolivia* (Apicomplexa: Haemogregarinidae) from ticks of North African *Testudo graeca* (Testudines: Testudinidae) and an estimation of their phylogenetic relationships using 18S rRNA sequences. *Comp. Parasitol.* **2013**, *80*, 292–296. [CrossRef]

94. Rossow, J.A.; Hernandez, S.M.; Sumner, S.M.; Altman, B.R.; Crider, C.G.; Gammage, M.B.; Segal, K.M.; Yabsley, M.J. Haemogregarine infections of three species of aquatic freshwater turtles from two sites in Costa Rica. *Int. J. Parasitol. Parasites Wildl.* **2013**, *2*, 131–135. [CrossRef]
95. Soares, P.; de Brito, E.S.; Paiva, F.; Pavan, D.; Viana, L.A. *Haemogregarina* spp. in a wild population from *Podocnemis unifilis* Troschel, 1848 in the Brazilian Amazonia. *Parasitol. Res.* **2014**, *113*, 4499–4503. [CrossRef]
96. Molla, S.H.; Bandyopadhyay, P.K.; Gürelli, G. Description of a new Haemogregarine, *Haemogregarina sundarbanensis* n. sp. (Apicomplexa: Haemogregarinidae) from Mud Turtle of Sundarban Regions, West Bengal, India. *Turkiye. Parazitol. Derg.* **2015**, *39*, 131–134. [CrossRef]
97. Picelli, A.M.; Carvalho, A.V.; Viana, L.A.; Malvasio, A. Prevalence and parasitemia of *Haemogregarina* sp. in *Podocnemis expansa* (Testudines: Podocnemididae) from the Brazilian Amazon. *Rev. Bras. Parasitol. Vet.* **2015**, *24*, 191–197. [CrossRef] [PubMed]
98. Arizza, V.; Sacco, F.; Russo, D.; Scardino, R.; Arculeo, M.; Vamberger, M.; Marrone, F. The good, the bad, and the ugly: *Emys trinacris*, *Placobdella costata* and *Haemogregarina stepanowi* in Sicily (Testudines, Annelida and Apicomplexa). *Folia Parasit.* **2016**, *63*, 029. [CrossRef] [PubMed]
99. Rakhshandehroo, E.; Sharifiyazdi, H.; Ahmadi, A. Morphological and molecular characterisation of *Haemogregarina* sp. (Apicomplexa: Adeleina: Haemogregarinidae) from the blood of the Caspian freshwater turtle *Mauremys caspica* (Gmelin) (Geoemydidae) in Iran. *Syst. Parasitol.* **2016**, *93*, 517–524. [CrossRef] [PubMed]
100. Alhaboubi, A.R.; Pollard, D.A.; Holman, P.J. Molecular and morphological characterization of a haemogregarine in the alligator snapping turtle, *Macrochelys temminckii* (Testudines: Chelydridae). *J. Parasitol.* **2017**, *116*, 207–215. [CrossRef] [PubMed]
101. Goes, V.C.; Brito, E.S.; Valadao, R.M.; Gutierrez, C.O.; Picelli, A.M.; Viana, L.A. Haemogregarine (Apicomplexa: Adeleorina) infection in Vanderhaege's toadheaded turtle, *Mesoclemmys vanderhaegei* (Chelidae), from a Brazilian Neotropical savanna region. *Folia Parasitol.* **2018**, *65*, 012. [CrossRef] [PubMed]
102. Úngari, L.P.; Santos, A.L.Q.; O'Dwyer, L.H.; da Silva, M.R.L.; Santos, T.C.R.; da Cunha, M.J.R.; de Melo Costa Pinto, R.; Cury, M.C. Molecular characterization and identification of *Hepatozoon* species Miller, 1908 (Apicomplexa: Adeleina: Hepatozoidae) in captive snakes from Brazil. *Parasitol. Res.* **2018**, *117*, 3857–3865.
103. Börner, C. Untersuchungen über Hämospridien. I-Ein Beitrag zur kenntnis des genus Haemogregarina Danilewsky. *Z. Wiss. Zool. Abt. A* **1901**, *69*, 398–416.
104. Pessôa, S.B.; De Biasi, P. Nota taxonomica sobre cistos esporôgônicos de algumas espécies de Hepatozoon (Sporozoa, Haemogregarinidae) parasites de serpents brasileiras. *Mem. Inst. Butantan (São Paulo)* **1973**, *37*, 299–307.
105. Hoare, C.A. On protozoal blood parasites collected in Uganda with an account of the life cycle of the croccdile haemogregarines. *Parasitology* **1932**, *24*, 210–224. [CrossRef]
106. Viana, L.A.; Marques, E.J. Haemogregarine parasites (Apicomplexa: Hepatozoidae) in *Caiman crocodilus yacare* (Crocodilia: Alligatoridae) from Pantanal, Corumba, MS, Brazil. *Rev. Bras. Parasitol. Vet.* **2005**, *14*, 173–175.
107. Viana, L.A.; Paiva, F.; Coutinho, M.E.; Lourenço-de-Oliveira, R. *Hepatozoon caimani* (Apicomplexa: Hepatozoidae) in Wild Caiman, *Caiman yacare*, from the Pantanal region, Brazil. *J. Parasitol.* **2010**, *96*, 83–88. [CrossRef] [PubMed]
108. Bennett, G.F.; Earle, R.A.; Penzhorn, B. *Ornithodoros peringueyi* (Argasidae) and *Xenopsylla trispinis* (Siphonaptera), probable intermediate hosts of *Hepatozzon atticoare* of the South African Cliff swallow, *Hirundo spilodera*. *Can. J. Zool.* **1992**, *70*, 188–190. [CrossRef]
109. Bennett, G.F.; Earle, R.A. New species of *Haemoproteus*, *Hepatozoon* and *Leucocytozoon* from South African birds. *S. Afr. J. Wildl. Res.* **1992**, *22*, 114–118.
110. Desser, S.S. Tissue "Cyst" of *Hepatozoon griseisciuri* in the Grey Squirrel, *Sciurus carolinensis*: The significance of these cysts in species of Hepatozoon. *J. Parasitol.* **1990**, *76*, 257–259. [CrossRef]
111. Göbel, E.; Krampitz, H.E. Histologische Untersuchungean zur Gamogonie und Sporogonie von *Hepatozoon erhardovae* in experimental infizierten rattenflohen (Xenopsylla cheopis). *Z. Parasitenkd.* **1982**, *67*, 261–271. [CrossRef]
112. Frank, C. Über die Bedeutung von Laelaps agilis CL Koch 1836 (Mosostigmata: Parasitiformae) fur die Ubertragung von *Hepatozoon sylvatici* Coles 1914 (Sporozoa: Haemogregarinidae). *Z. Parasitenkd.* **1977**, *53*, 307–310. [CrossRef]
113. Forlano, M.D.; Teixeira, K.R.S.; Scolfield, A.; Elisei, C.; Yotoko, K.S.C.; Fernandes, K.R.; Linhares, G.F.C.; Ewing, S.A.; Massard, C.L. Molecular characterization of *Hepatozoon* sp. from Brazilian dogs and its phylogenetic relationship with other *Hepatozoon* spp. *Vet. Parasitol.* **2007**, *145*, 21–30. [CrossRef]
114. Otranto, D.; Dantas-Torres, F.; Weigl, S.; Latrofa, M.S.; Stanneck, D.; Decaprariis, D.; Capelli, G.; Baneth, G. Diagnosis of *Hepatozoon canis* in young dogs by cytology and PCR. *Parasite. Vector.* **2011**, *4*, 55. [CrossRef]
115. Baneth, G.; Sheiner, A.; Eyal, O.; Hahn, S.; Beaufils, J.P.; Anug, Y.; Talmi-Frank, D. Redescription of *Hepatozoon felis* (Apicomplexa: Hepatozoidae) based on phylogenetic analysis, tissue and blood form morphology, and possible transplacental transmission. *Parasite. Vector.* **2013**, *6*, 102. [CrossRef]
116. Ramos, C.A.N.; Babo-Terra, V.J.; Pedroso, T.C.; Filho, A.F.S.; Araújo, F.R.; Cleveland, H.P.K. Molecular identification of *Hepatozoon canis* in dogs from Campo Grande, Mato Grosso do Sul, Brazil. *Braz. J. Vet. Parasitol. Jaboticabal* **2015**, *24*, 247–250. [CrossRef]
117. Paiz, L.M.; Silva, R.C.; Satake, F.; Fraga, T.L. Hematological disorders detected in dogs infected by *Hepatozoon canis* in a municipality in Mato Grosso do Sul State, Brazil. *Arq. Bras. Med. Vet. Zootec.* **2016**, *68*, 1187–1194. [CrossRef]

118. De Sousa, K.C.M.; Fernandes, M.P.; Herrera, H.M.; Benevenute, J.L.; Santos, F.M.; Rocha, F.L.; Barreto, W.T.G.; Macedo, G.C.; Campos, J.B.; Martins, T.F.; et al. Molecular detection of *Hepatozoon* spp. in domestic dogs and wild mammals in southern Pantanal, Brazil with implications in the transmission route. *Vet. Parasitol.* **2017**, *237*, 37–46. [CrossRef] [PubMed]
119. Bhusri, B.; Sariya, L.; Mongkolphan, C.; Suksai, P.; Kaewchot, S.; Changbunjong, T. Molecular characterization of *Hepatozoon felis* in *Rhipicephalus sanguineus* ticks infested on captive lions (*Panthera leo*). *J. Parasit. Dis.* **2017**, *41*, 903–907. [CrossRef]
120. Mitkova, B.; Hrazdilova, K.; Novotna, M.; Jurankova, J.; Hofmannova, L.; Forejtek, P.; Modry, D. Autochthonous *Babesia canis*, *Hepatozoon canis* and imported *Babesia gibsoni* infection in dogs in the Czech Republic. *Vet. Med.* **2017**, *62*, 138–146. [CrossRef]
121. Barati, A.; Razmi, G.R. A parasitologic and molecular survey of *Hepatozoon canis* infection in stray dogs in northeastern Iran. *J. Parasitol.* **2018**, *104*, 413–417. [CrossRef]
122. Tuna, G.E.; Bakırcı, S.; Dinler, C.; Battal, G.; Ulutaş, B. Molecular Identification and Clinicopathological Findings of *Hepatozoon* sp. Infection in a Cat: First Report from Turkey. *Turkiye Parazitol. Derg.* **2018**, *42*, 286–289. [CrossRef] [PubMed]
123. Attipa, C.; Maguire, D.; Solano-Gallego, L.; Szladovits, B.; Barker, E.N.; Farr, A.; Baneth, G.; Tasker, S. *Hepatozoon canis* in three imported dogs: A new tickborne disease reaching the United Kingdom. *Vet. Rec.* **2018**, *183*, 716. [CrossRef]
124. Harris, D.J.; Sergiadou, D.; Halajian, A.; Swanepoel, L.; Roux, F. Molecular screening indictes high prevalence and mixed infections of *Hepatozoon* parasites in wild felines from South Africa. *J. S. Afr. Vet. Assoc.* **2020**, *91*, a2055. [CrossRef]
125. Van As, M.; Netherlands, E.C.; Smit, N.J. Molecular characterization and morphological description of two new species of *Hepatozoon* Miller, 1908 (Apicomplexa: Adeleorina: Hepatozoidae) infecting leukocytes of African leopards *Panthera pardus pardus* (L.). *Parasite. Vector.* **2020**, *13*, 222. [CrossRef]
126. Baticados, A.M.; Baticados, W.N.; Carlos, E.T.; Carlos, S.M.; Villarba, L.A.; Subiaga, S.G.; Magcalas, J.M. Parasitological detection and molecular evidence of *Hepatozoon canis* from canines in Manila, Philippines. *Vet. Med. Res. Rep.* **2011**, *1*, 7–10. [CrossRef]
127. Bray, R.S. A check-list of the parasitic protozoa of West Africa with some notes on their classification. *Bull. Inst. Fr. Afr. Noire.* **1964**, *26*, 238–315.
128. Yanai, T.; Tomita, A.; Masegi, T.; Ishikawa, K.; Iwasaki, T.; Yamazoe, K.; Ueda, K. Histopathologic features of naturally occurring hepatozoonosis in wild martens (*Martes melampus*) in Japan. *J. Wildl. Dis.* **1996**, *31*, 233–237. [CrossRef] [PubMed]
129. Saoud, M.F.A.; Ramadan, N.F.; Mohammed, S.H.; Fawzi, S.M. Haemogregarines of geckos in Egypt, together with a description of *Haemogregarina helmymohammedi* n. sp. *Qatar Univ. Sci. J.* **1995**, *15*, 131–146.
130. Smith, T.G.; Desser, S.S. Ultrastructural features of cystic and merogonic stages of *Hepatozoon sipedon* (Apicomplexa: Adeleorina) in northern leopard frogs (*Rana pipiens*) and northern water snakes (*Narodia sipedon*) from Ontario, Canada. *J. Eukaryot. Microbiol.* **1998**, *45*, 419–425. [CrossRef] [PubMed]
131. Nadler, S.A.; Miller, J.H. A redescription of *Hepatozoon mocassini* (Laveran, 1902) n. comb. from *Agkistrodon piscivorus leucostoma* Troost 1836. *J. Protozool.* **1984**, *31*, 321–324. [CrossRef]
132. Abdel-Baki, A.S.; Mansour, L.; Al-Malki, E.S.; Al-Quraishy, S.; Abdel-Halim, H.M. Morphometric and molecular characterisation of *Hepatozoon bashtari* n. sp. in painted saw-scaled viper, *Echis coloratus* (Ophidia, Viperidae). *Parasitol. Res.* **2020**, *119*, 3793–3801. [CrossRef]
133. Hussein, A.N.A. Light and transmission electron microscopic studies of a haemogregarine in naturally infected fan-footed gecko (*Ptyodactylus hasselquistii*). *Parasitol. Res.* **2006**, *98*, 468–471. [CrossRef]
134. Reichenow, E. *Karyolysus lacerate*, ein wirtwechselndes Coccidium der Eidechse *Laverta muralis* und der Milbe *Liponyssus saurarum*. *Arb. Gesundh. Amt. Berl.* **1913**, *45*, 317–363.
135. Honigberg, B.M.; Chairman of Committee. A revised classification of the phylum Protozoa. *J. Protozool.* **1964**, *11*, 7–20. [CrossRef]
136. Rubini, D.S.; Paduan, K.S.; Perez, R.R.; Ribolla, P.E.M.; O'Dwyer, L.H. Molecular characterization of feline *Hepatozoon* species from Brazil. *Vet. Parasitol.* **2006**, *137*, 168–171. [CrossRef]
137. Ortuño, A.; Castella, J.; Criado-Fornelio, A.; Buling, A.; Barba-Carretero, J.C. Molecular detection of a *Hepatozoon* species in stray cats from a feline colony in North-eastern Spain. *Vet. J.* **2008**, *177*, 134–135. [CrossRef] [PubMed]
138. Vilcins, I.E.; Ujvari, B.; Old, J.M.; Deane, E. Molecular and morphological description of a *Hepatozoon* species in reptiles and their ticks in the Northern Territory, Australia. *J. Parasitol.* **2009**, *95*, 434–442. [CrossRef] [PubMed]
139. Maia, J.P.M.C.; Perera, A.; Harris, D.J. Molecular survey and microscopic examination of *Hepatozoon* Miller, 1908 (Apicomplexa: Adeleorina) in lacertid lizards from the western Mediterranean. *Folia Parasitol.* **2012**, *59*, 241–248. [CrossRef] [PubMed]
140. Tomé, B.M.; Maia, J.P.M.C.; Harris, D.J. Molecular assessment of apicomplexan parasites in the snake *Psammophis* from north Africa: Do multiple parasite lineages reflect the final vertebrate host diet? *J. Parasitol.* **2013**, *99*, 883–887. [CrossRef]
141. Xavier, R.; Severino, R.; Pérez-Losada, M.; Gestal, C.; Freitas, R.; Harris, D.J.; Verissino, A.; Rosado, D.; Cable, J. Phylogenetic analysis of apicomplexan parasites infecting commercially valuable species from the North-East Atlantic reveals high levels of diversity and insights into the evolution of the group. *Parasite. Vector.* **2018**, *11*, 63. [CrossRef]
142. Waeschenbach, A.; Webster, B.L.; Bray, R.A.; Littlewood, D.T.J. Added resolution among ordinal level relationships of tapeworms (Platyhelminthes: Cestoda) with complete small and large subunit nuclear ribosomal RNA genes. *Mol. Phylogenet. Evol.* **2007**, *45*, 311–325. [CrossRef]
143. Ahmad, A.S.; Saeed, M.A.; Rashid, I.; Ashraf, K.; Shehzad, W.; Traub, R.J.; Baneth, G.; Jabbar, A. Molecular characterization of *Hepatozoon canis* from farm dogs in Pakistan. *Parasitol. Res.* **2018**, *117*, 1131–1138. [CrossRef]
144. Hayes, P.M.; Smit, N.J. Molecular insights into the identification and phylogenetics of the cosmopolitan marine fish blood parasite, *Haemogregarina bigemina* (Adeleorina: Haemogregarinidae). *Int. J. Parasitol. Parasites. Wildl.* **2019**, *8*, 216–220. [CrossRef]

145. Nordmeyer, S.C.; Henry, G.; Guerra, T.; Rodriquez, D.; Forstner, M.R.J.; Hahn, D. Identification of blood parasites in individuals fromsix families of freshwater turtles. *Chelonian Conserv. Biol.* **2020**, *19*, 85–94. [CrossRef]
146. Mathew, J.S.; Van Den Bussche, R.A.; Ewing, S.A. Phylogenetic relationships of *Hepatozoon* (Apicomplexa Adeleorina) based on molecular, morphologic, and life-cycle characters. *J. Parasitol.* **2000**, *86*, 366–372. [CrossRef]
147. Perkins, S.L.; Keller, A.K. Phylogeny of nuclear small subunit rRNA genes of haemogregarines amplified with specific primers. *J. Parasitol.* **2001**, *87*, 870–876. [CrossRef]
148. Inokuma, H.; Okuda, M.; Ohno, K.; Shimoda, K.; Onishi, T. Analysis of the 18S rRNA gene sequence of a *Hepatozoon* detected in two Japanese dogs. *Vet. Parasitol.* **2002**, *106*, 265–271. [CrossRef]
149. Criado-Fornelio, A.; Buling, A.; Cunha-Filho, N.A.; Ruas, J.L.; Farias, N.A.; Rey-Valeiron, C.; Pingret, J.L.; Etievant, M.; Barba-Carretero, M.J.C. Development and evaluation of a quantitative PCR assay for detection of *Hepatozoon* sp. *Vet. Parasitol.* **2007**, *150*, 352–356. [CrossRef]
150. Tabar, M.D.; Altet, L.; Francino, O.; Sánchez, A.; Ferrer, L.; Roura, X. Vector-borne infections in cats: Molecular study in Barcelona area (Spain). *Vet. Parasitol.* **2008**, *151*, 332–336. [CrossRef]
151. Kledmanee, K.; Suwanpakdee, S.; Krajangwong, S.; Chatsiriwech, J.; Suksai, P.; Suwannachat, P.; Sariya, L.; Buddhirongawatr, R.; Charoonrut, P.; Chaichoun, K. Development of multiplex polymerase chain reaction for detection of *Ehrlichia canis, Babesia* spp. and *Hepatozoon canis* in canine blood. *Southeast Asian J. Trop. Med. Public Health* **2009**, *40*, 35–39.
152. Zintl, A.; Finnerty, E.J.; Murphy, T.M.; De Waal, T.; Gray, J.S. Babesias of red deer (*Cervus elaphus*) in Ireland. *Vet. Res.* **2011**, *42*, 7. [CrossRef]
153. Hodžić, A.; Alić, A.; Fuehrer, H.P.; Harl, J.; Wille-Piazzai, W.; Duscher, G.G. A molecular survey of vector-borne pathogens in red foxes (*Vulpes vulpes*) from Bosnia and Herzegovina. *Parasite. Vector.* **2015**, *8*, 88. [CrossRef]

animals

Review

Systematic Review of Hepatitis E Virus in Brazil: A One-Health Approach of the Human-Animal-Environment Triad

Danny Franciele da Silva Dias Moraes [1,2,3], João R. Mesquita [3,4,*], Valéria Dutra [1] and Maria São José Nascimento [5]

1 Faculty of Veterinary Medicine, Federal University of Mato Grosso, Cuiabá 78060-900, Brazil; dannyfsdm@gmail.com (D.F.d.S.D.M.); valdutra@ufmt.br (V.D.)
2 Secretaria de Estado do Meio Ambiente de Mato Grosso (SEMA), Cuiabá 78050-970, Brazil
3 Abel Salazar Institute of Biomedical Sciences (ICBAS), University of Porto, 4050-313 Porto, Portugal
4 Epidemiology Research Unit (EPIUnit), Instituto de Saúde Pública da Universidade do Porto, 4050-600 Porto, Portugal
5 Faculty of Pharmacy, University of Porto (FFUP), 4050-313 Porto, Portugal; saojose@ff.up.pt
* Correspondence: jrmesquita@icbas.up.pt

Simple Summary: Hepatitis E virus (HEV) is an important causative agent of acute and chronic hepatitis worldwide. Originally identified in epidemics associated with flooding in Asia, it nowadays shows very distinct genetic and epidemiological patterns. While HEV genotypes (HEV-) 1 and 2 are associated with the original outbreaks (waterborne diseases), HEV-3 and HEV-4 present a zoonotic pattern (associated with consumption of meat from infected animals), HEV-5 and 6 have been found only in wild boar in Japan, and HEV-7 and 8 have been detected in camels and dromedary seldom affecting humans. Brazil, with a precarious sanitary structure and being an important world meat producer, was the focus of this study in order to identify patterns of occurrence of HEV. After reviewing scientific studies, it was identified that the only genotype found in Brazil is HEV-3 and the area where there were more reports was the South region of the country. This is the region that produces more pork. These results indicate that HEV-3 is widespread in the country and sanitary surveillance is essential in the national production of pigs, as well as the implementation of monitoring protocols in hospitals.

Abstract: Brazil is the fifth largest country in the world with diverse socioeconomic and sanitary conditions, also being the fourth largest pig producer in the world. The aim of the present systematic review was to collect and summarize all HEV published data from Brazil (from 1995 to October 2020) performed in humans, animals, and the environment, in a One Health perspective. A total of 2173 papers were retrieved from five search databases (LILACs, Mendeley, PubMed, Scopus, and Web of Science) resulting in 71 eligible papers after application of exclusion/inclusion criteria. Data shows that HEV genotype 3 (HEV-3) was the only retrieved genotype in humans, animals, and environment in Brazil. The South region showed the highest human seroprevalence and also the highest pig density and industry, suggesting a zoonotic link. HEV-1 and 2 were not detected in Brazil, despite the low sanitary conditions of some regions. From the present review we infer that HEV epidemiology in Brazil is similar to that of industrialized countries (only HEV-3, swine reservoirs, no waterborne transmission, no association with low sanitary conditions). Hence, we alert for the implementation of HEV surveillance systems in swine and for the consideration of HEV in the diagnostic routine of acute and chronic hepatitis in humans.

Keywords: Brazil; HEV; zoonotic; One Health

Citation: Moraes, D.F.d.S.D.; Mesquita, J.R.; Dutra, V.; Nascimento, M.S.J. Systematic Review of Hepatitis E Virus in Brazil: A One-Health Approach of the Human-Animal-Environment Triad. *Animals* **2021**, *11*, 2290. https://doi.org/10.3390/ani11082290

Academic Editor: Fabio Ostanello

Received: 16 June 2021
Accepted: 29 July 2021
Published: 3 August 2021

1. Introduction

In the last years, hepatitis E virus (HEV) has captured widespread attention when autochthonous hepatitis E cases started to be reported in industrialized countries [1]. Until then, hepatitis E was considered a rare disease in these countries and only associated with travelers returning from HEV endemic areas in Africa and Asia [2]. All the autochthonous cases reported in industrialized countries were caused by two HEV genotypes, namely HEV genotypes 3 (HEV-3) and 4 (HEV-4), that showed to have distinct epidemiological and clinical characteristics from the HEV genotype 1 (HEV-1) and HEV genotype 2 (HEV-2) circulating in developing countries. HEV-1 and HEV-2 are restricted to humans, transmitted by orofecal route through contaminated waters (usually linked to the lack of basic sanitation), and associated with large waterborne outbreaks of acute hepatitis in underdeveloped regions [3]. HEV-3 and HEV-4 are zoonotic viruses, common in domestic and wild pigs that infect humans as an accidental host through the consumption of uncooked contaminated pork products, being associated with sporadic human hepatitis cases [2,4]. Clinical features of these genotypes are also unique, with infections mostly asymptomatic in immunocompetent but with the capacity to progress to chronic hepatitis with liver cirrhosis in immunocompromised patients (such as organ transplant recipients and HIV patients), being also associated to diverse extra-hepatic manifestations (neurological and haematological) [2].

HEV is a non-enveloped positive-sense single-stranded RNA virus, belonging to *Hepeviridae* family, genera *Orthohepevirus*, species A, with eight genotypes currently recognized (HEV-1 to HEV-8) [3]. HEV-1 and HEV-4 have been detected in human cases, while HEV-5 and HEV-6 are genotypes strictly found in wild boar, HEV-7 and HEV-8 found in dromedary and Bactrian-camels [3]. There is only one report of HEV-7 in humans [5]. Currently, HEV-3 is subdivided into at least 11 subtypes (3a–3j, 3ra) [6].

Since swine are the main reservoir of HEV-3 as well as the main source of human infection and given that Brazil is the fourth largest pig producer in the world [7], a high HEV-3 circulation in the country is expected. Brazil is divided into 5 regions, namely North, Northeast, Midwest, Southeast and South, 26 states and a Federal District, with a total, of 5570 municipalities [8]. The South region has the highest pig production in the territory, accounting for 66.12% of the national production [7]. Moreover, Brazil is a country with continental dimensions, being the 5th largest country in the world with a population of circa 211 million, having a great extension of rural and urban areas with extremely diverse socioeconomic and sanitary conditions that influence infectious diseases dynamics [9]. There is today an increased awareness to monitor and survey the interfaces of human, animal, and environment in order to manage global health. Hence, the present systematic review aimed to collect and summarize all HEV published data from Brazil (from 1995 to October 2020) performed in humans, swine, other animals, and the environment, from a One Health perspective.

2. Materials and Methods

Exhaustive searches were carried out in the electronic databases: Latin American and Caribbean Health Sciences Literature (LILACs), Mendeley, PubMed, Scopus, and Web of Science. Two independent investigators (DFSDM and JRM) searched the databases, and included all studies published until October 2020. The study followed the protocol of the Preferred Reporting of Systematic Reviews and Meta-Analysis (PRISMA) [10], and the studies included should necessarily be published, indexed, and peer reviewed. No filters or other forms of search restrictions were used to achieve the greatest possible reach.

The literary search was made in the databases already mentioned above using the keywords (HEV OR Hepatitis E Virus) AND (Brazil). After reading the title and the abstract, papers that did not address Brazil as a scope or part of the scope, papers that did not study HEV, duplicate studies, review articles and experimental studies were excluded from this systematic review. Papers that did not make clear the information in the title and abstract were read in full and only those that contained the target content were included.

For the purpose of constructing this systematic review, all studies found in the databases that aimed at the parsing HEV in Brazil on their study scope were included, regardless of language, studied population or sample size. All authors independently screened the databases, and relevant information was extracted. Differences in opinions about whether to include an article were solved by consensus between all the authors.

3. Results

A total of 2173 papers were retrieved from the 5 databases used for the search (Figure 1). After removal of duplicated papers (n = 542), exclusion criteria were applied to eliminate non-related papers, namely papers classified as "non-Brazilian" (n = 24), "non-HEV" (n = 1519), as well as review articles and in vivo animal experimental studies.

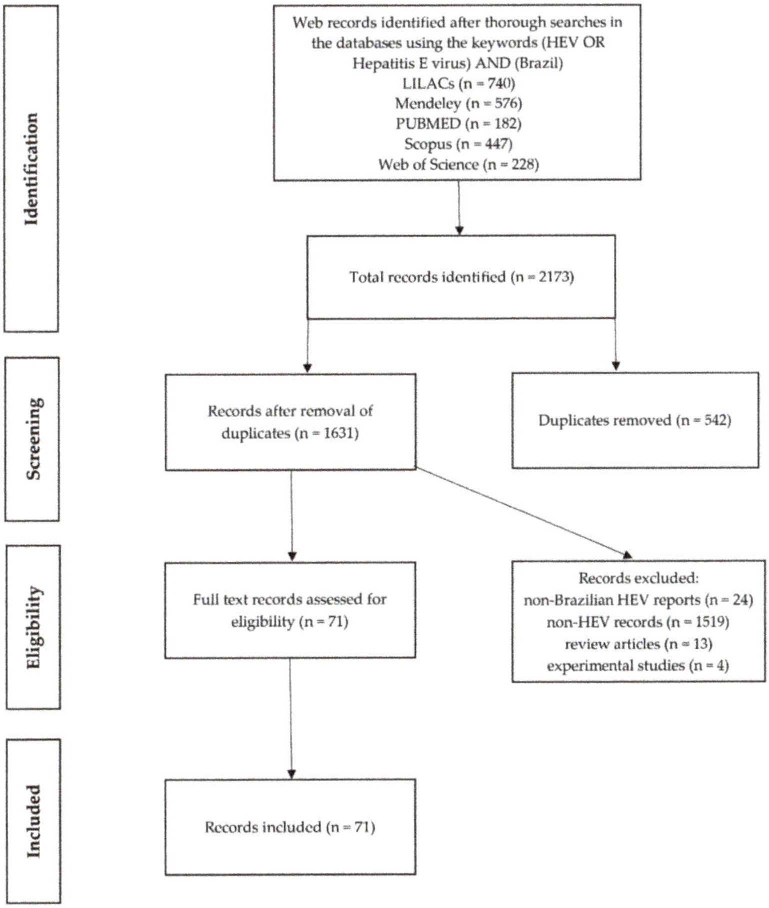

Figure 1. PRISMA Flow diagram showing the steps of the record selection procedure and reporting the strategies of inclusion/exclusion (explaining their reasons).

Application of inclusion and exclusion criteria generated a total of 71 eligible papers. They were all included in the study after being assessed by full-reading. The distribution of published papers by regions of Brazil and type of study can be observed in Figure 2. HEV studies in humans, swine and animal products, animals other than swine, and environment are summarized in Tables 1–4, respectively.

Table 1. HEV in humans, Brazil.

Region of Brazil	Sampling Location	Sampling Date	Population Details	Type of Samples	Hev Diagnostic Assay	Number of Positive/Total (%)	Hev Genotype	Additional Data	Reference
North	Acre	2004	Rural settlements	Sera	IgG/IgM (only on IgG positive cases) (EIA [1,2] + immunoblot [4])	IgG 50/388 (12.9%), IgM 7/43 (16.3%)	-	The odds for HEV seropositivity increased by 3.3% for each additional year of age	[11]
	Acre	1997	Riverine communities of amazon basin	Sera	IgG (EIA [3])	14/349 (4%)	-	-	[12]
	Amazonas	-	Blood donors, hemodialyzed, pregnant women	Sera	IgG (EIA [3])	Blood donors 1/227 (0.45%), hemodialyzed 1/192 (0.52%), pregnant women 0/100 (0%)	-	-	[13]
	Pará	2015	Rural afro-descendant communities	Sera	IgM/IgG (EIA [2] + immunoblot [4]), RNA (RT-qPCR)	IgM 2/535 (0.3%), IgG 2/535 (0.3%), RNA 0/9 (0%)	-	Afro-descendant rural communities from the eastern Brazilian Amazon had low HEV infection	[14]
	Pará	1993–2014	Non-A-C hepatitis or suspected cases of HEV infection	Sera	IgM/IgG (EIA [2] + immunoblot [4]), RNA (RT-qPCR)	IgM 11/318 (3.4%), IgG 19/318 (5.9%), RNA 0/318 (0%)	-	HEV low circulation rate even between suspected cases in the Eastern Brazilian Amazon	[15]
Northeast	Bahia	1995–1999	Acute hepatitis cases	Sera	IgG/IgM (only on IgG positive cases) (EIA [3,5])	Anti-HEV in hepatitis A cases: IgG 15/40 (38%), IgM 4/15 (26.67%); anti-HEV in hepatitis B cases: IgG 4/42 (10%), IgM 0/4 (0%); anti-HEV in hepatitis non-A-C: IgG 2/12 (8.34%), IgM 1/2 (50%)	-	IgG prevalence was significantly higher in patients with hepatitis A (38%) compared to the hepatitis B group (10%) ($p < 0.01$)	[16]
	Bahia	1992–1996	Acute hepatitis cases	Sera	IgM/IgG (EIA [3])	IgM 0/43 (0%), IgG 5/43 (12%)	-	-	[17]

Table 1. *Cont.*

Region of Brazil	Sampling Location	Sampling Date	Population Details	Type of Samples	Hev Diagnostic Assay	Number of Positive/Total (%)	Hev Genotype	Additional Data	Reference
Northeast	Bahia	1992–1994	Blood donors, hemodialyzed, acute viral hepatitis, schistosomiasis cases	Sera	IgG (EIA [3])	Blood donors 4/200 (2%), hemodialyzed 0/392 (0%), acute viral hepatitis 14/79 (17.7%), schistosomiasis 3/30 (10%)	-	Among acute viral hepatitis cases, those with hepatitis A had a higher frequency of positivity compared with all other hepatotropic viruses ($p < 0.003$)	[18]
	Pernambuco	2016–2017	HIV patients	Sera	IgG (EIA [2]), RNA (RT-PCR)	IgG 15/366 (4.1%), RNA 0/366 (0%)	-	Several risk factors were evaluated: age, years of school, sexual orientation, oral-anal sex, use of injectable drugs and piped water availability. Piped water showed to be a protective factor for HEV infection ($p = 0.018$)	[19]
	Pernambuco	-	Schistosomiasis cases	Sera	IgM/IgG (EIA [6]), RNA (RT-qPCR)	IgM 0/80 (0%), IgG 15/80 (18.8%), RNA 0/80 (0%)	-	-	[20]
Midwest	Goiás	2014	Renal transplant recipients	Sera	IgM/IgG (EIA [2]), RNA (RT-qPCR)	IgM 0/316 (0%), IgG 8/316 (2.5%), RNA 0/316 (0%)	-	HEV infection was infrequent in kidney transplant recipients in Central Brazil	[21]
	Goiás	2012–2014	Non-A-C hepatitis cases	Sera	IgM/IgG (EIA [2] + immunoblot [4]), RNA (RT-qPCR)	IgM 1/379 (0.3%), IgG 20/379 (5.3%), RNA 0/379 (0%)		Sociodemographic characteristics were evaluated: sex, age, marital status, ethnicity, schooling	

Table 1. *Cont.*

Region of Brazil	Sampling Location	Sampling Date	Population Details	Type of Samples	Hev Diagnostic Assay	Number of Positive/Total (%)	Hev Genotype	Additional Data	Reference
								and monthly income. Low education level ($p = 0.005$) and living in rural areas ($p = 0.056$) were found to be associated with HEV seropositivity	[22]
	Goiás and Mato Grosso do Sul	2011–2012	Rural settlements	Sera	IgM/IgG (EIA [2])	Anti-HEV (total) 36/923 (3.9%)	-	-	[23]
Midwest	Goiás	2010–2011	Recyclable waste pickers	Sera	IgM/IgG (EIA [2] + immunoblot [4]), RNA (Nested RT-PCR)	IgM 3/431 (0.7%), IgG 22/431 (5.1%), RNA 0/3 (0%)	-	Sociodemographic characteristics were evaluated: sex, age, marital status, ethnicity, schooling and monthly income. Age > 40 years wsa found to be associated ($p < 0.01$) with HEV seropositivity	[24]
	Goiás	2011	Rural settlements	Sera	IgM/IgG (EIA [2] + immunoblot [4]), RNA (RT-qPCR)	IgM 0/464, IgG 16/464 (3.4%), RNA 0/464 (0%)	-	Sociodemographic characteristics were evaluated: sex, age, marital status, ethnicity, schooling and monthly income. Dwelling in a rural settlement for >5 years was associated ($p = 0.025$) with HEV seropositivity	[25]

Table 1. *Cont.*

Region of Brazil	Sampling Location	Sampling Date	Population Details	Type of Samples	Hev Diagnostic Assay	Number of Positive/Total (%)	Hev Genotype	Additional Data	Reference
Midwest	Mato Grosso	2009–2010	Blood donors, rural settlements	Sera	IgG (EIA 7)	Blood donors 4/101 (4%), rural settlements 26/310 (8.4%)	-	Living in rural settlements was not found to be a risk factor for HEV infection ($p = 0.206$)	[26]
	Mato Grosso	1998	Children (3–9 years old)	Sera	IgG (EIA 3)	3 years 0/8 (0%), 4 years 0/13 (0%), 5 years 5/48 (10.4%), 6 years 5/87 (5.7%), 7 years 1/106 (0.9%), 8 years 8/124 (6.4%), 9 years 3/101 (3%)	-	The overall HEV seroprevalence in children (3–9 years old) was 4.5%	[27]
	Mato Grosso	1995	Community of Amazon non-A-C acute hepatitis and asymptomatic cases	Sera	IgM/IgG (EIA 3)	Non-A-C 2/16 (12.5%), asymptomatic 7/66 (10.60%)	-	Authors claim to be the first study reporting evidence for HEV infection in brazilian Amazon	[28]
	Mato Grosso	1993	Gold miners	Sera	IgG (EIA 5)	6/97 (6.18%)	-	Authors claim to be the first HEV survey in Brazil	[29]
	Mato Grosso	-	Amazon poor community	Sera	IgG (EIA 3)	10/299 (3.3%)	-	-	[30]
	Mato Grosso do Sul	2013–2015	Crack cocaine users	Sera	IgG/IgM (EIA 6), RNA (RT-qPCR)	IgM 2/698 (0.28%), IgG 99/698 (14.2%), RNA 0/2 (0%)	-	-	[31]
Southeast	Rio de Janeiro	2012–2014	HIV positive	Sera	IgM/IgG (EIA 2), RNA (RT-qPCR)	IgM 0/280 (0%), IgG 0/280 (0%), RNA 11/280 (3.6%)	3	The RNA load ranged from 10^2–10^8 copies/mL	[32]

Table 1. *Cont.*

Region of Brazil	Sampling Location	Sampling Date	Population Details	Type of Samples	Hev Diagnostic Assay	Number of Positive/Total (%)	Hev Genotype	Additional Data	Reference
Southeast	Rio de Janeiro	2004–2008	Non-A-C hepatitis	Sera	IgM/IgG (EIA [1]), RNA (RT-qPCR)	IgM 1/64 (1.56%), IgG 1/64 (1.56%), HEV RNA 1/64 (1.56%)	3b	Authors claim to be the first report of an autochthonous HEV infection in Brazil. A single sample tested positive for both IgM/IgG and HEV-RNA (viral load of 10^5 copies/mL)	[33]
	Rio de Janeiro	1999	Poor community	Sera	IgG (EIA [3])	17/699 (2.4%)	-	-	[34]
	Rio de Janeiro	1994–1998	Blood donors, pregnant women, non-A-C hepatitis cases, hemodialyzed, intravenous drug users (IVDU), individuals living in the rural and urban areas	Sera	IgG (EIA [3])	Blood donors 4/93 (4.3%), pregnant women 3/304 (1%), non-A-C 3/146 (2.1%), hemodialyzed 4/65 (6.2%), IVDU 12/102 (11.8%), rural area 3/145 (2.1%), urban area 0/260 (0%)	-	-	[35]
	Rio de Janeiro	-	Pig handlers	Sera	IgG (EIA [8a])	2/32 (6.3%)	-	-	[11]
	São Paulo	2015–2016	Chronic hepatitis C cases	Sera	IgG/IgM (only on IgG positive and inconclusive cases) (EIA [6])	IgG 63/618 (10.2%), IgM 0/66 (0%)	-	HEV seroprevalence in patients with cirrhosis was significantly higher than in patients without cirrhosis (13.2% vs 8%, $p = 0.04$)	[36]

Table 1. *Cont.*

Region of Brazil	Sampling Location	Sampling Date	Population Details	Type of Samples	Hev Diagnostic Assay	Number of Positive/Total (%)	Hev Genotype	Additional Data	Reference
Southeast	São Paulo	2014	Blood donors	Sera	IgG/IgM (only on IgG positive cases) (EIA [6]), RNA (RT-qPCR)	IgG 49/500 (9.8%), IgM 1/49 (2.04%), RNA 0/49 (0%)	-	-	[37]
	São Paulo	2013	Transfusion-dependent thalassemia or sickle cell disease (SCD)	Sera	IgG (EIA [6]), RNA (RT-PCR)	IgG: Thalassemia 8/40 (20%), SCD 4/52 (7.7%); RNA 0/92 (0%)	-	The overall anti-HEV IgG seroprevalence in patients with thalassemia and SCD was 13.0%	[38]
	São Paulo	2013	Liver transplant recipients	Sera	IgM/IgG (EIA [2])	IgM 6/284 (2.6%), IgG 23/284 (8.1%)	-	-	[39]
	São Paulo	2012	Pediatric liver transplant case	Sera	IgM/IgG (EIA [2]), RNA (RT-qPCR)	IgM(+), IgG (+), RNA (+)	3b	Authors claim to be the first report of chronic and/or pediatric HEV infection in Latin America. RNA showed a load of 4.5 log_{10} copies/mL	[40]
	São Paulo	2011–2013	Urban and rural residents	Sera	IgM/IgG (EIA [2,6] + immunoblot [7],) RNA (RT-qPCR)	IgG 50/242 (20.7%), RNA 0/244	-	-	[41]
	São Paulo	2007–2013	HIV positive	Sera	IgM/IgG (EIA [2] + immunoblot [4]), RNA (RT-qPCR)	IgM 5/354 (1.4%), IgG 38/354 (10.7%), RNA 0/354 (0%)	-	-	[42]
	São Paulo	2001–2011	Renal transplant recipients	Sera	IgG (EIA [2]), RNA (Nested RT-PCR)	IgG 28/192 (15%), RNA 20/192 (10%)	-	Exposure to HEV during hemodialysis suggested as the cause of the high prevalence	[43]

Table 1. *Cont.*

Region of Brazil	Sampling Location	Sampling Date	Population Details	Type of Samples	Hev Diagnostic Assay	Number of Positive/Total (%)	Hev Genotype	Additional Data	Reference
Southeast	São Paulo	1998–2013	Non-A-C hepatitis cases	Sera	IgM/IgG (EIA [9])	IgM (from 2006 to 2013) 27/552 (4.1%), IgG (from 1998 to 2013) 47/2.271 (2.1%)	-	The highest IgM/IgG seroprevalences were observed in latest years, namely 2011 to 2013: IgM (8.8% in 2011, 5.8% in 2012, 7.4% in 2013); IgG (5.9% in 2011, 8.6% in 2012, 6.1% in 2013)	[44]
	São Paulo	1998–2007	Renal transplant recipients	Sera	IgG (EIA [2]), RNA (Nested RT-PCR)	IgG 0/96 (0%), RNA 3/96 (3.1%)	3i	Authors claim to be the first report of HEV infection with subtype 3i in Brazil	[45]
	São Paulo	-	Blood donors	Sera	HEV-specific T-cell, RNA (RT-PCR)	T-cell response 570/33,582 (1.7%), RNA 4/29 (13.79%)	-	-	[46]
	São Paulo	-	Group I (Blood donors) A: normal ALT levels; B: high ALT levels; Group II (Women test for HIV) C: prostitutes; D: non-prostitutes; Group III (hospital employees) E; care workers; F: cleaning service workers	Sera	IgG (EIA [3])	Group I 8/205 (4%): A 5/165 (3%), B 3/40 (7.5%). Group II 38/214 (17.7%): C 3/21 (14.2%), D 35/193 (18.1%). Group III 10/170 (5.9%): E 3/117 (2.6%), F 7/53 (13.2%)	-	-	[47]

Table 1. *Cont.*

Region of Brazil	Sampling Location	Sampling Date	Population Details	Type of Samples	Hev Diagnostic Assay	Number of Positive/Total (%)	Hev Genotype	Additional Data	Reference
	São Paulo	-	Hospital settings, hemodialyzed	Sera	IgG (EIA ^{3})	Hospital settings 1/23 (4.34%), hemodialyzed 2/38 (5.26%)	-	The overall anti-HEV IgG seroprevalence was 4.9%	[48]
South	Paraná	2002–2003	Pregnant women, female blood donors	Sera	IgG (EIA ^{6}), RNA (Nested RT-PCR)	IgG: Pregnant women 40/209 (19%), female blood donors 51/199 (26%); RNA 0/408 (0%)	-	The overall IgG positivity of pregnant women and female blood donors was 22.5%. No significant difference (p= 0.11) in the HEV seroprevalence was observed between the two groups	[49]
	Paraná	1999	Blood donors	Sera	IgG (EIA ^{3})	23/996 (2.3%)	-	-	[50]
	Paraná	-	Young patient with neurological disorders	Sera	IgM/IgG, RNA (Nested RT-PCR)	IgM (+), IgG (+), RNA (+)	3	Case report about young patient with severe chronic hepatitis and presenting Epstein-Barr virus (EBV) in their cerebrospinal fluid	[51]
	Rio Grande do Sul	2015	Blood donors	Sera	IgG (EIA ^{8b})	314/780 (40.25%)	-	An *in house* ELISA with 91.4% sensitivity and 95.9% specificity was developed and used	[52]
	Rio Grande do Sul	2012–2015	Blood donors, HIV positive	Sera	IgM/IgG (EIA ^{2} + immunoblot ^{4}), RNA (RT-qPCR)	Blood donors: IgM 1/281 (0.35%), IgG 20/281 (7.1%), RNA 1/281 (0.35%); HIV positive: IgM 3/360 (0.83%), IgG 24/360 (6.7%), RNA 8/360 (2.23%)	3	The RNA load ranged from 2500–4000 copies/mL	[53]

Table 1. *Cont.*

Region of Brazil	Sampling Location	Sampling Date	Population Details	Type of Samples	Hev Diagnostic Assay	Number of Positive/Total (%)	Hev Genotype	Additional Data	Reference
	Santa Catarina	2014	Blood donors	Sera	IgM/IgG (EIA [6]), RNA (RT-qPCR)	IgM 1/300 (0.33%), IgG 30/300 (10%), RNA 0/300 (0%)	-	-	[54]
Brazil (nationwide)		2014–2018	Viral hepatitis cases	Sera	HEV assays not defined	0/216,397 (0%)	-	Data compiled from official national notifications	[55]
		2010–2012	Children with acute flaccid paralysis or Guillain-Barré syndrome	Stools	RNA (RT-qPCR)	0/325 (0%)	-	HEV infection could not be associated with the neurological disorders	[56]

[1] bioELISA® HEV IgG/IgM (Biokit™, Barcelona, Spain); [2] *recom*Well® HEV IgM/*recom*Well® HEV IgG (Mikrogen, Diagnostik, Munich, Germany); [3] IgG Abbott Diagnostika™(Wiesbaden, Germany); [4] *recom*Line® HEV IgG/IgM (Mikrogen, Diagnostik, Munich, Germany); [5] GLD HEV (Genelabs Diagnostics®, Singapore, Singapore); [6] Wantai™ HEV-IgG ELISA kit (Wantai Biological, Beijing, China); [7] MPD® HEV ELISA (MP Diagnostics™, MP Biomedicals, CA, USA); [8] in-house: [a] two HEV recombinant proteins, a mosaic protein (MP-II) and a protein containing region 452–617 aa of the ORF2 of the HEV Burma strain were used as coating antigens; [b] ORF2 recombinant protein was used as coating antigen; [9] Hepatitis E Virus (HEV) Antibody (IgG) Quest Diagnostics® (New York, NY, USA);

Table 2. HEV in swine and animal products, Brazil.

Region of Brazil	Sampling Location	Sampling Date	Animal & Production Details	Type of Samples	HEV Diagnostic Assay	Number of Positive Samples/Total Tested (%)	HEV Genotype	Additional Data	References
HEV in swine									
North	Pará	2010	Slaughtered (6 months old)	Sera, livers, stools	IgM/IgG (ELISA [1] + immunoblot [2], RNA (Nested RT-PCR)	IgM 0/151 (0%), IgG 13/151 (8.6%); RNA: serum 4/151 (2.64%), livers 6/151 (3.97%), stools 12/151 (7.94%)	3c, 3f	The global rate of HEV infection was 9.9%. Coinfection with two subtypes was observed in one pig	[57]
Northeast	Pernambuco	2017	From intensive/semi-intensive herd systems (2–6 months old)	Stools	RNA (RT-PCR)	2/119 (1.7%)	3f	-	[58]

Table 2. *Cont.*

Region of Brazil	Sampling Location	Sampling Date	Animal & Production Details	Type of Samples	HEV Diagnostic Assay	Number of Positive Samples/Total Tested (%)	HEV Genotype	Additional Data	References
Northeast	Pernambuco	-	Slaughtered, intensive/semi-intensive herd systems	Sera	IgG (EIA [3])	Slaughtered 78/96 (81.3%), herds 188/229 (82.1%)	-	Not performing disinfection (after cleaning) and mixed drinking water (stagnant and running) were risk factors for IgG prevalence while semi-intensive production system had a protective effect	[59]
Midwest	Federal District	2014	Young (6–10 months old) and adults (11–48 months old) from 234 family herds	Sera	IgG (EIA [3])	Young 85/122 (69.7%), adults 219/327 (67.0%)	-	No difference was observed in IgG seropositivity by gender or age	[60]
	Mato Grosso	2015	Family-scale herds	Sera, stools	RNA (Nested RT-PCR)	Sera 0/150 (0%), stools 12/150 (8%)	3d, 3i, 3h	From the 15 herds tested, 8 (53.3%) had pigs infected with HEV	[61]
	Mato Grosso	-	Large and family scale herds	Livers, gallbladder, small & large intestines, bile, stools	HEV antigen (Immunohisto-chemistry with polyclonal primary antibody-4), RNA (Nested RT-PCR)	Large-scale herds/RNA and HEV antigen: livers 0/25 (0%), bile 0/25 (0%), stools 0/25 (0%). Family scale/RNA: livers 6/25 (24%), bile 7/25 (28%), stools 6/25 (24%).	3b, 3f	HEV was not detected in pigs from large-scale farms, only in family herds	[62]

Table 2. *Cont.*

Region of Brazil	Sampling Location	Sampling Date	Animal & Production Details	Type of Samples	HEV Diagnostic Assay	Number of Positive Samples/Total Tested (%)	HEV Genotype	Additional Data	References
Midwest						Family scale/HEV antigen: livers 1/25 (0.25%), small intestine 7/25 (28%), large intestine 4/25 (16%)			
	Mato Grosso	-	Piglets (from IgG positive sows)	Sera	IgG (EIA[5a])	8/47 (17%)	3	Piglets were monitored after weaning and seroconversion (due to natural infection) was observed in 17% of 6–8 weeks old. Genotyping was performed in a stool pool (from piglets 10–12 weeks old)	[63]
	Mato Grosso	2002–2003	Slaughtered (28 weeks old)	Sera	IgG (EIA [5a])	211/260 (81.2%)	-	-	[64]
Southeast	Minas Gerais	2012	Slaughtered	Bile	RNA (RT-qPCR)	51/335 (15.2%)	3c, 3i	Authors suggest intragenotype HEV recombination	[65]
	Rio de Janeiro	2008	Slaughtered	Bile	RNA (RT-qPCR)	11/115 (9.6%)	3b	Viral loads varied from 10^1–10^5 copies/mL	[66]
	Rio de Janeiro	-	Piglets (from IgG positive sows)	Sera	IgM/IgG (EIA [5a]), RNA (Nested RT-PCR)	Sera (16 weeks old): IgM 1/26 (3.84%), IgG 0/26 (0%); sera (22 weeks old): IgM 0/26 (0%), IgG 23/26 (88.4%); sera (13 weeks old): RNA 8/26 (30.76%)	3	Piglets were monitored after weaning and seroconversion (due to natural infection) was observed in 88.4% of 22 weeks old.	

Table 2. *Cont.*

Region of Brazil	Sampling Location	Sampling Date	Animal & Production Details	Type of Samples	HEV Diagnostic Assay	Number of Positive Samples/Total Tested (%)	HEV Genotype	Additional Data	References
Southeast								Transferred antibodies from colostrum were observed in 92.3% piglets, decreasing weekly until 16 week-old	[63]
	Rio de Janeiro	-	Two large herds, A and B (age range 1 to >25 weeks old in B)	Sera	IgG (EIA [5a])	Herd A 17/70 (24.3%), herd B 227/357 (63.7%)	-	-	[11]
	São Paulo	-	Young (40–60 days old)	Stools	RNA (RT-PCR)	7/8 (87.5%)	3	-	[67]
South	Paraná	2014	Family scale herds (22 weeks old)	Stools	RNA (Nested RT-PCR/RT-qPCR)	34/170 (20%)	3b	Among the 34 positive samples, only 4 (11.8%) presented viral loads higher than 10^3 copies/mL	[68]
	Paraná	2010	Slaughtered	Liver, bile	RNA (Nested RT-PCR)	Liver 2/118 (1.7%), bile 1/118 (0.84%)	3b	-	[69]
	Paraná	2009	Herds with animals of different ages	Stools	RNA (Nested RT-PCR)	1–4-week-old 2/25 (8%), 5–8 weeks old 1/33 (3%), 9–24 weeks old 26/170 (15.3%), >1-year-old 3/99 (3%)	3b	-	[70]
	Rio Grande do Sul	2012–2014	Family-scale herds	Sera	IgG (EIA [5b]), RNA (Nested RT-PCR)	IgG (2012) 567/731 (77.6%), IgG (2014) 467/713 (65.5%), RNA (2014) 6/713 (0.8%)	3b, 3c, 3h	-	[71]

Table 2. *Cont.*

Region of Brazil	Sampling Location	Sampling Date	Animal & Production Details	Type of Samples	HEV Diagnostic Assay	Number of Positive Samples/Total Tested (%)	HEV Genotype	Additional Data	References
South	Rio Grande do Sul	-	Large-scale herds	Stools	RNA (Nested RT-PCR)	8/9 (88.9%)	3b	-	[72]
	Rio Grande do Sul	2012–2016	Family scale pig herds and wild boars	Sera	Antibodies (EIA [3])	Pigs 139/261 (53.26%), wild boar 8/56 (14.29%)	-	This study shows pigs from family scale can play a more important role as a HEV reservoirs than wild boars ($p < 0.001$)	[73]
	Santa Catarina	2017–2018	Wild boars	Sera	Antibodies (EIA [3])	8/61 (13.1%)	-	-	[74]
	Santa Catarina	2012–2016	Family scale pig herds and wild boars	Sera	Antibodies (EIA [3])	Pigs 39/121 (32.23%), wild boar 3/193 (1.55%)	-	This study shows pigs from family scale can play a more important role as a HEV reservoirs than wild boars ($p < 0.001$)	[73]
HEV in animal products									
South	Rio Grande do Sul	2015–2016	Edible products of animal origin	Bovine, swine, chicken and capybara raw meats, processed meats (mortadella, sausage, salami, ham, pâté)	RNA (Nested RT-PCR)	Bovine 0/57 (0%), swine 0/30 (0%), chicken 0/29 (0%), capybara 0/1 (0%), mortadella 0/8 (0%), sausage 0/12 (0%), salami 0/14 (0%), ham 0/4 (0%), pâté 0/4 (0%)	-	-	[75]
	Rio Grande do Sul	2015	Pork products	Pâtés, blood sausage (*morcilla*)	RNA (Nested RT-PCR)	18/50 (36%)	3	-	[76]

[1] *recom*Well® HEV IgM/ *recom*Well® HEV IgG (Mikrogen, Diagnostik, Munich, Germany); [2] *recom*Line® HEV IgG/IgM (Mikrogen, Diagnostik, Munich, Germany); [3] PrioCHECK™ AB HEV antibody ELISA kit (Thermo Fisher, Zurich, Switzerland); [4] HEV antibody (Abbiotec™, California, USA); [5] in-house: [a] two HEV recombinant proteins, a mosaic protein (MP-II) and a protein containing region 452–617 aa of the ORF2 of the HEV Burma strain used as coating antigens; [b] in-house indirect ELISA containing recombinant HEV-ORF2p antigen.

Table 3. HEV in animals other than swine, Brazil.

Region of Brazil	Sampling Location	Sampling Date	Animal Species	Type of Samples	HEV Diagnostic Assay	Number of Positive Samples/Total Tested (%)	HEV Genotype	Additional Data	Reference
Southeast	Rio de Janeiro	2012–2016	Golden-headed lion tamarin (*Leontopithecus chrysomelas*)	Stools, livers	RNA (RT-PCR)	stools 0/101 (0%), livers 0/95 (0%)	-	-	[77]
	Rio de Janeiro	-	Captive New World monkeys (*Callithrix jacchus*, *C. kuhli*, *C. asiurus*, *C. penicilata*, *C. argenta*, *Aotus* sp.), dogs, cows, sheeps, goats, chickens, wild rodents (*Nectomus* sp.)	Sera	IgG (EIA [1])	Monkeys 0/42 (0%), dogs 3/43 (6.97%), cows 1/70 (1.42%), sheeps 0/12 (0%), goats 0/5 (0%), chickens 5/25 (20%), wild rodents 2/4 (50%)	-	-	[11]
	São Paulo	2008–2013	Wild rodents (*Akodon montensis*, *Calomys tener*, *Oligoryzomys nigripes*, *Necromys asiurus*, *Mus musculus*)	Sera	RNA (RT-PCR)	*A. montensis* 0/199 (0%), *C. tener* 4/109 (3.66%), *O. nigripes* 0/63 (0%), *N. asiurus* 3/252 (1.19%), *M. musculus* 0/24 (0%)	A new orthohepevirus species was proposed	Novel strains were termed *Calomys* HEV (CaHEV) and *Necromys* HEV (NeHEV)	[78]

[1] in-house, two HEV recombinant proteins, a mosaic protein (MP-II) and a protein containing region 452–617 aa of the ORF2 of the HEV Burma strain were used as coating antigens.

Table 4. HEV in environmental samples, Brazil.

Region of Brazil	Sampling Location	Sampling Date	Matrices	Detection Method (RNA)	Number of Positive Samples/Total Tested (%)	HEV Genotype	Additional Data	References
South	Rio Grande do Sul—Vale do Taquari	2016–2017	Water	Nested RT-PCR	0/32 (0%)	-	Samples were from area that drains effluents from numerous pig farms	[79]

Table 4. *Cont.*

Region of Brazil	Sampling Location	Sampling Date	Matrices	Detection Method (RNA)	Number of Positive Samples/Total Tested (%)	HEV Genotype	Additional Data	References
South	Rio Grande do Sul—Northern coast	2016–2017	Water and bivalves (*Donax hanleyanus*)	Nested RT-PCR	Water 0/42 (0%), bivalves 0/42 (0%)	-	Samples were from recreation beaches	[80]
	Rio Grande do Sul—Sinos river	2012–2014	Water and sediment	Nested RT-PCR	Water 0/250 (0%), sediment 0/68 (0%)	-	Sampling site had poor water quality, very close to human settlements	[76]
	Rio Grande do Sul—Vale do Taquari	-	Swine slurry lagoon water	Nested RT-PCR	8/8 (100%)	3b	Samples were from one of the largest swine producers in Rio Grande do Sul and a great public initiative for decontamination of water bodies was initiated at the time of this study	[72]
Southeast	Rio de Janeiro—North and hill region	2008	Swine slaughterhouse effluent	RT-qPCR	3/6 (50%)	3b	RNA was found with mean viral load of 10^2 genome copies/mL in effluent	[66]

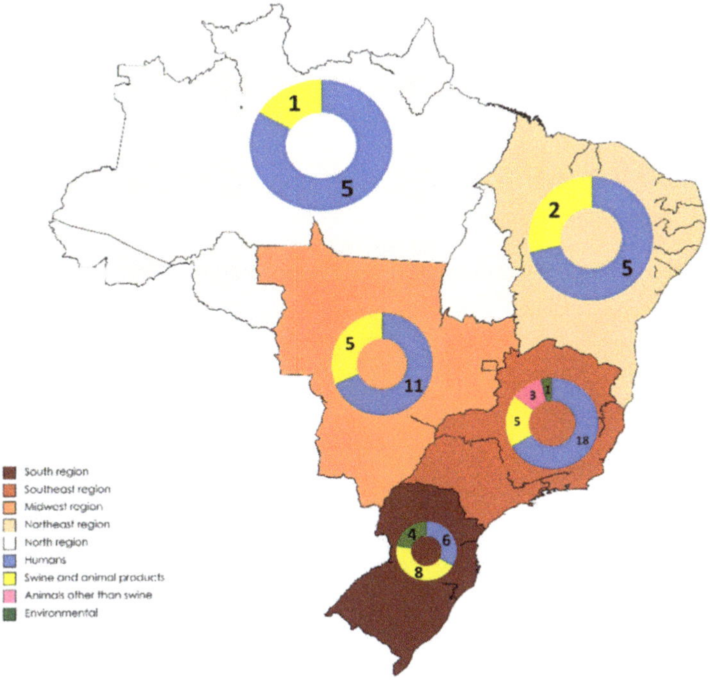

Figure 2. Distribution (number) of HEV studies according to the regions of Brazil and the origin (human, swine and animal products, animals other than swine, and environmental).

3.1. HEV in Humans

HEV studies performed in humans in Brazil (Table 1) were focused on a variety of population groups and most were serological surveys.

Studies performed in populations from regions with lower sanitation and hygiene conditions in the North region found an anti-HEV IgG seroprevalence of 0.3% in afro descendants [14]. Studies done in poor communities in the Midwest region found an anti-HEV IgG seroprevalence of 3.3% and 10.66% in adults [28,30] and 4.5% in children [27]. In the Southeast region, a seroprevalence of 2.4% was found also in poor communities [34].

Seroprevalence studies focusing on rural settlements (Table 1) found anti-HEV IgG seroprevalences of 12.9% in the North [11], 3.4% [25], 3.9% [23], and 8.4% [26] in the Midwest, and 2.1% [35] and 20.7% [41] in the Southeast. Three of these studies performed in rural settlements were also focused on current and/or recent infections. The study of the Midwest region found 0% of anti-HEV IgM and HEV RNA [25] and the study of the North found 0.3% of anti-HEV IgM [14].

Several investigations were conducted in HIV patients from Brazil and found anti-HEV IgG seroprevalence of 4.1% [19] in the North, 0% [32], 6.7% [53] and 10.7% [42] in the Southeast. Anti-HEV IgM and HEV RNA in HIV patients was searched only in the Southeast region and found anti-HEV IgM in 0% [32], 0.83% [53], and 1.4% [42], while HEV RNA was detected in 2.23% [53] and 3.6% [32].

HEV studies in Brazil have also focused on transplant recipients (Table 1). Among those with kidney transplants, anti-HEV IgG seroprevalence was found to be of 2.5% [21] in the Midwest, and 3.1% [45] and 15% [43] in the Southeast. HEV RNA was found in 3.1% [45] and 10% [43] of kidney transplant recipients. Only two studies investigated HEV infection in liver transplant recipients, namely a case report in a pediatric patient [40] and a study in the Southeast region that found a seroprevalence of anti-HEV IgG and IgM of 8.1% and 2.6%, respectively [39].

Several investigations in Brazil were conducted in healthy blood donors and pregnant women (Table 1). Anti-HEV IgG seroprevalence in blood donors was found to be 0.45% [13] in the North, 2% [18] in the Northeast, 4% [26] in the Midwest, 4% [47], 4.3% [35] and 9.8% [37] in the Southeast, and 2.3% [50], 7.1% [53], 10% [54], 26% [49], and 40.25% [52] in the South. Of these studies, three also investigated current and/or recent infections by detecting anti-HEV IgM/HEV RNA, having found 0.33% and 0% [54], and 0.35% and 0.35% [53] respectiely, in the South. In the study of Southeast, anti-HEV IgM/RNA was 2.4% and 0%, but only IgG positive samples were tested [37].

Seroprevalence studies were also conducted in populations with occupational, exposure risk to HEV infection. In hospital employees anti-HEV IgG seroprevalences of 4.34% [48] and 5.9% [47] were found, while in recyclable waste pickers [24] and pig handlers [11] seroprevalences were 5.1% and 6.3%, respectively.

Molecular characterization of the HEV strains detected in humans in Brazil showed that all belonged to HEV-3 [32,33,40,45,53]. Further characterization of some of the strains identified subtypes 3b [33,40] and 3i [45].

3.2. HEV in Swine and in Animal Products

All studies performed in swine (Table 2) found evidence of HEV infection, either by using the detection of anti-HEV IgG and/or HEV RNA. Seroprevalence studies in younger pigs (<10 months) found an anti-HEV IgG prevalence of 8.6% in North region of Brazil [57] and 69.7% in the Midwest region [60]. The detection of HEV RNA in stools in this age group was 1.7% in the Northeast region [58] 7.94% in the North region [57] and 87.5% in Southwest [67].

In pigs from family-scale the anti-HEV IgG prevalence was 0% [61] and 67% [60] in the Midwest region, and 77.6% in the South region [71]. Regarding the detection of HEV RNA in stools of pigs from family-scale farms, 8% [61] and 24% [62] were found positive in the Midwest region, and 20% [68] in the South region.

Seroprevalence studies on slaughtered pigs showed anti-HEV IgG in 81.2% in Midwest [64] and 81.3% in the Northeast [59]. The detection of HEV RNA in bile from slaughtered pigs showed to be positive in 9.6% [66] and 15.2% [65] in Southeast and 0.84% in South [69].

The molecular characterization of the HEV found in pigs showed several subtypes (Table 2), namely 3b [62,66,68–72] 3c [57,65,71], 3d [61], 3f [57,58,62], 3h [61,71], and 3i [61,65].

Concerning wild boar, only two HEV seroprevalence studies were performed, both in the South region, having found a seroprevalence of 14.29% in Rio Grande do Sul state [73] while in Santa Catarina state, 1.55% [73] and 13.1% [74] seroprevalences were observed.

Regarding the HEV contamination of meat and meat products derived from swine and other animals (Table 2), HEV RNA was detected in 36% of the pig pâtés and blood sausages (morcilla) derived from pork [76]. In another study, no HEV was detected either in pig processed meats such as mortadella, sausage, salami, ham, and pate, or in the raw meat of bovine, swine, chicken, and capybara [75].

3.3. HEV in Animals Other Than Swine

None of the studies performed in free-living monkeys has found evidence of HEV infection, either by using the detection of anti-HEV IgG [11] or HEV RNA [77] (Table 3). Anti-HEV IgG was detected in cows (1.42%), dogs (6.97%), chickens (20%), and wild rodents (50%), but not in sheep and goats [11]. Two new viruses were detected in wild rodents, *Calomys* HEV (CaHEV) and *Necromys* HEV (NeHEV), and a new orthohepevirus species was proposed [78] (Table 3).

3.4. HEV in Environment

The detection of HEV RNA in waters (bathing/recreation waters, pig farm draining waters, settlement influenced waters), bivalve molluscs, and sediments was negative [55,76,79] (Table 4). In the two studies performed on pig slurry lagoons, HEV RNA was detected in 50% [66] and 100% [72] of the samples.

4. Discussion

The HEV studies in humans in Brazil started in the early 90s. The majority of these initial investigations were conducted in rural areas, possibly motivated by the HEV-1 and HEV-2 data from endemic regions in developing countries with similar poor sanitary conditions. The first HEV reports in Brazil focused on communities with low levels of sanitation, such as gold miners [29] and poor communities [28,30] from the Amazon area of the Midwest region, and from the Southeast region [34]. In these reports, the fecally contaminated water was pointed as a potential route of HEV transmission and the seroprevalences within these communities ranged from 0.45% in children to 10.66% in adults [27,28].

After the recognition of HEV-3 as being responsible for autochthonous hepatitis E in industrialized countries [81,82], HEV studies in Brazil started to focus on cases of acute non-A-C viral hepatitis in order to clarify the potential role of HEV in these undiagnosed cases [17,28,35], efforts that still motivate publications nowadays [15,36]. In general, markers of current and/or recent HEV infection (anti-IgM HEV and HEV RNA) have been detected but at a low prevalence, indicating that HEV was not the causal agent of the majority of these acute hepatitis cases.

Based on the knowledge that HEV-3 infection may progress to a chronic hepatitis in immunocompromised patients [3], some HEV studies in Brazil have focused on organ transplant recipients [39] and HIV patients [42]. In kidney transplants, HEV seroprevalence varied from infrequent (2.5%) [21] to frequent (15%) [43]. In liver transplant recipients the prevalence of anti-HEV antibodies showed to be higher than immunocompetent populations in Brazil, suggesting HEV infection as a possible cause of liver injury [39]. Concerning HIV patients, studies showed similar HEV seroprevalences when compared with blood donors indicating that HIV patients are not at risk for HEV infection [19,53].

Hepatitis E caused by HEV-1 and HEV-2 has been associated with morbidity and mortality in pregnant women [3]. Possibly motivated by this, some HEV seroprevalence studies have been performed in pregnant women in Brazil, however no risk for HEV seropositivity has been shown in this particular group when compared with the general population [13,35,49].

Several studies have evaluated the HEV seroprevalence in the general population of Brazil, with the majority using blood donors as the sampled group. A great range of HEV seroprevalence was observed, with the lowest detected in the North (0.45%) [13] and Northeast regions (2%) [18]. Mid-range levels of HEV seroprevalence were observed in the Midwest (4%) and Southeast (4%, 9.8%) regions [26,37,47]. In the South region, the five seroprevalence studies showed values of 2.3% [50], 7.1% [53], 10% [54], 26% [49], and 40.25% [52]. The high seroprevalence detected in the South has been justified for being the region in Brazil with the highest density of pig farms and the largest consumption of pig meat and related products [52]. In fact, pig breeding has been suggested to influence human HEV seroprevalence in other countries [83,84]. Epidemiologic surveys performed in rural population of Brazil, namely in the North [11] and in the Southeast regions, have found higher seroprevalences in these populations (12.9% and 20.7%, respectively) when compared to those previously reported on blood donors from the same regions [11,41]. This difference has been attributed to the lower sanitary conditions of the rural populations. Overall, the range of seroprevalences observed in Brazil has to be interpreted with caution since some studies were performed several decades apart and using different immunoassays. It is widely known that the different anti-HEV IgG immunoassays and their performance characteristics strongly influence HEV seroprevalence data [85].

Despite the strong evidence of widespread HEV circulation in Brazil, the recent report of the official governmental databases presented no notification of hepatitis E among the notified 216,379 hepatitis cases [86]. This draws attention to an underdiagnosis and/or underreporting of hepatitis E in Brazil. The underdiagnosing of hepatitis E cases has been reported elsewhere and is partly attributed to the fact that HEV testing has not been traditionally included in hepatitis differential diagnostic algorithms [87].

Many HEV studies in Brazil have focused on swine, which is understandable given the fact that this country is the 4th largest pig producer in the world, with more than 2 million breeders and producing 3975 thousand tons/year of pork meat, with the South region representing 66.12% of the national production [88]. Circulation of HEV in pigs of Brazil was observed either in large or family-scale herds, and in all age groups, based on HEV RNA presence in stools/biological fluids/organs (0.8–88.9%) or anti-HEV IgG seroprevalence (0–77.6%) [61,62,68,72]. Evidence for HEV infection in slaughtered pigs was also shown by the high seroprevalence (>80%) detected [59,64]. The circulation of HEV was also demonstrated in wild boars of Brazil with seroprevalences ranging from 1.55% to 14.29% [73,74]. HEV was inclusively found in pig pâtés and blood sausages derived from pork [76]. Overall, HEV is highly disseminated in the swine population throughout Brazil and might present a risk to animal handlers and pork consumers, mainly if pork meat and meat products are eaten raw or undercooked. The presence of HEV in pigs and derived pig products has been widely reported in other countries [84,88–90].

In the past years there has been an interest in studying HEV infection in non-human primates, inclusively *Macaca fascicularis* were used on experimental in vivo studies performed in Brazil to evaluate HEV pathogenesis [91–93]. HEV seroprevalences have been reported in farmed *Rhesus* monkeys in China (70.8%) [94] and in captive non-human primates in Italy (4.2%) [95] but the only seroprevalence study performed in Brazil in wild non-human primates did not detect any (0%) anti-HEV antibodies [11]. Furthermore, no HEV RNA was detected in the stools and livers of Golden-headed lion tamarins of Brazil [77].

Serological studies in Brazil also focused on other animals, having reported the presence of antibodies anti-HEV in cows, dogs, chicken, and wild rodents, but not in sheep and goats [11]. Antibodies against HEV have also been detected in dogs in the United Kingdom [96], in chicken, cows, wild rodents, sheep, and goats in China [97–100], chickens in Korea [101], sheep in Italy [102], but the zoonotic importance of these animals concerning HEV remain to be clarified. Noteworthy, two novel HEV strains were discovered in wild rodents from Brazil (*Calomys tener* and *Necromys asiurus*) [78].

Concerning the HEV studies that focused on the environment in Brazil, only water samples under the influence of swine farm effluents, namely slurry lagoons, were found positive for HEV [66,72]. Samples from the southern region of Brazil, with a high density of swine production, detected HEV in up to 100% of the samples analyzed [72]. This same region coincides with the highest rates of human seropositivity for HEV and is also the region with the highest concentration of pig production in the country. This fact, analyzed from the One Health perspective, highlights the zoonotic character of this virus. Swine-influenced waters contaminated by HEV have been frequently detected and reported in other countries [103,104]. In the studies of Brazil, HEV was not detected in bivalve molluscs, recreation waters, or even in waters that drained effluents from pig farms or waters of poor quality, very close to human settlements [76,79,80]. However, studies in other countries have reported HEV in bivalve molluscs [105–107], seawater [108], and wastewater [109,110]. These discrepancies of detection of HEV in environment samples could be in part due to the low concentration of HEV and complexity of the matrices, two well-known limiting factors of the detection of enteric viruses in environmental samples.

Concerning the molecular characterization of HEV strains detected in Brazil, studies showed that all HEVs found in Brazil were classified as HEV-3 (6 studies in humans, 15 in swine and animal products, and 2 on environmental samples). HEV-3 is known to have a zoonotic (swine) origin and the subtypes 3b and 3i were detected in humans [33,40,45] and pigs [61,62,65,66,68–72], while the subtypes 3c [57,65,71], subtype 3d [61], subtype 3f [57,58,62] and subtypes 3h [61,71] have been only detected in pigs. As molecular studies have been performed using several molecular assays and primer choices, different regions of HEV have been targeted and characterized. This clearly hampers the robust classification of HEV subtypes and, consequently, a solid comparison between subtypes, hence caution must be taken when analyzing this data. In fact, attention should be paid to several factors that could bias the interpretation of results here presented. A clear focus has been given to human samples with little attention to animal or environmental matrices, most likely due to the initial understanding of this disease, not known to be zoonotic at that time. Additionally, not only a higher number of studies have also focused on the South where the highest density of pig farms is present but also a vast diversity of sample sizes has been used throughout the studies, making it difficult to robustly compare results. Further studies spatially dispersed are for these reasons recommended.

The present systematic review is not the first that targets HEV in Brazil. The two published so far have centered only on human infection [111,112] while here we present for the first time a perspective focusing on the One Health triad, having included HEV studies on humans, animals, and environment. A One Health approach makes it possible to look at issues such as zoonotic diseases, food safety, and food security, as well as environmental contamination and other aspects. In this perspective this review evidenced that the scientific community has approached the topic of HEV on every aspect of environment, human, and animal systems individually, however when compiled, this translates into data that broadens the scope to One Health.

5. Conclusions

Overall, this systematic review shows that HEV-3 was the only retrieved genotype in humans, animals, and environment in Brazil. The South region showed the highest HEV seroprevalence in humans, which curiously is also the region with the highest pig density, swine industry, and pig HEV circulation, suggesting a zoonotic link. HEV- 1 and HEV-2 were not detected in any of the studies performed in Brazil, even in those focusing on low sanitary condition communities. This allowed us to infer that HEV epidemiology in Brazil is similar to that of industrialized countries (only HEV-3 circulation, swine reservoirs, no waterborne transmission, no association with low sanitary conditions). Hence, we alert for the implementation of HEV surveillance systems in swine and for the inclusion of HEV in the diagnostic routine of acute and chronic hepatitis in humans. More sequence data are needed on HEV strains circulating in humans, animals, and the environment to further evidence the zoonotic origin of HEV infection in Brazil.

Author Contributions: D.F.d.S.D.M.: Conceptualization, data curation and investigation (search of articles in electronic databases and their respective cataloguing), formal analysis, methodology, and writing original draft preparation; J.R.M.: Conceptualization, data curation and investigation (search of articles in electronic databases and their respective cataloguing), review of the writing and substance of this article, supervision, and validation; V.D.: Conceptualization, methodology, revised this paper, supervision, and validation; M.S.J.N.: Conceptualization, data curation and investigation, wrote full text and revised the article improving the technical quality of the manuscript, supervision, and validation. All authors have read and agreed to the published version of the manuscript.

Funding: This research received no external funding.

Institutional Review Board Statement: Not applicable.

Data Availability Statement: Not applicable.

Conflicts of Interest: The authors declare that they have no conflict of interest.

References

1. Lewis, H.C.; Wichmann, O.; Duizer, E. Transmission routes and risk factors for autochthonous hepatitis E virus infection in Europe: A systematic review. *Epidemiol. Infect.* **2010**, *138*, 145–166. [CrossRef]
2. Kamar, N.; Dalton, H.R.; Abravanel, F.; Izopet, J. Hepatitis E Virus Infection. *Clin. Microbiol. Rev.* **2014**, *27*, 116–138. [CrossRef]
3. Wang, B.; Meng, X.-J. Hepatitis E virus: Host tropism and zoonotic infection. *Curr. Opin. Microbiol.* **2021**, *59*, 8–15. [CrossRef] [PubMed]

4. Meng, X.J.; Purcell, R.H.; Halbur, P.G.; Lehman, J.R.; Webb, D.M.; Tsareva, T.S.; Haynes, J.S.; Thacker, B.J.; Emerson, S.U. A novel virus in swine is closely related to the human hepatitis E virus. *Proc. Natl. Acad. Sci. USA* **1997**, *94*, 9860–9865. [CrossRef] [PubMed]
5. Lee, G.H.; Tan, B.H.; Teo, E.C.; Lim, S.G.; Dan, Y.Y.; Wee, A.; Aw, P.P.; Zhu, Y.; Hibberd, M.L.; Tan, C.K.; et al. Chronic infection with camelid hepatitis E virus in a liver transplant recipient who regularly consumes camel meat and milk. *Gastroenterology* **2016**, *150*, 355–357. [CrossRef]
6. Smith, D.B.; Simmonds, P.; Izopet, J.; Oliveira-Filho, E.F.; Ulrich, R.G.; Johne, R.; Koenig, M.; Jameel, S.; Harrison, T.J.; Meng, X.J.; et al. Proposed reference sequences for hepatitis E virus subtypes. *J. Gen. Virol.* **2016**, *97*, 537–542. [CrossRef] [PubMed]
7. Embrapa. Estatística e Desempenho da Produção Nacional. Available online: https://www.embrapa.br/suinos-e-aves/cias/estatisticas (accessed on 17 July 2020).
8. Cidades, Instituto Brasileiro de Geografia e Estatística. Available online: https://cidades.ibge.gov.br/ (accessed on 16 July 2020).
9. Souza, P.F.; Xavier, D.R.; Suarez Mutis, M.C.; da Mota, J.C.; Peiter, P.C.; de Matos, V.P.; Magalhães, M.; Barcellos, C. Spatial spread of malaria and economic frontier expansion in the Brazilian Amazon. *PLoS ONE* **2019**, *14*, e0217615. [CrossRef] [PubMed]
10. Liberati, A.; Altman, D.G.; Tetzlaff, J.; Mulrow, C.; Gotzsche, P.C.; Ioannidis, J.P.; Clarke, M.; Devereaux, P.J.; Kleijnen, J.; Moher, D. The PRISMA statement for reporting systematic reviews and meta-analyses of studies that evaluate health care interventions: Explanation and elaboration. *PLoS Med.* **2009**, *6*, 1–35. [CrossRef]
11. Vitral, C.L.; Silva-Nunes, M.; Pinto, M.A.; Oliveira, J.M.; Gaspar, A.M.; Pereira, R.C.; Ferreira, M.U. Hepatitis A and E seroprevalence and associated risk factors: A community-based cross-sectional survey in rural Amazonia. *BMC Infect. Dis.* **2014**, *14*, 458. [CrossRef]
12. Paula, V.S.; Arruda, M.E.; Vitral, C.L.; Gaspar, A.M.C. Seroprevalence of viral hepatitis in riverine communities from the western region of the brazilian amazon basin. *Memórias Inst. Oswaldo Cruz* **2001**, *96*, 1123–1128. [CrossRef] [PubMed]
13. Kiesslich, D.; Júnior, J.E.R.; Crispim, M.A. Prevalence of hepatitis E virus antibodies among different groups in the Amazonian basin. *R. Soc. Trop. Med. Hyg. Trans.* **2002**, *96*, 215. [CrossRef]
14. Souza, A.J.S.; Oliveira, C.M.A.; Sarmento, V.P.; Chagas, A.; Nonato, N.S.; Brito, D.C.N.; Barbosa, K.M.V.; Soares, M.; Nunes, H.M. Hepatitis E virus infection among rural Afro-descendant communities from the eastern Brazilian Amazon. *Rev. Soc. Bras. Med. Trop.* **2018**, *51*, 803–807. [CrossRef] [PubMed]
15. Souza, A.J.S.; Malheiros, A.P.; Sarmento, V.P.; Resende, F.S.; Alves, M.M.; Nunes, H.M.; Soares, M.C.P.; Sa, L.R.M. Serological and molecular retrospective analysis of hepatitis E suspected cases from the Eastern Brazilian Amazon 1993–2014. *Rev. Soc. Bras. Med. Trop.* **2019**, *52*, 1–4. [CrossRef]
16. Lyra, A.C.; Pinho, J.R.; Silva, L.K.; Sousa, L.; Saraceni, C.P.; Braga, E.L.; Pereira, J.E.; Zarife, M.A.; Reis, M.G.; Lyra, L.G.; et al. HEV, TTV and GBV-C/HGV markers in patients with acute viral hepatitis. *Braz. J. Med. Biol. Res.* **2005**, *38*, 767–775. [CrossRef] [PubMed]
17. Paraná, R.; Vitvitski, L.; Andrade, Z.; Trepo, C.; Cotrim, H.; Bertillon, P.; Silva, F.; Silva, L.; Oliveira, I.R.; Lyra, L. Acute sporadic non-A, non-B hepatitis in Northeastern Brazil: Etiology and natural history. *Hepatology* **1999**, *30*, 289–293. [CrossRef]
18. Paraná, R.; Cotrim, H.P.; Cortey-Boennec, M.L.; Trepo, C.; Lyra, L. Prevalence of hepatitis E virus IgG antibodies in patients from a referral unit of liver diseases in Salvador, Bahia, Brazil. *Am. J. Trop. Med. Hyg.* **1997**, *57*, 60–61. [CrossRef]
19. Bezerra, L.A.; Oliveira-Filho, E.F.; Júnior, J.V.J.S.; Morais, V.M.S.; Gonçales, J.P.; Silva, D.M.; Coêlho, M.R.C.D. Risk analysis and seroprevalence of HEV in people living with HIV/AIDS in Brazil. *Acta Trop.* **2019**, *189*, 65–68. [CrossRef]
20. Passos-Castilho, A.M.; Sena, A.; Domingues, A.L.C.; Lopes-Neto, E.P.; Medeiro, T.B.; Granato, C.F.H.; Ferraz, M.L. Hepatitis E virus seroprevalence among schistosomiasis patients in Northeastern Brazil. *Braz. J. Infect. Dis.* **2016**, *20*, 262–266. [CrossRef] [PubMed]
21. Oliveira, J.; Freitas, N.R.; Teles, S.A.; Bottino, F.O.; Lemos, A.S.; Oliveira, J.M.; Paula, V.; Pinto, M.A.; Martins, R.M.B. Prevalence of hepatitis E virus RNA and antibodies in a cohort of kidney transplant recipients in Central Brazil. *Int. J. Infect. Dis.* **2018**, *69*, 41–43. [CrossRef]
22. Freitas, N.R.; Santana, E.B.; Silva, A.M.; Silva, S.M.; Teles, S.A.; Gardinali, N.R.; Pinto, M.A.; Martins, R.M. Hepatitis E virus infection in patients with acute non-A, non-B, non-C hepatitis in Central Brazil. *Memórias Inst. Oswaldo Cruz* **2016**, *111*, 692–696. [CrossRef]
23. Caetano, K.A.A.; Bergamaschi, F.P.R.; Carneiro, M.A.S.; Pinheiro, R.S.; Araujo, L.A.; Matos, M.A.; Carvalho, P.M.R.S.; Souza, M.M.; Matos, M.A.; Del-Rios, N.H.A.; et al. Hepatotropic viruses (hepatitis A, B, C, D and E) in a rural Brazilian population: Prevalence, genotypes, risk factors and vaccination. *Trans. R. Soc. Trop. Med. Hyg.* **2019**, *114*, 91–98. [CrossRef]
24. Martins, R.M.; Freitas, N.R.; Kozlowski, A.; Reis, N.R.; Lopes, C.L.; Teles, S.A.; Gardinali, N.R.; Pinto, M.A. Seroprevalence of hepatitis E antibodies in a population of recyclable waste pickers in Brazil. *J. Clin. Virol.* **2014**, *59*, 188–191. [CrossRef]
25. Freitas, N.R.; Caetano, K.A.A.; Teles, S.A.; Matos, M.A.; Carneiro, M.A.S.; Gardinali, N.R.; Pinto, M.A.; Martins, R.M.B. Hepatitis E seroprevalence and associated factors in rural settlers in Central Brazil. *Rev. Soc. Bras. Med. Trop.* **2017**, *50*, 675–679. [CrossRef]
26. Silva, S.M.; Oliveira, J.M.; Vitral, C.L.; de Almeida Vieira, K.; Pinto, M.A.; Souto, F.J. Prevalence of hepatitis E virus antibodies in individuals exposed to swine in Mato Grosso, Brazil. *Memórias Inst. Oswaldo Cruz* **2012**, *107*, 338–341. [CrossRef] [PubMed]
27. Assis, S.B.; Souto, F.J.; Fontes, C.J.; Gaspar, A.M. Prevalence of hepatitis A and E virus infection in school children of an Amazonian municipality in Mato Grosso State. *Rev. Soc. Bras. Med. Trop.* **2002**, *35*, 155–158. [CrossRef] [PubMed]

28. Souto, F.J.; Fontes, C.J.; Parana, R.; Lyra, L.G. Short report: Further evidence for hepatitis E in the Brazilian Amazon. *Am. J. Trop. Med. Hyg.* **1997**, *57*, 149–150. [CrossRef] [PubMed]
29. Pang, L.; Alencar, F.E.; Cerutti, C.; Milhous, W.K.; Andrade, A.L.; Oliveira, R.; Kanesa-Thasan, N.; MaCarthy, P.O.; Hoke, C.H. Short report: Hepatitis E infection in the Brazilian Amazon. *Am. J. Trop. Med. Hyg.* **1995**, *52*, 347–348. [CrossRef]
30. Souto, F.J.; Fontes, C.J. Prevalence of IgG-class antibodies against hepatitis E virus in a community of the southern Amazon: A randomized survey. *Ann. Trop. Med. Parasitol.* **1998**, *92*, 623–625. [CrossRef]
31. Castro, V.O.L.; Tejada-Strop, A.; Weis, S.M.S.; Stabile, A.C.; Oliveira, S.; Teles, S.A.; Kamili, S.; Motta-Castro, A.R.C. Evidence of hepatitis E virus infections among persons who use crack cocaine from the Midwest region of Brazil. *J. Med. Virol.* **2019**, *91*, 151–154. [CrossRef]
32. Salvio, A.L.; Lopes, A.O.; Almeida, A.J.; Gardinali, N.R.; Lima, L.R.P.; Oliveira, J.M.; Sion, F.S.; Ribeiro, L.C.P.; Pinto, M.A.; Paula, V.S. Detection and quantification of hepatitis E virus in the absence of IgG and IgM anti-HEV in HIV-positive patients. *J. Appl. Microbiol.* **2018**, *125*, 1208–1215. [CrossRef] [PubMed]
33. Santos, D.R.L.D.; Lewis-Ximenez, L.L.; Silva, M.F.; Sousa, P.S.; Gaspar, A.M.; Pinto, M.A. First report of a human autochthonous hepatitis E virus infection in Brazil. *J. Clin. Virol.* **2010**, *47*, 276–279. [CrossRef]
34. Santos, D.C.; Souto, F.J.; Santos, D.R.; Vitral, C.L.; Gaspar, A.M. Seroepidemiological markers of enterically transmitted viral hepatitis A and E in individuals living in a community located in the North Area of Rio de Janeiro, RJ, Brazil. *Memórias Inst. Oswaldo Cruz* **2002**, *97*, 637–640. [CrossRef]
35. Trinta, K.S.; Liberto, M.I.; Paula, V.S.; Yoshida, C.F.; Gaspar, A.M. Hepatitis E virus infection in selected Brazilian populations. *Memórias Inst. Oswaldo Cruz* **2001**, *96*, 25–29. [CrossRef] [PubMed]
36. Bricks, G.; Senise, J.F.; Pott, H., Jr.; Grandi, G.; Carnaúba, D., Jr.; de Moraes, H.A.B.; Granato, C.F.H.; Castelo, A. Previous hepatitis E virus infection, cirrhosis and insulin resistance in patients with chronic hepatitis C. *Braz. J. Infect. Dis.* **2019**, *23*, 45–52. [CrossRef]
37. Passos-Castilho, A.M.; Reinaldo, M.R.; Sena, A.; Granato, C.F.H. High prevalence of hepatitis E virus antibodies in Sao Paulo, Southeastern Brazil: Analysis of a group of blood donors representative of the general population. *Braz. J. Infect. Dis.* **2017**, *21*, 535–539. [CrossRef]
38. Slavov, S.N.; Maconetto, J.D.M.; Martinez, E.Z.; Silva-Pinto, A.C.; Covas, D.T.; Eis-Hubinger, A.M.; Kashima, S. Prevalence of hepatitis E virus infection in multiple transfused Brazilian patients with thalassemia and sickle cell disease. *J. Med. Virol.* **2019**, *91*, 1693–1697. [CrossRef]
39. Gomes-Gouvêa, M.S.; Ferreira, A.C.; Feitoza, B.; Pessoa, M.G.; Abdala, E.; Terrabuio, D.R.; Moraes, A.C.; Bonazzi, P.R.; D'Albuquerque, L.C. Evidence of hepatitis E virus infection in liver transplant recipients from Brazil. *Hepatology* **2013**, *58*, 1052A.
40. Passos-Castilho, A.M.; Porta, G.; Miura, I.K.; Pugliese, R.P.; Danesi, V.L.; Porta, A.; Guimaraes, T.; Seda, J.; Antunes, E.; Granato, C.F. Chronic hepatitis E virus infection in a pediatric female liver transplant recipient. *J. Clin. Microbiol.* **2014**, *52*, 4425–4427. [CrossRef]
41. Almeida, E.A.D.; de Oliveira, J.M.; Haddad, S.K.; da Roza, D.L.; Bottino, F.O.; Faria, S.; Bellíssimo-Rodrigues, F.; Costa Passos, A.D. Declining prevalence of hepatitis A and silent circulation of hepatitis E virus infection in southeastern Brazil. *Int J. Infect. Dis* **2020**, *101*, 17–23. [CrossRef]
42. Ferreira, A.C.; Gomes-Gouvea, M.S.; Lisboa-Neto, G.; Mendes-Correa, M.C.J.; Picone, C.M.; Salles, N.A.; Mendrone, A., Jr.; Carrilho, F.J.; Pinho, J.R.R. Serological and molecular markers of hepatitis E virus infection in HIV-infected patients in Brazil. *Arch. Virol.* **2017**, *163*, 43–49. [CrossRef]
43. Hering, T.; Passos, A.M.; Perez, R.M.; Bilar, J.; Fragano, D.; Granato, C.; Medina-Pestana, J.O.; Ferraz, M.L. Past and current hepatitis E virus infection in renal transplant patients. *J. Med. Virol.* **2014**, *86*, 948–953. [CrossRef] [PubMed]
44. Passos-Castilho, A.M.; Sena, A.; Reinaldo, M.R.; Granato, C.F. Hepatitis E virus infection in Brazil: Results of laboratory-based surveillance from 1998 to 2013. *Rev. Soc. Bras. Med. Trop.* **2015**, *48*, 468–470. [CrossRef] [PubMed]
45. Passos, A.M.; Heringer, T.P.; Medina-Pestana, J.O.; Ferraz, M.L.; Granato, C.F. First report and molecular characterization of hepatitis E virus infection in renal transplant recipients in Brazil. *J. Med. Virol.* **2013**, *85*, 615–619. [CrossRef]
46. Araujo, P.; Latini, F.; Cortez, A.; Diaz, R.S.; Palazzo, P. Current Epidemiology of Hepatitis E Virus Infection in Sao Paulo, Brazil: Preliminary Results. *Transfusion* **2015**, *55*, 188A–189A. [CrossRef]
47. Gonçales, N.S.; Pinho, J.R.; Moreira, R.C.; Saraceni, C.P.; Spina, A.M.; Stucchi, R.B.; Filho, A.D.; Magna, L.A.; Júnior, F.L.G. Hepatitis E virus immunoglobulin G antibodies in different populations in Campinas, Brazil. *Clin. Vaccine Immunol.* **2000**, *7*, 813–816. [CrossRef]
48. Focaccia, R.; Sette, H., Jr.; Conceição, O.J.G. Hepatitis E in Brazil. *Lancet* **1995**, *346*, 1165. [CrossRef]
49. Hardtke, S.; Rocco, R.; Ogata, J.; Braga, S.; Barbosa, M.; Wranke, A.; Doi, E.; Cunha, D.; Maluf, E.; Wedemeyer, H.; et al. Risk factors and seroprevalence of hepatitis E evaluated in frozen-serum samples (2002–2003) of pregnant women compared with female blood donors in a Southern region of Brazil. *J. Med. Virol.* **2018**, *90*, 1856–1862. [CrossRef]
50. Bortoliero, A.L.; Bonametti, A.M.; Morimoto, H.K.; Matsuo, T.; Reiche, E.M. Seroprevalence for hepatitis E virus (HEV) infection among volunteer blood donors of the Regional Blood Bank of Londrina, State of Paraná, Brazil. *Rev. Inst. Med. Trop. São Paulo* **2006**, *48*, 87–92. [CrossRef]
51. Oliveira, J.M.D.; Junior, A.P.; Gardinali, N.R.; Pinto, M.A. Severe chronic hepatitis in a young immunossupressed Brazilian patient co-infected with Hepatitis E Virus (HEV) and Epstein-Barr Virus (EBV): A case report. *J. Viral Hepat.* **2018**, *25*, 91–92. [CrossRef]

52. Pandolfi, R.; Almeida, D.R.; Pinto, M.A.; Kreutz, L.C.; Frandoloso, R. In house ELISA based on recombinant ORF2 protein underline high prevalence of IgG anti-hepatitis E virus amongst blood donors in south Brazil. *PLoS ONE* **2017**, *12*, e176409. [CrossRef]
53. Silva, C.M.; Oliveira, J.M.; Mendoza-Sassi, R.A.; Figueiredo, A.S.; Mota, L.D.D.; Nader, M.M.; Gardinali, N.R.; Kevorkian, Y.B.; Salvador, S.B.S.; Pinto, M.A.; et al. Detection and characterization of hepatitis E virus genotype 3 in HIV-infected patients and blood donors from southern Brazil. *Int. J. Infect. Dis.* **2019**, *86*, 114–121. [CrossRef]
54. Passos-Castilho, A.M.; Sena, A.; Geraldo, A.; Spada, C.; Granato, C.F. High prevalence of hepatitis E virus antibodies among blood donors in Southern Brazil. *J. Med. Virol.* **2016**, *88*, 361–364. [CrossRef] [PubMed]
55. Timóteo, M.V.F.; Araujo, F.J.D.R.; Martins, K.C.P.; Silva, H.R.D.; Neto, G.A.D.S.; Pereira, R.A.C.; Paulino, J.D.S.; Pessoa, G.T.; Alvino, V.D.S.; Costa, R.H.F. Perfil epidemiológico das hepatites virais no Brasil. *Res. Soc. Dev.* **2020**, *9*, 1–13. [CrossRef]
56. Morgado, L.N.; Oliveira, J.M.; Pinto, M.A.; Burlandy, F.M.; Silva, E.E.; Silva, J.P.; Vitral, C.L. Hepatitis E virus is not detected in association with neurological disorders among Brazilian children. *Microbes Infect.* **2018**, *21*, 133–135. [CrossRef] [PubMed]
57. Souza, A.J.; Gomes-Gouvea, M.S.; Soares, M.D.C.P.; Pinho, J.R.R.; Malheiros, A.P.; Carneiro, L.A.; Santos, D.R.; Pereira, W.L. HEV infection in swine from Eastern Brazilian Amazon: Evidence of co-infection by different subtypes. *Comp. Immunol. Microbiol. Infect. Dis.* **2012**, *35*, 477–485. [CrossRef]
58. Oliveira-Filho, E.F.; Santos, D.R.D.; Duraes-Carvalho, R.; Silva, A.; Lima, G.B.; Filho, A.F.B.B.; Pena, L.J.; Gil, L.H. Evolutionary study of potentially zoonotic hepatitis E virus genotype 3 from swine in Northeast Brazil. *Memórias Inst. Oswaldo Cruz* **2019**, *114*, 1–5. [CrossRef] [PubMed]
59. Oliveira-Filho, E.F.; Lopes, K.G.S.; Cunha, D.S.; Silva, V.S.; Barbosa, C.N.; Brandespim, D.F.; Pinheiro, J.W., Jr.; Bertani, G.R.; Gil, L.H.V.G. Risk Analysis and Occurrence of Hepatitis E Virus (HEV) in Domestic Swine in Northeast Brazil. *Food Environ. Virol.* **2017**, *9*, 256–259. [CrossRef]
60. Vilanova, L.F.L.S.; Rigueira, L.L.; Perecmanis, S. Seroprevalence of hepatitis E virus infection in domestic pigs in the Federal District, Brazil. *Arq. Bras. Med. Veterinária Zootec.* **2018**, *70*, 469–474. [CrossRef]
61. De Campos, C.G.; Silveira, S.; Schenkel, D.M.; Carvalho, H.; Teixeira, E.A.; Souza, M.A.; Dutra, V.; Nakazato, L.; Canal, C.W.; Pescador, C.A. Detection of hepatitis E virus genotype 3 in pigs from subsistence farms in the state of Mato Grosso, Brazil. *Comp. Immunol. Microbiol. Infect. Dis.* **2018**, *58*, 11–16. [CrossRef] [PubMed]
62. Lana, M.V.C.; Gardinali, N.R.; Cruz, R.A.; Lopes, L.L.; Silva, G.S.; Caramori, J.G., Jr.; Oliveira, A.C.; Souza, M.A.; Colodel, E.M.; Alfieri, A.A.; et al. Evaluation of hepatitis E virus infection between different production systems of pigs in Brazil. *Trop. Anim. Health Prod.* **2014**, *46*, 399–404. [CrossRef]
63. Santos, D.R.; Vitral, C.L.; Paula, V.S.; Marchevsky, R.S.; Lopes, J.F.; Gaspar, A.M.; Saddi, T.M.; de Mesquita, N.C., Jr.; Guimarães, F.R.; Caramori, J.G., Jr.; et al. Serological and molecular evidence of hepatitis E virus in swine in Brazil. *Vet. J.* **2009**, *182*, 474–480. [CrossRef]
64. Guimarães, F.R.; Saddi, T.M.; Vitral, C.L.; Pinto, M.A.; Gaspar, A.M.C.; Souto, F.J.D. Hepatitis e virus antibodies in swine herds of mato grosso, state, central brazil. *Braz. J. Microbiol.* **2005**, *36*, 223–226. [CrossRef]
65. Amorim, A.R.; Mendes, G.S.; Pena, G.P.A.; Santos, N. Hepatitis E virus infection of slaughtered healthy pigs in Brazil. *Zoonoses Public Health* **2018**, *65*, 501–504. [CrossRef]
66. Santos, D.R.; Paula, V.S.; Oliveira, J.M.; Marchevsky, R.S.; Pinto, M.A. Hepatitis E virus in swine and effluent samples from slaughterhouses in Brazil. *Vet. Microbiol.* **2011**, *149*, 236–241. [CrossRef] [PubMed]
67. Paiva, H.H.; Tzaneva, V.; Haddad, R.; Yokosawa, J. Molecular characterization of swine hepatitis E virus from Southeastern Brazil. *Braz. J. Microbiol.* **2007**, *38*, 693–698. [CrossRef]
68. Passos-Castilho, A.M.; Granato, C.F.H. High frequency of hepatitis E virus infection in swine from South Brazil and close similarity to human HEV isolates. *Braz. J. Microbiol.* **2017**, *48*, 373–379. [CrossRef]
69. Gardinali, N.R.; Barry, A.F.; Otonel, R.A.; Alfieri, A.F.; Alfieri, A.A. Hepatitis E virus in liver and bile samples from slaughtered pigs of Brazil. *Memórias Inst. Oswaldo Cruz* **2012**, *107*, 935–939. [CrossRef]
70. Gardinali, N.R.; Barry, A.F.; Silva, P.F.; Souza, C.; Alfieri, A.F.; Alfieri, A.A. Molecular detection and characterization of hepatitis E virus in naturally infected pigs from Brazilian herds. *Res. Vet. Sci.* **2012**, *93*, 1515–1519. [CrossRef] [PubMed]
71. Silva, M.S.; Silveira, S.; Caron, V.S.; Mosena, A.C.S.; Weber, M.N.; Cibulski, S.P.; Medeiros, A.A.R.; Silva, G.S.; Corbellini, L.G.; Klein, R.; et al. Backyard pigs are a reservoir of zoonotic hepatitis E virus in southern Brazil. *Trans. R. Soc. Trop. Med. Hyg.* **2018**, *112*, 14–21. [CrossRef]
72. Vasconcelos, J.; Soliman, M.C.; Staggemeier, R.; Heinzelmann, L.; Weidlich, L.; Cimirro, R.; Esteves, P.A.; Silva, A.D.; Spilki, F.R. Molecular detection of hepatitis E virus in feces and slurry from swine farms, Rio Grande do Sul, Southern Brazil. *Arq. Bras. Med. Veterinária Zootec.* **2015**, *67*, 777–782. [CrossRef]
73. Silva, V.S.; Lopes, K.G.S.; Bertani, G.R.; Oliveira-Filho, E.F.; Trevisol, I.M.; Kramer, B.; Coldebella, A.; Gil, L.H.V.G. Seroprevalence of Hepatitis E virus (HEV) in domestic non-commercial pigs reared in small-scale farms and wild boar in South of Brazil. In Proceedings of the International Conference on the Epidemiology and Control of Biological, Chemical and Physical Hazards in Pigs and Pork, Foz do Iguaçu, Brasil, 21–24 August 2017; pp. 72–75.
74. Severo, D.R.T.; Werlang, R.A.; Mori, A.P.; Baldi, K.R.A.; Mendes, R.E.; Surian, S.R.S.; Coldebella, A.; Kramer, B.; Trevisol, I.M.; Gomes, T.M.A.; et al. Health profile of free-range wild boar (*Sus scrofa*) subpopulations hunted in Santa Catarina State, Brazil. *Transbound. Emerg. Dis.* **2020**, *68*, 857–869. [CrossRef] [PubMed]

75. Pereira, J.G.; Soares, V.M.; Souza, F.G.; Tadielo, L.E.; Santos, E.A.R.; Brum, M.C.S.; Henzel, A.; Duval, E.H.; Spilki, F.R.; da Silva, W.P. Hepatitis A Virus, Hepatitis E Virus, and Rotavirus in Foods of Animal Origin Traded at the Borders of Brazil, Argentina, and Uruguay. *Food Environ. Virol.* **2018**, *10*, 365–372. [CrossRef]
76. Heldt, F.H.; Staggmeier, R.; Gularte, J.S.; Demoliner, M.; Henzel, A.; Spilki, F.R. Hepatitis E Virus in surface water, sediments, and pork products marketed in Southern Brazil. *Food Environ. Virol.* **2016**, *8*, 200–205. [CrossRef] [PubMed]
77. Molina, C.V.; Heinemann, M.B.; Kierulff, C.; Pissinatti, A.; Silva, T.F.; Freitas, D.G.; Souza, G.O.; Miotto, B.A.; Cortez, A.; Semensato, B.P.; et al. Leptospira spp., rotavirus, norovirus, and hepatitis E virus surveillance in a wild invasive golden-headed lion tamarin (*Leontopithecus chrysomelas*; Kuhl, 1820) population from an urban park in Niterói, Rio de Janeiro, Brazil. *Am. J. Primatol.* **2019**, *81*, 1–11. [CrossRef] [PubMed]
78. Souza, W.M.; Romeiro, M.F.; Sabino-Santos, G.; Maia, F.G.M.; Fumagalli, M.J.; Modha, S.; Nunes, M.R.T.; Murcia, P.R.; Figueiredo, L.T.M. Novel orthohepeviruses in wild rodents from São Paulo State, Brazil. *Virology* **2018**, *519*, 12–16. [CrossRef]
79. Souza, F.G.; Gularte, J.S.; Demoliner, M.; Lima, A.F.; Siebert, J.C.; Rigotto, C.; Henzel, A.; Eisen, A.K.A.; Spilki, F.R. Teschovirus and other swine and human enteric viruses in Brazilian watersheds impacted by swine husbandry. *Braz. J. Microbiol.* **2020**, *51*, 711–717. [CrossRef]
80. Gularte, J.S.; Girardia, V.; Demolinera, M.; Souza, F.G.; Filippia, M.; Eisena, A.K.A.; Menac, K.D.; Quevedo, D.M.; Rigottoa, C.; Barros, M.P.; et al. Human mastadenovirus in water, sediment, sea surface microlayer, and bivalve mollusk from southern Brazilian beaches. *Mar. Pollut. Bull.* **2019**, *142*, 335–349. [CrossRef]
81. Dalton, H.R.; Bendall, R.; Ijaz, S.; Banks, M. Hepatitis E: An emerging infection in developed countries. *Lancet Infect. Dis.* **2008**, *8*, 698–709. [CrossRef]
82. Arends, J.E.; Ghisetti, V.; Irving, W.; Dalton, H.R.; Izopet, J.; Hoepelman, A.I.; Salmon, D. Hepatitis E: An emerging infection in high income countries. *J. Clin. Virol.* **2014**, *59*, 81–88. [CrossRef]
83. Meng, X.J.; Wiseman, B.; Elvinger, F.; Guenette, D.K.; Toth, T.E.; Engle, R.E.; Emerson, S.U.; Purcell, R.H. Prevalence of antibodies to hepatitis E virus in veterinarians working with swine and in normal blood donors in the United States and other countries. *J. Clin. Microbiol.* **2002**, *40*, 117–122. [CrossRef]
84. Nascimento, M.S.J.; Pereira, S.S.; Teixeira, J.; Abreu-Silva, J.; Oliveira, R.M.S.; Myrmel, M.; Stene-Johansen, K.; Øverbø, J.; Gonçalves, G.; Mesquita, J.R. A nationwide serosurvey of hepatitis E virus antibodies in the general population of Portugal. *Eur. J. Public Health* **2018**, *28*, 720–724. [CrossRef]
85. Izopet, J.; Tremeaux, P.; Marion, O.; Migueres, M.; Capelli, N.; Chapuy-Regaud, S.; Mansuy, J.M.; Abravanel, F.; Kamar, N.; Lhomme, S. Hepatitis E virus infections in Europe. *J. Clin. Virol* **2019**, *120*, 20–26. [CrossRef]
86. Harvala, H.; Wong, V.; Simmonds, P.; Johannessen, I.; Ramalingam, S. Acute viral hepatitis—Should the current screening strategy be modified? *J. Clin. Virol.* **2014**, *59*, 184–187. [CrossRef]
87. Embrapa. Estatística de produção suína no Brasil. Available online: https://www.embrapa.br/suinos-e-aves/cias/estatisticas (accessed on 16 July 2020).
88. Moor, D.; Liniger, M.; Baumgartner, A.; Felleisen, R. Screening of Ready-to-Eat Meat Products for Hepatitis E Virus in Switzerland. *Food Environ. Virol.* **2018**, *10*, 263–271. [CrossRef]
89. Boxman, I.L.A.; Jansen, C.C.C.; Hägele, G.; Zwartkruis-Nahuis, A.; Tijsma, A.S.L.; Vennema, H. Monitoring of pork liver and meat products on the Dutch market for the presence of HEV RNA. *Int. J. Food Microbiol.* **2019**, *296*, 58–64. [CrossRef]
90. Montone, A.M.I.; De Sabato, L.; Suffredini, E.; Alise, M.; Zaccherini, A.; Volzone, P.; Di Maro, O.; Neola, B.; Capuano, F.; Di Bartolo, I. Occurrence of HEV-RNA in Italian Regional Pork and Wild Boar Food Products. *Food Environ. Virol.* **2019**, *11*, 420–426. [CrossRef] [PubMed]
91. Carvalho, L.G.; Marchevsky, R.S.; Santos, D.R.; Oliveira, J.M.; Paula, V.S.; Lopes, L.M.; Poel, W.H.V.; González, J.E.; Munné, M.S.; Moran, J.; et al. Infection by Brazilian and Dutch swine hepatitis E virus strains induces haematological changes in Macaca fascicularis. *BMC Infect. Dis.* **2013**, *13*, 495. [CrossRef] [PubMed]
92. Gardinali, N.R.; Guimaraes, J.R.; Melgaco, J.G.; Kevorkian, Y.B.; Bottino, F.O.; Vieira, Y.R.; Silva, A.C.; Pinto, D.P.; Fonseca, L.B.; Vilhena, L.S.; et al. Cynomolgus monkeys are successfully and persistently infected with hepatitis E virus genotype 3 (HEV-3) after long-term immunosuppressive therapy. *PLoS ONE* **2017**, *12*, e0174070. [CrossRef]
93. Bottino, F.O.; Gardinali, N.R.; Salvador, S.B.S.; Figueiredo, A.S.; Cysne, L.B.; Francisco, J.S.; Oliveira, J.M.; Machado, M.P.; Pinto, M.A. Cynomolgus monkeys (*Macaca fascicularis*) experimentally and naturally infected with hepatitis E virus: The bone marrow as a possible new viral target. *PLoS ONE* **2018**, *13*, e0205039. [CrossRef] [PubMed]
94. Yang, F.; Duan, S.; Guo, Y.; Li, Y.; Yoshizaki, S.; Takeda, N.; Wakita, T.; Muramatsu, M.; Zhao, Y.; He, Z.; et al. Current status of hepatitis E virus infection at a rhesus monkey farm in China. *Vet. Microbiol.* **2019**, *230*, 244–248. [CrossRef] [PubMed]
95. Melegari, I.; Di Profio, F.; Marsilio, F.; Sarchese, V.; Palombieri, A.; Friedrich, K.G.; Coccia, F.; Di Martino, B. Serological and molecular investigation for hepatitis E virus (HEV) in captive non-human primates, Italy. *Virus Res.* **2018**, *251*, 17–21. [CrossRef]
96. McElroy, A.; Hiraide, R.; Bexfield, N.; Jalal, H.; Brownlie, J.; Goodfellow, I.; Caddy, S.L. Detection of Hepatitis E Virus Antibodies in Dogs in the United Kingdom. *PLoS ONE* **2015**, *10*, e0128703. [CrossRef]
97. Geng, J.B.; Fu, H.W.; Wang, L.; Wang, X.J.; Guan, J.M.; Chang, Y.B.; Li, L.J.; Zhu, Y.H.; Zhuang, H.; Liu, Q.H.; et al. Hepatitis E virus (HEV) genotype and the prevalence of anti-HEV in 8 species of animals in the suburbs of Beijing. *Zhonghua Liu Xing Bing Xue Za Zhi* **2010**, *31*, 47–50.

98. Huang, F.; Li, Y.; Yu, W.; Jing, S.; Wang, J.; Long, F.; He, Z.; Yang, C.; Bi, Y.; Cao, W.; et al. Excretion of infectious hepatitis E virus into milk in cows imposes high risks of zoonosis. *Hepatology* **2016**, *64*, 350–359. [CrossRef] [PubMed]
99. Li, S.; Liu, M.; Cong, J.; Zhou, Y.; Miao, Z. Detection and Characterization of Hepatitis E Virus in Goats at Slaughterhouse in Tai'an Region, China. *Biomed. Res. Int.* **2017**, *2017*, 3723650. [CrossRef] [PubMed]
100. Wang, B.; Cai, C.L.; Li, B.; Zhang, W.; Zhu, Y.; Chen, W.H.; Zhuo, F.; Shi, Z.L.; Yang, X.L. Detection and characterization of three zoonotic viruses in wild rodents and shrews from Shenzhen city, China. *Virol. Sin.* **2017**, *32*, 290–297. [CrossRef]
101. Kwon, H.M.; Sung, H.W.; Meng, X.J. Serological prevalence, genetic identification, and characterization of the first strains of avian hepatitis E virus from chickens in Korea. *Virus Genes* **2012**, *45*, 237–245. [CrossRef]
102. Sarchese, V.; Di Profio, F.; Melegari, I.; Palombieri, A.; Sanchez, S.B.; Arbuatti, A.; Ciuffetelli, M.; Marsilio, F.; Martella, V.; Di Martino, B. Hepatitis E virus in sheep in Italy. *Transbound. Emerg. Dis.* **2019**, *66*, 1120–1125. [CrossRef]
103. La Rosa, G.; Della Libera, S.; Brambilla, M.; Bisaglia, C.; Pisani, G.; Ciccaglione, A.R.; Bruni, R.; Taffon, S.; Equestre, M.; Iaconelli, M. Hepatitis E Virus (Genotype 3) in Slurry Samples from Swine Farming Activities in Italy. *Food Environ. Virol.* **2017**, *9*, 219–229. [CrossRef]
104. Cuevas-Ferrando, E.; Randazzo, W.; Pérez-Cataluña, A.; Sánchez, G. HEV Occurrence in Waste and Drinking Water Treatment Plants. *Front. Microbiol.* **2019**, *10*, 2937. [CrossRef]
105. Crossan, C.; Baker, P.J.; Craft, J.; Takeuchi, Y.; Dalton, H.R.; Scobie, L. Hepatitis E virus genotype 3 in shellfish, United Kingdom. *Emerg. Infect. Dis.* **2012**, *18*, 2085–2087. [CrossRef] [PubMed]
106. Mesquita, J.R.; Oliveira, D.; Rivadulla, E.; Abreu-Silva, J.; Varela, M.F.; Romalde, J.L.; Nascimento, M.S. Hepatitis E virus genotype 3 in mussels (*Mytilus galloprovinciallis*), Spain. *Food Microbiol.* **2016**, *58*, 13–15. [CrossRef] [PubMed]
107. Rivadulla, E.; Varela, M.F.; Mesquita, J.R.; Nascimento, M.S.J.; Romalde, J.L. Detection of Hepatitis E Virus in Shellfish Harvesting Areas from Galicia (Northwestern Spain). *Viruses* **2019**, *11*, 618. [CrossRef] [PubMed]
108. Ishida, S.; Yoshizumi, S.; Ikeda, T.; Miyoshi, M.; Goto, A.; Matsubayashi, K.; Ikeda, H. Detection and molecular characterization of hepatitis E virus in clinical, environmental and putative animal sources. *Arch. Virol.* **2012**, *157*, 2363–2368. [CrossRef]
109. Masclaux, F.G.; Hotz, P.; Friedli, D.; Savova-Bianchi, D.; Oppliger, A. High occurrence of hepatitis E virus in samples from wastewater treatment plants in Switzerland and comparison with other enteric viruses. *Water Res.* **2013**, *47*, 5101–5109. [CrossRef] [PubMed]
110. Matos, A.; Mesquita, J.R.; Gonçalves, D.; Abreu-Silva, J.; Luxo, C.; Nascimento, M.S. First detection and molecular characterization of hepatitis E virus in water from wastewater treatment plants in Portugal. *Ann. Agric. Environ. Med.* **2018**, *25*, 364–367. [CrossRef]
111. Horvatits, T.; Ozga, A.K.; Westholter, D.; Hartl, J.; Manthey, C.F.; Lutgehetmann, M.; Rauch, G.; Kriston, L.; Lohse, A.W.; Bendall, R.; et al. Hepatitis E seroprevalence in the Americas: A systematic review and meta-analysis. *Liver Int.* **2018**, *38*, 1951–1964. [CrossRef]
112. Tengan, F.M.; Figueiredo, G.M.; Nunes, A.K.S.; Manchiero, C.; Dantas, B.P.; Magri, M.C.; Prata, T.V.G.; Nascimento, M.; Mazza, C.C.; Abdala, E.; et al. Seroprevalence of hepatitis E in adults in Brazil: A systematic review and meta-analysis. *Infect. Dis. Poverty* **2019**, *8*, 1–10. [CrossRef]

animals MDPI

Opinion

High-Fat Diet-Induced Trefoil Factor Family Member 2 (TFF2) to Counteract the Immune-Mediated Damage in Mice

Abdelaziz Ghanemi [1,2], Mayumi Yoshioka [2] and Jonny St-Amand [1,2,*]

1 Department of Molecular Medicine, Faculty of Medicine, Laval University, Québec, QC G1V 0A6, Canada; abdelaziz.ghanemi@crchudequebec.ulaval.ca
2 Functional Genomics Laboratory, Endocrinology and Nephrology Axis, CHU de Québec-Université Laval Research Center, Québec, QC G1V 4G2, Canada; mayumi.yoshioka@crchudequebec.ulaval.ca
* Correspondence: jonny.st-amand@crchudequebec.ulaval.ca; Tel.: +1-(418)-525-4444 (ext. 46448); Fax: +1-(418)-654-2298

Simple Summary: High-fat (HF) diet induces both immune-mediated damage and trefoil factor family member 2 (*Tff2*) expression. As TFF2 has tissue repair and protection properties, this suggests that HF diet-induced *Tff2* production and the resulting TFF2 mucosal protective effects would be a mechanism to counteract the HF diet-induced tissue damage. On the other hand, the induction of *Tff2* by HF diet could indicate that TFF2 is a food intake regulator (appetite control) since *Tff2* is also expressed in the brain. This highlights the importance of exploring TFF2-related pathways in the context of obesity management towards potential therapies.

Abstract: Physiological homeostasis requires a balance between the immunological functions and the resulting damage/side effects of the immunological reactions including those related to high-fat (HF) diet. Within this context, whereas HF diet, through diverse mechanisms (such as inflammation), leads to immune-mediated damage, trefoil factor family member 2 (*Tff2*) represents a HF diet-induced gene. On the other hand, TFF2 both promotes tissue repair and reduces inflammation. These properties are towards counteracting the immune-mediated damage resulting from the HF diet. These observations suggest that the HF diet-induction of *Tff2* could be a regulatory pathway aiming to counteract the immune-mediated damage resulting from the HF diet. Interestingly, since *Tff2* expression increases with HF diet and with *Tff2* also expressed in the brain, we also hypothesize that TFF2 could be a HF diet-induced food intake-control signal that reduces appetite. This hypothesis fits with counteracting the immune damage since reducing the food intake will reduce the HF intake and therefore, reduces the HF diet-induced tissue damage. Such food intake signaling would be an indirect mechanism by which TFF2 promotes tissue repair as well as a pathway worth exploring for potential obesity management pharmacotherapies.

Keywords: trefoil factor family member 2 (TFF2); high-fat diet; immunity; damage; mice

Citation: Ghanemi, A.; Yoshioka, M.; St-Amand, J. High-Fat Diet-Induced Trefoil Factor Family Member 2 (TFF2) to Counteract the Immune-Mediated Damage in Mice. *Animals* **2021**, *11*, 258. https://doi.org/10.3390/ani11020258

Received: 22 December 2020
Accepted: 19 January 2021
Published: 21 January 2021

Animal physiological homeostasis requires a balance between the immunological functions and the damage/side effects of those immunological reactions. Knowing that immunological reactions can be triggered by diverse factors, the homeostasis supposes that parallel or secondary pathways are activated or stimulated with these immunological reactions to repair the damage. The immune system is a complex network of cells and circulating fluids that is modulated by the nervous system [1], endocrine system [2], infections [3], and even diet. Indeed, different types of diets, such as high-sucrose and high-fat (HF) diets, have been shown to impact immune functions [4,5], among other factors and genes [6,7]. HF diets characterize our modern life, and are associated with diverse diseases and health problems, such as obesity, dyslipidemia, diabetes, fatty liver disease and cardiovascular diseases [7–10]. However, such HF diet-induced immune modulations, which could be implicated in the HF diet-induced risks and diseases, are yet to be fully understood. Within this context, the molecules and signals that are either upregulated or downregulated with HF diets could be the mechanistic answer, as per the examples we provide below from studies on mice.

For instance, trefoil factor family member 2 (TFF2), known as spasmolytic peptide [11], is well involved in mucosal repair, protection and proliferation, as it represents an important stabilizer of the gastric mucus, with roles in tissue remodeling [12]. Herein, we go beyond its mucosal protective role to explore the hypothesis linking this diet-induced molecule, TFF2, to the diet-induced immunomodulation. Indeed, whereas *Tff2* has been reported as a gene that is specifically induced by HF diets in mice [13,14], its knockout protected mice from HF diet-induced obesity [15] through a metabolic phenotype that contributes to more energy expenditure and reduced energy storage [16]. The importance of the studies that identified *Tff2* as a gene specifically induced by HF diets is that the control groups were, unlike in other studies, fasted mice [13,14]. Based on the HF induction of TFF2, we notice a correlation between the HF diet-induced immunological changes and the TFF2-related immunological effects and benefits (as illustrated below). This correlation suggests that TFF2 would be involved in mediating the protective effects against such HF diet damage.

On one side, a HF diet has important immunological impacts. For instance, a HF diet increases TNFα and IL1β in young mice's hippocampus [17], and leads to chronic systemic inflammation [18]. Moreover, a chronic HF diet is also associated with obesity [19,20], which also affects the immunity [21] and might explain some of the impacts obesity has on regeneration impairment through diverse processes, including inflammation [22], which is important in the context of TFF2′s roles in tissues repair.

On the other hand, TFF2, beyond its well-known roles in injured mucosa healing [23–25], has a noticeable role in the immune response [25,26], as suggested by its expression in immune organs [27] and its expression during inflammations [12]. Indeed, *Helicobacter* infection upregulated it in gastric tissues, macrophages and lymphocytes [11], whereas *Helicobacter pylori* eradication decreased TFF2 level in patients' sera [28]. Furthermore, TFF2 deficiency leads to a deregulation of macrophages' and lymphocytes' proliferative responses [11], and an accelerated gastritis progression [29] during *Helicobacter* infection. This correlates with both the ulceration role of *Helicobacter pylori* [30] and the tissue repair/protections roles of TFF2 in animal selected tissues [12].

TFF2 expression during such immunological changes seems to be an attempt to limit the negative impacts of these immune reactions, such as inflammation [12], due to the HF diet. For instance, TFF2 could both limit the recruitment of leukocytes and the monocyte production of nitric oxide [25], and decrease macrophage responsiveness [27], which would contribute to promoting the tissue repair environment. Therefore, this TFF2-induced downregulation of selected immunological responses would be a step required to accomplish the healing and protecting effects TFF2 governs.

These illustrative examples present TFF2 as a mediator of the HF diet-triggered mechanisms attempting to correct the HF diet's negative impacts, mediated through the immune system. Interestingly, unlike glucose, which causes insulin as a hormone to be secreted immediately following meal ingestion [31], there is no equivalent hormone for lipid ingestion. TFF2 could be that missing signal within animal endocrinology, since in the studies in which *Tff2* was shown to be unregulated at 3 h following a low-fat meal ingestion, it was upregulated with a HF meal [13,14]. The acute character of this expression indicates an immediate effect of the HF diet on Tff2 expression. Therefore, TFF2 could be a short-term lipid-specific signal that controls lipid intake by limiting lipid ingestion through a TFF2-dependant feedback acting on food intake centers. This is supported by the differential *Tff2* expression in the hypothalamus of fasted, and low-fat and HF diet-fed, mice (lipid ratio-dependent expression) [15]. This hypothesis is further supported by the increase in the drive to consume a HF meal, as well as the appetite enhancement as a consequence of TFF2 deficiency [15]. This would suggest that TFF2 counteracts HF diet-induced damage indirectly through reducing the HF intake. The other remarkable link is that TFF2 is mostly expressed in the digestive system [32,33], which represents the site whereat the animal's neuroendocrine receptors first interact with the ingested food, including HF meals; this further suggests the acute responsiveness of the HF diet's induction of TFF2 in the mouse intestine. Always within the digestive system, the HF diet impacts the local microbiome [34,35], which could be another key link between the diet and the immunological changes, especially with the known interactions between the immune system and the microbiome [36–38], the microbiota richness reduction [39], and dysbiosis, in all of which the HF diet has been implicated [40]. In addition, since several effects of a HF diet are mediated by microbiota [18] with probiotics that upregulate TFF2 [41], these microbiota-mediated effects of the HF diet could be through TFF2 expression changes.

These elements highlight TFF2 expression (HF diet-induced) as a feedback aiming to counteract the immune-mediated HF diet-induced damage. However, the correcting potential and efficacy of TFF2 would depend on the severity and the chronic or acute character of such a HF diet. This explains why during obesity (such as in HF diet-induced obesity in animal models), those TFF2-correcting mechanisms are less efficient due to the strong immune-mediated damage that overcomes the TFF2-counteracting ability. Further explorations of diets' impacts on TFF2 expression, such as high-salt diets [42], within an immunological context would expand this emerging field linking the type of diet to the immunological changes via identifying the linking factors. Importantly, combining these metabolic and immunological properties of TFF2 would allow us to further understand how mice immunologically react to a HF diet, and elucidate more diet-induced effects on immunology, infections and inflammation. Importantly, extrapolating these concepts from mice to humans and building clinical trials based on animal experiments could lead to developing novel TFF2-based therapies for diseases and conditions, such as inflammation, and, most importantly, a potential control for lipid intake (appetite control) towards a better obesity management strategy, which requires urgent solutions due obesity's epidemiological profile and its impacts on health and the economy [43–46].

Author Contributions: A.G. drafted the manuscript; A.G., M.Y. and J.S.-A. critically revised the manuscript. All authors have read and agreed to the published version of the manuscript.

Funding: This research received no external funding.

Institutional Review Board Statement: Not applicable.

Informed Consent Statement: Not applicable.

Data Availability Statement: Not applicable.

Acknowledgments: Abdelaziz Ghanemi received a merit scholarship for foreign students from the Ministry of Education and Higher Education of Quebec, Canada. The Fonds de recherche du Québec—Nature et technologies (FRQNT) is responsible for managing the program (Bourses d'excellence pour étudiants étrangers du Ministère de l'Éducation et de l'Enseignement supérieur du Québec, Le Fonds de recherche du Québec—Nature et technologies (FRQNT) est responsable de la gestion du programme). The graphical abstract was created using images from: http://smart.servier.com. Servier Medical Art by Servier is licensed under a Creative Commons Attribution 3.0 Unported License.

Conflicts of Interest: The authors declare no conflict of interest.

References

1. Habek, M. Immune and autonomic nervous system interactions in multiple sclerosis: Clinical implications. *Clin. Auton. Res.* **2019**, *29*, 267–275. [CrossRef] [PubMed]
2. Renner, U.; Sapochnik, M.; Lucia, K.; Stalla, G.K.; Arzt, E. Intrahypophyseal Immune-Endocrine Interactions: Endocrine Integration of the Inflammatory Inputs. *Front. Horm. Res.* **2017**, *48*, 37–47. [CrossRef] [PubMed]
3. Brizić, I.; Hiršl, L.; Britt, W.J.; Krmpotić, A.; Jonjić, S. Immune responses to congenital cytomegalovirus infection. *Microbes. Infect.* **2018**, *20*, 543–551. [CrossRef] [PubMed]
4. Brown, K.; DeCoffe, D.; Molcan, E.; Gibson, D.L. Diet-Induced Dysbiosis of the Intestinal Microbiota and the Effects on Immunity and Disease. *Nutrients* **2012**, *4*, 1095–1119. [CrossRef]

5. Sato Mito, N.; Suzui, M.; Yoshino, H.; Kaburagi, T.; Sato, K. Long term effects of high fat and sucrose diets on obesity and lymphocyte proliferation in mice. *J. Nutr. Health Aging* **2009**, *13*, 602–606. [CrossRef]
6. Ghanemi, A.; Melouane, A.; Yoshioka, M.; St-Amand, J. Exercise and High-Fat Diet in Obesity: Functional Genomics Perspectives of Two Energy Homeostasis Pillars. *Genes* **2020**, *11*, 875. [CrossRef]
7. Keleher, M.R.; Zaidi, R.; Shah, S.; Oakley, M.E.; Pavlatos, C.; El Idrissi, S.; Xing, X.; Li, D.; Wang, T.; Cheverud, J.M. Maternal high-fat diet associated with altered gene expression, DNA methylation, and obesity risk in mouse offspring. *PLoS ONE* **2018**, *13*, e0192606. [CrossRef]
8. Heydemann, A. An Overview of Murine High Fat Diet as a Model for Type 2 Diabetes Mellitus. *J. Diabetes Res.* **2016**, *2016*, 2902351. [CrossRef]
9. Udomkasemsab, A.; Prangthip, P. High fat diet for induced dyslipidemia and cardiac pathological alterations in Wistar rats compared to Sprague Dawley rats. *Clin. Investig. Arterioscler.* **2019**, *31*, 56–62. [CrossRef]
10. Recena Aydos, L.; Aparecida do Amaral, L.; Serafim de Souza, R.; Jacobowski, A.C.; Freitas Dos Santos, E.; Rodrigues Macedo, M.L. Nonalcoholic Fatty Liver Disease Induced by High-Fat Diet in C57bl/6 Models. *Nutrients* **2019**, *11*, 3067. [CrossRef]
11. Kurt-Jones, E.A.; Cao, L.; Sandor, F.; Rogers, A.B.; Whary, M.T.; Nambiar, P.R.; Cerny, A.; Bowen, G.; Yan, J.; Takaishi, S.; et al. Trefoil family factor 2 is expressed in murine gastric and immune cells and controls both gastrointestinal inflammation and systemic immune responses. *Infect. Immun.* **2007**, *75*, 471–480. [CrossRef] [PubMed]
12. Ghanemi, A.; Yoshioka, M.; St-Amand, J. Trefoil Factor Family Member 2 (TFF2) as an Inflammatory-Induced and Anti-Inflammatory Tissue Repair Factor. *Animals* **2020**, *10*, 1646. [CrossRef] [PubMed]
13. Mucunguzi, O.; Melouane, A.; Ghanemi, A.; Yoshioka, M.; Boivin, A.; Calvo, E.L.; St-Amand, J. Identification of the principal transcriptional regulators for low-fat and high-fat meal responsive genes in small intestine. *Nutr. Metab.* **2017**, *14*, 1–10. [CrossRef] [PubMed]
14. Yoshioka, M.; Bolduc, C.; Raymond, V.; St-Amand, J. High-fat meal-induced changes in the duodenum mucosa transcriptome. *Obesity (Silver Spring)* **2008**, *16*, 2302–2307. [CrossRef]
15. De Giorgio, M.R.; Yoshioka, M.; Riedl, I.; Moreault, O.; Cherizol, R.G.; Shah, A.A.; Blin, N.; Richard, D.; St-Amand, J. Trefoil factor family member 2 (Tff2) KO mice are protected from high-fat diet-induced obesity. *Obesity (Silver Spring)* **2013**, *21*, 1389–1395. [CrossRef]
16. Ghanemi, A.; Melouane, A.; Mucunguzi, O.; Yoshioka, M.; St-Amand, J. Energy and metabolic pathways in trefoil factor family member 2 (Tff2) KO mice beyond the protection from high-fat diet-induced obesity. *Life Sci.* **2018**, *215*, 190–197. [CrossRef]
17. Nakandakari, S.; Muñoz, V.R.; Kuga, G.K.; Gaspar, R.C.; Sant'Ana, M.R.; Pavan, I.C.B.; da Silva, L.G.S.; Morelli, A.P.; Simabuco, F.M.; da Silva, A.S.R.; et al. Short-term high-fat diet modulates several inflammatory, ER stress, and apoptosis markers in the hippocampus of young mice. *Brain Behav. Immun.* **2019**, *79*, 284–293. [CrossRef]
18. Schachter, J.; Martel, J.; Lin, C.S.; Chang, C.J.; Wu, T.R.; Lu, C.C.; Ko, Y.F.; Lai, H.C.; Ojcius, D.M.; Young, J.D. Effects of obesity on depression: A role for inflammation and the gut microbiota. *Brain Behav. Immun.* **2018**, *69*, 1–8. [CrossRef]
19. Lissner, L.; Levitsky, D.A.; Strupp, B.J.; Kalkwarf, H.J.; Roe, D.A. Dietary fat and the regulation of energy intake in human subjects. *Am. J. Clin. Nutr.* **1987**, *46*, 886–892. [CrossRef]
20. Schutz, Y.; Flatt, J.P.; Jéquier, E. Failure of dietary fat intake to promote fat oxidation: A factor favoring the development of obesity. *Am. J. Clin. Nutr.* **1989**, *50*, 307–314. [CrossRef]
21. Andersen, C.J.; Murphy, K.E.; Fernandez, M.L. Impact of Obesity and Metabolic Syndrome on Immunity. *Adv. Nutr.* **2016**, *7*, 66–75. [CrossRef] [PubMed]
22. Ghanemi, A.; Yoshioka, M.; St-Amand, J. Regeneration during Obesity: An Impaired Homeostasis. *Animals* **2020**, *10*, 2344. [CrossRef] [PubMed]
23. Taupin, D.; Podolsky, D.K. Trefoil factors: Initiators of mucosal healing. *Nat. Rev. Mol. Cell Biol.* **2003**, *4*, 721–732. [CrossRef] [PubMed]
24. Tran, C.P.; Cook, G.A.; Yeomans, N.D.; Thim, L.; Giraud, A.S. Trefoil peptide TFF2 (spasmolytic polypeptide) potently accelerates healing and reduces inflammation in a rat model of colitis. *Gut* **1999**, *44*, 636–642. [CrossRef] [PubMed]
25. Baus-Loncar, M.; Kayademir, T.; Takaishi, S.; Wang, T. Trefoil factor family 2 deficiency and immune response. *Cell Mol. Life Sci.* **2005**, *62*, 2947–2955. [CrossRef]
26. Baus-Loncar, M.; Schmid, J.; Lalani el, N.; Rosewell, I.; Goodlad, R.A.; Stamp, G.W.; Blin, N.; Kayademir, T. Trefoil factor 2 (TFF2) deficiency in murine digestive tract influences the immune system. *Cell Physiol. Biochem.* **2005**, *16*, 31–42. [CrossRef] [PubMed]
27. Judd, L.M.; Chalinor, H.V.; Walduck, A.; Pavlic, D.I.; Däbritz, J.; Dubeykovskaya, Z.; Wang, T.C.; Menheniott, T.R.; Giraud, A.S. TFF2 deficiency exacerbates weight loss and alters immune cell and cytokine profiles in DSS colitis, and this cannot be rescued by wild-type bone marrow. *Am. J. Physiol. Gastrointest. Liver. Physiol.* **2015**, *308*, G12–G24. [CrossRef]
28. Kaise, M.; Miwa, J.; Fujimoto, A.; Tashiro, J.; Tagami, D.; Sano, H.; Ohmoto, Y. Influence of Helicobacter pylori status and eradication on the serum levels of trefoil factors and pepsinogen test: Serum trefoil factor 3 is a stable biomarker. *Gastric Cancer* **2013**, *16*, 329–337. [CrossRef]
29. Fox, J.G.; Rogers, A.B.; Whary, M.T.; Ge, Z.; Ohtani, M.; Jones, E.K.; Wang, T.C. Accelerated progression of gastritis to dysplasia in the pyloric antrum of TFF2 -/- C57BL6 x Sv129 Helicobacter pylori-infected mice. *Am. J. Pathol.* **2007**, *171*, 1520–1528. [CrossRef]
30. Mobley, H.L. The role of Helicobacter pylori urease in the pathogenesis of gastritis and peptic ulceration. *Aliment. Pharmacol. Ther.* **1996**, *10* (Suppl. 1), 57–64. [CrossRef]

31. Kalwat, M.A.; Cobb, M.H. Mechanisms of the amplifying pathway of insulin secretion in the β cell. *Pharmacol. Ther.* **2017**, *179*, 17–30. [CrossRef] [PubMed]
32. Madsen, J.; Nielsen, O.; Tornøe, I.; Thim, L.; Holmskov, U. Tissue localization of human trefoil factors 1, 2, and 3. *J. Histochem. Cytochem.* **2007**, *55*, 505–513. [CrossRef] [PubMed]
33. Hoffmann, W.; Jagla, W.; Wiede, A. Molecular medicine of TFF-peptides: From gut to brain. *Histol. Histopathol.* **2001**, *16*, 319–334. [CrossRef]
34. Hasebe, K.; Rivera, L.R.; Smith, C.M.; Allnutt, T.; Crowley, T.; Nelson, T.M.; Dean, O.M.; McGee, S.L.; Walder, K.; Gray, L. Modulation of high fat diet-induced microbiome changes, but not behaviour, by minocycline. *Brain Behav. Immun.* **2019**, *82*, 309–318. [CrossRef] [PubMed]
35. Hassan, A.M.; Mancano, G.; Kashofer, K.; Fröhlich, E.E.; Matak, A.; Mayerhofer, R.; Reichmann, F.; Olivares, M.; Neyrinck, A.M.; Delzenne, N.M.; et al. High-fat diet induces depression-like behaviour in mice associated with changes in microbiome, neuropeptide Y, and brain metabolome. *Nutr. Neurosci.* **2019**, *22*, 877–893. [CrossRef] [PubMed]
36. Lambring, C.B.; Siraj, S.; Patel, K.; Sankpal, U.T.; Mathew, S.; Basha, R. Impact of the Microbiome on the Immune System. *Crit. Rev. Immunol.* **2019**, *39*, 313–328. [CrossRef] [PubMed]
37. Shi, N.; Li, N.; Duan, X.; Niu, H. Interaction between the gut microbiome and mucosal immune system. *Mil. Med. Res.* **2017**, *4*, 14. [CrossRef]
38. Ticinesi, A.; Lauretani, F.; Tana, C.; Nouvenne, A.; Ridolo, E.; Meschi, T. Exercise and immune system as modulators of intestinal microbiome: Implications for the gut-muscle axis hypothesis. *Exerc. Immunol. Rev.* **2019**, *25*, 84–95.
39. Cândido, F.G.; Valente, F.X.; Grześkowiak, Ł.M.; Moreira, A.P.B.; Rocha, D.; Alfenas, R.C.G. Impact of dietary fat on gut microbiota and low-grade systemic inflammation: Mechanisms and clinical implications on obesity. *Int. J. Food Sci. Nutr.* **2018**, *69*, 125–143. [CrossRef]
40. Netto Candido, T.L.; Bressan, J.; Alfenas, R.C.G. Dysbiosis and metabolic endotoxemia induced by high-fat diet. *Nutr. Hosp.* **2018**, *35*, 1432–1440. [CrossRef]
41. Khoder, G.; Al-Yassir, F.; Al Menhali, A.; Saseedharan, P.; Sugathan, S.; Tomasetto, C.; Karam, S.M. Probiotics Upregulate Trefoil Factors and Downregulate Pepsinogen in the Mouse Stomach. *Int. J. Mol. Sci.* **2019**, *20*, 3901. [CrossRef] [PubMed]
42. Chen, X.; Hu, Y.; Xie, Y.; Wang, Y. High salt diet can down-regulate TFF2 expression level in gastric mucosa of MGs after H. pylori infection. *Microb. Pathog.* **2018**, *118*, 316–321. [CrossRef] [PubMed]
43. Ghanemi, A.; St-Amand, J. Redefining obesity toward classifying as a disease. *Eur. J. Intern. Med.* **2018**, *55*, 20–22. [CrossRef] [PubMed]
44. Ghanemi, A.; Yoshioka, M.; St-Amand, J. Broken Energy Homeostasis and Obesity Pathogenesis: The Surrounding Concepts. *J. Clin. Med.* **2018**, *7*, 453. [CrossRef] [PubMed]
45. Ghanemi, A.; Yoshioka, M.; St-Amand, J. Will an obesity pandemic replace the coronavirus disease-2019 (COVID-19) pandemic? *Méd. Hypotheses* **2020**, *144*, 110042. [CrossRef]
46. Ghanemi, A.; Yoshioka, M.; St-Amand, J. Obesity as a Neuroendocrine Reprogramming. *Medicina* **2021**, *57*, 66. [CrossRef]

animals

MDPI

Letter

Trefoil Factor Family Member 2 (TFF2) as an Inflammatory-Induced and Anti-Inflammatory Tissue Repair Factor

Abdelaziz Ghanemi [1,2], Mayumi Yoshioka [2] and Jonny St-Amand [1,2,*]

1 Department of Molecular Medicine, Faculty of Medicine, Laval University, Québec, QC G1V 0A6, Canada; abdelaziz.Ghanemi@crchudequebec.ulaval.ca

2 Endocrinology and Nephrology Axis, Functional Genomics Laboratory, CHU de Québec-Université Laval Research Center, Québec, QC G1V 4G2, Canada; mayumi.yoshioka@crchudequebec.ulaval.ca

* Correspondence: jonny.st-amand@crchudequebec.ulaval.ca; Tel.: +1-(418)-654-2296; Fax: +1-(418)-654-2761

Received: 24 August 2020; Accepted: 11 September 2020; Published: 14 September 2020

check for updates

Abstract: Trefoil factor family member 2 (TFF2) is known for its involvement in mucosal repair. Whereas it is overexpressed during inflammatory processes, adding TFF2 leads to an anti-inflammatory effect that would contribute to create the microenvironment required for tissue repair. These properties present TFF2 with a homeostatic pattern during inflammatory processes as illustrated by selected examples.

Keywords: trefoil factor family member 2 (TFF2); inflammation; tissue repair

Dear Editor,

Compared to the diverse physiological entities, digestive and respiratory systems represent the tissues that interact the most with exogenous organisms and molecules, as they represent the two "entrances" of the body. This anatomical property exposes these systems to diverse stimuli and injuries leading to inflammatory reactions, especially with their rich blood flow and close interactions with the immune system. In addition, their mucosa have a relatively high regenerative and repair activity. Within the context of mucosal repair, trefoil factor family member 2 (TFF2), also known as spasmolytic polypeptide and isolated in 1982 [1], is a biological factor known for its involvement in mucosal repair, protection and proliferation especially within both digestive and respiratory systems [2–8]. TFF2 represents an important component and a stabilizer of the gastric mucus with the property of binding to the mucin MUC6 [9] and is also involved in tissue remodeling [2,10]. It is expressed in different species such as mouse [11], cow [12], rat [13], pork [9] and human [14]. In veterinary science, the animal models of TFF2-modified expression illustrate the importance of this protein in animal health as shown by studies investigating obesity, gastric secretion, asthma, etc [2,3,10,11].

These TFF2 properties are reflected by the increased susceptibility to injury seen in TFF2-deficient mice. Indeed, TFF2-deficient mice have an increased gastric ulceration degree compared to wild-type mice following indomethacin administration [3]. Since there is numerous inflammatory diseases [4,15–17] that develop in the digestive and respiratory systems, we would like to summarize hypothetic links between the TFF2 and selected inflammatory-related processes [2,18–20].

TFF2 has been shown to be overexpressed (or upregulated) following inflammations or inflammatory conditions [18] such as in asthma [2], gastrointestinal ulcerative disease [19] and allergic airway inflammation [20]. Furthermore, knowing that some interleukins (IL) have been linked to tissue repair [21–23], such regulation could also be under the control of selected cytokines since, for instance, IL-4 and IL-13 induce TFF2 in the lung [20]. Other treatments, also leading to cell damage, upregulate TFF2 or *TFF2* expression, such as hypoxia [24] and aspirin in which the damages are also associated with hypoxia [24,25]. This suggests that the upregulation would be a response of the inflammation-induced damage rather than the inflammation itself, which correlates with aspirin damage-induced activation of *Tff2* gene in rats [13]. This would mean that TFF2 would not be required to develop the inflammation but would rather increase with inflammation, either induced by inflammation or the factor triggering the inflammation. This TFF2 induction would initiate the healing and repairing process that counteracts the inflammation-induced damage, which could be a protective mechanism such as during chronic superficial gastritis [26].

Interestingly, other studies have pointed TFF2 with a potential anti-inflammatory effect. For instance, a recombinant human TFF2 was shown to reduce colitis inflammation in a rat model; it increases the colonic epithelial repair rate [27]. Within the same line, applying TFF2 does reduce inflammatory indexes in a hapten colitis rodent model and has even been suggested as a therapeutic scaffold for inflammatory bowel disease treatment [28]. Importantly, TFF2 treatment reduces fibrosis (subepithelial collagen deposition) in a murine model of chronic allergic airways disease [2], which could indicate a reduced fibrogenesis in tissues undergoing inflammation [29,30]. Thus, TFF2 effects are not limited to an anti-inflammatory effect but would also reduce the tissue fibrosis. Both effects are towards tissue repair and counteract the deteriorating inflammatory consequences (damage and fibrosis) as well. This could explain the TFF2 beneficial effect on intestinal inflammation in animal models, which would involve reducing both macrophage responsiveness [28] and leukocyte recruitment [31], regulating the NO-mediated inflammation (monocyte) [32] and blocking inflammatory cell recruitment [28] within its mechanism. On the same path, TFF2 is also expressed during gastric cancer [33,34]. This could indicate that the presence of TFF2 aims to limit the cancer-induced inflammatory damages. It could also represent an attempt to limit cancer growth as suggested by an in vitro study that shows the inhibition of the growth of gastric cancer cells by TFF2 expression [35].

It is worth precising that the anti-inflammatory effect or fibrosis reduction have been observed when exogenous TFF2 was added in different conditions [2,27,32] rather than when the inflammation-related endogenous TFF2 was overexpressed (since inflammation develops although the inflammation-induced upregulation of TFF2 expression [2,18–20]). This highlights TFF2 overexpression as an attempt to limit the inflammation and its consequences (such as fibrogenesis). Such an anti-inflammatory effect or fibrosis reduction would be among the main mechanisms underlying the pathways via which TFF2 mediates its mucosal protection. Although the inflammatory-induced TFF2 overexpression (not its exogenous addition) would not lead to a measurable effect on inflammation or fibrosis, inflammatory-related TFF2 expression would probably contribute to create the biological environment required for tissue repair, but not only through recruiting selected factors and interacting with biomolecules such as mucins [18,36].

Interestingly, probiotics have been shown to increase the production of TFF2 in the mouse stomach [37]. Probiotics also have, in addition to roles in tissue repair [38], anti-inflammatory effects especially in the intestine [39], which is one of the key tissues of TFF2 expression. Thus, TFF2 might be among the pathways linking probiotics to the anti-inflammatory and tissue repair effects, probably involving immunological mechanisms impacted by probiotics [40]. In addition, the reported antibiotic activity of TFF2 [14] could be complimentary in both inflammation and immunological regulation towards reducing inflammation-related damages.

Tff2 has been recently characterized as a high-fat diet-induced gene in the intestinal mucosa [41] and the knock out of this gene lead to a protection from high-fat diet-induced obesity [11,42]. Both these facts could be further considered for the future exploration of the links between inflammation and metabolics. Indeed, obesity, for which a high-fat diet increases its development, also represents a risk factor for both inflammation and cancer development. Therefore, the metabolic implications of TFF2 could be behind a part of the inflammatory and cancer processes, especially based on known links between metabolic activities and the factors related to inflammation and cancer [43–45]. Within this context, IL could complete TFF2 roles during tissue repair. For instance, tissue injuries induce IL-6 production [46], which is required for gastric homeostasis [47] and has been shown to play metabolic roles [43]. This would indicate complementarity roles between TFF2 and IL during tissue repair by contributing to create the microenvironment as well as the metabolic conditions required for post-injury repair and counteracting the tissue damages. Within the context of diet, it is also worth mentioning that a diet rich in antioxidants would have a beneficial effect on inflammation development [48]. Moreover, the high-fat diet-induced *Tff2* gene expression could be related to counteracting inflammation damages, since high-fat diet induces oxidative stress [49] and is usually associated with obesity [50,51] which has both oxidative stress [52] and inflammation [53,54] in its context.

Moreover, the other TFFs (TFF1 and TFF3) would require additional exploration within the context of inflammation because of their implication in the inflammation process [4] as well as the possible expression interdependence linking TFF2, TFF1 and TFF3 [55,56]. Furthermore, the inflammatory properties of TFFs correlate with their immunological roles [28]. This could also justify the expression of TFFs (minute amounts) in the immune and central nervous systems [57] as well as in cancers [12,58] as regulatory factors. Deeper understudying of TFF2 implications in inflammation or inflammatory-related diseases and conditions would allow developing new methods to confirm diagnosis, make prognosis or follow a therapy efficiency based on TFF2 expression variation as a biological marker, such as in tumors [33]. Moreover, these implications of TFF2 in inflammation would suggest the potential usage of TFF2 or targeting TFF2-related pathways to develop novel therapies or optimize those in usage for diseases and conditions involving an inflammatory component. The "homeostatic property" of TFF2 exposed is similar to the one we reported for the secreted protein acidic and rich in cysteine (SPARC) during inflammation [59] and cancer [60]. Interestingly, SPARC is also involved in response to injury and tissue remodeling [61,62]. Such opposing effects may broaden the application horizons and these two examples of TFF2 and SPARC illustrate mechanistic links between the need to control inflammation as well as adapting cellular patterns (metabolism, structural shape, etc.) during tissue repair and regeneration processes. Elucidating these links will expand therapeutic perspectives based on molecular pathways of diseases in animals and humans.

Author Contributions: A.G. drafted the manuscript; A.G., M.Y. and J.S.-A. critically revised the manuscript. All authors have read and agreed to the published version of the manuscript.

Funding: This research received no external funding.

Acknowledgments: Abdelaziz Ghanemi is a recipient of a Merit scholarship program for foreign students from the Ministry of Education and Higher Education of Quebec, Canada, The Fonds de recherche du Québec—Nature et technologies (FRQNT) is responsible for managing the program (Bourses d'excellence pour étudiants étrangers du Ministère de l'Éducation et de l'Enseignement supérieur du Québec, Le Fonds de recherche du Québec—Nature et technologies (FRQNT) est responsable de la gestion du programme). The graphical abstract was created using images from: http://smart.servier.com. Servier Medical Art by Servier is licensed under a Creative Commons Attribution 3.0 Unported License.

Conflicts of Interest: The authors declare no conflict of interest.

References

1. Jørgensen, K.H.; Thim, L.; Jacobsen, H.E. Pancreatic spasmolytic polypeptide (PSP): I. Preparation and initial chemical characterization of a new polypeptide from porcine pancreas. *Regul. Pept.* **1982**, *3*, 207–219. [CrossRef]
2. Royce, S.G.; Lim, C.; Muljadi, R.C.; Samuel, C.S.; Ververis, K.; Karagiannis, T.C.; Giraud, A.S.; Tang, M.L. Trefoil factor-2 reverses airway remodeling changes in allergic airways disease. *Am. J. Respir. Cell Mol. Biol.* **2013**, *48*, 135–144. [CrossRef] [PubMed]
3. Farrell, J.J.; Taupin, D.; Koh, T.J.; Chen, D.; Zhao, C.-M.; Podolsky, D.K.; Wang, T.C. TFF2/SP-deficient mice show decreased gastric proliferation, increased acid secretion, and increased susceptibility to NSAID injury. *J. Clin. Investig.* **2002**, *109*, 193–204. [CrossRef] [PubMed]
4. Aamann, L.; Vestergaard, E.M.; Grønbæk, H. Trefoil factors in inflammatory bowel disease. *World J. Gastroenterol.* **2014**, *20*, 3223–3230. [CrossRef] [PubMed]

5. Playford, R.J.; Marchbank, T.; Chinery, R.; Evison, R.; Pignatelli, M.; Boulton, R.A.; Thim, L.; Hanby, A.M. Human spasmolytic polypeptide is a cytoprotective agent that stimulates cell migration. *Gastroenterology* **1995**, *108*, 108–116. [CrossRef]
6. McKenzie, C.; Marchbank, T.; Playford, R.J.; Otto, W.; Thim, L.; Parsons, M.E. Pancreatic spasmolytic polypeptide protects the gastric mucosa but does not inhibit acid secretion or motility. *Am. J. Physiol.* **1997**, *273 Pt 1*, G112–G117. [CrossRef]
7. Aihara, E.; Engevik, K.A.; Montrose, M.H. Trefoil Factor Peptides and Gastrointestinal Function. *Annu. Rev. Physiol.* **2017**, *79*, 357–380. [CrossRef]
8. Greeley, M.A.; Van Winkle, L.S.; Edwards, P.C.; Plopper, C.G. Airway trefoil factor expression during naphthalene injury and repair. *Toxicol. Sci.* **2010**, *113*, 453–467. [CrossRef]
9. Heuer, F.; Stürmer, R.; Heuer, J.; Kalinski, T.; Lemke, A.; Meyer, F.; Hoffmann, W. Different Forms of TFF2, A Lectin of the Human Gastric Mucus Barrier: In Vitro Binding Studies. *Int. J. Mol. Sci.* **2019**, *20*, 5871. [CrossRef]
10. Royce, S.G.; Lim, C.; Muljadi, R.C.; Tang, M.L. Trefoil factor 2 regulates airway remodeling in animal models of asthma. *J. Asthma* **2011**, *48*, 653–659. [CrossRef]
11. Ghanemi, A.; Melouane, A.; Mucunguzi, O.; Yoshioka, M.; St-Amand, J. Energy and metabolic pathways in trefoil factor family member 2 (Tff2) KO mice beyond the protection from high-fat diet-induced obesity. *Life Sci.* **2018**, *215*, 190–197. [CrossRef]
12. Katoh, M. Trefoil factors and human gastric cancer (review). *Int. J. Mol. Med.* **2003**, *12*, 3–9. [CrossRef] [PubMed]
13. Konturek, P.C.; Brzozowski, T.; Pierzchalski, P.; Kwiecien, S.; Pajdo, R.; Hahn, E.G.; Konturek, S.J. Activation of genes for spasmolytic peptide, transforming growth factor alpha and for cyclooxygenase (COX)-1 and COX-2 during gastric adaptation to aspirin damage in rats. *Aliment. Pharm.* **1998**, *12*, 767–777. [CrossRef]
14. Hanisch, F.G.; Bonar, D.; Schloerer, N.; Schroten, H. Human trefoil factor 2 is a lectin that binds α-GlcNAc-capped mucin glycans with antibiotic activity against Helicobacter pylori. *J. Biol. Chem.* **2014**, *289*, 27363–27375. [CrossRef] [PubMed]
15. Sébert, M.; Sola-Tapias, N.; Mas, E.; Barreau, F.; Ferrand, A. Protease-Activated Receptors in the Intestine: Focus on Inflammation and Cancer. *Front. Endocrinol. (Lausanne)* **2019**, *10*, 717. [CrossRef] [PubMed]
16. Ma, K.; Lu, N.; Zou, F.; Meng, F.Z. Sirtuins as novel targets in the pathogenesis of airway inflammation in bronchial asthma. *Eur. J. Pharm.* **2019**, *865*, 172670. [CrossRef]
17. Schuliga, M. NF-kappaB Signaling in Chronic Inflammatory Airway Disease. *Biomolecules* **2015**, *5*, 1266–1283. [CrossRef]
18. Hoffmann, W. TFF2, a MUC6-binding lectin stabilizing the gastric mucus barrier and more (Review). *Int. J. Oncol.* **2015**, *47*, 806–816. [CrossRef]
19. Ortiz-Masiá, D.; Hernández, C.; Quintana, E.; Velázquez, M.; Cebrián, S.; Riaño, A.; Calatayud, S.; Esplugues, J.V.; Barrachina, M.D. iNOS-derived nitric oxide mediates the increase in TFF2 expression associated with gastric damage: Role of HIF-1. *FASEB J.* **2010**, *24*, 136–145. [CrossRef]
20. Nikolaidis, N.M.; Zimmermann, N.; King, N.E.; Mishra, A.; Pope, S.M.; Finkelman, F.D.; Rothenberg, M.E. Trefoil factor-2 is an allergen-induced gene regulated by Th2 cytokines and STAT6 in the lung. *Am. J. Respir. Cell Mol. Biol.* **2003**, *29*, 458–464. [CrossRef]
21. Knipper, J.A.; Willenborg, S.; Brinckmann, J.; Bloch, W.; Maaß, T.; Wagener, R.; Krieg, T.; Sutherland, T.; Munitz, A.; Rothenberg, M.E.; et al. Interleukin-4 Receptor α Signaling in Myeloid Cells Controls Collagen Fibril Assembly in Skin Repair. *Immunity* **2015**, *43*, 803–816. [CrossRef] [PubMed]
22. Balaji, S.; Wang, X.; King, A.; Le, L.D.; Bhattacharya, S.S.; Moles, C.M.; Butte, M.J.; de Jesus Perez, V.A.; Liechty, K.W.; Wight, T.N.; et al. Interleukin-10-mediated regenerative postnatal tissue repair is dependent on regulation of hyaluronan metabolism via fibroblast-specific STAT3 signaling. *FASEB J.* **2017**, *31*, 868–881. [CrossRef] [PubMed]
23. Hadian, Y.; Bagood, M.D.; Dahle, S.E.; Sood, A.; Isseroff, R.R. Interleukin-17: Potential Target for Chronic Wounds. *Mediat. Inflamm.* **2019**, *2019*, 1297675. [CrossRef] [PubMed]
24. Hernández, C.; Santamatilde, E.; McCreath, K.J.; Cervera, A.M.; Díez, I.; Ortiz-Masiá, D.; Martínez, N.; Calatayud, S.; Esplugues, J.V.; Barrachina, M.D. Induction of trefoil factor (TFF)1, TFF2 and TFF3 by hypoxia is mediated by hypoxia inducible factor-1: Implications for gastric mucosal healing. *Br. J. Pharmacol.* **2009**, *156*, 262–272. [CrossRef] [PubMed]

25. Azarschab, P.; Al-Azzeh, E.; Kornberger, W.; Gött, P. Aspirin promotes TFF2 gene activation in human gastric cancer cell lines. *FEBS Lett.* **2001**, *488*, 206–210. [CrossRef]
26. Hu, G.Y.; Yu, B.P.; Dong, W.G.; Li, M.Q.; Yu, J.P.; Luo, H.S.; Rang, Z.X. Expression of TFF2 and Helicobacter pylori infection in carcinogenesis of gastric mucosa. *World J. Gastroenterol.* **2003**, *9*, 910–914. [CrossRef]
27. Tran, C.P.; Cook, G.A.; Yeomans, N.D.; Thim, L.; Giraud, A.S. Trefoil peptide TFF2 (spasmolytic polypeptide) potently accelerates healing and reduces inflammation in a rat model of colitis. *Gut* **1999**, *44*, 636–642. [CrossRef]
28. Judd, L.M.; Chalinor, H.V.; Walduck, A.; Pavlic, D.I.; Däbritz, J.; Dubeykovskaya, Z.; Wang, T.C.; Menheniott, T.R.; Giraud, A.S. TFF2 deficiency exacerbates weight loss and alters immune cell and cytokine profiles in DSS colitis, and this cannot be rescued by wild-type bone marrow. *Am. J. Physiol. Gastrointest. Liver Physiol.* **2015**, *308*, G12–G24. [CrossRef]
29. Ellermann, M.; Gharaibeh, R.Z.; Fulbright, L.; Dogan, B.; Moore, L.N.; Broberg, C.A.; Lopez, L.R.; Rothemich, A.M.; Herzog, J.W.; Rogala, A.; et al. Yersiniabactin-Producing Adherent/Invasive Escherichia coli Promotes Inflammation-Associated Fibrosis in Gnotobiotic Il10(-/-) Mice. *Infect. Immun.* **2019**, *87*, e00587-19. [CrossRef]
30. Gordon, I.O.; Agrawal, N.; Willis, E.; Goldblum, J.R.; Lopez, R.; Allende, D.; Liu, X.; Patil, D.Y.; Yerian, L.; El-Khider, F.; et al. Fibrosis in ulcerative colitis is directly linked to severity and chronicity of mucosal inflammation. *Aliment. Pharmacol. Ther.* **2018**, *47*, 922–939. [CrossRef]
31. Soriano-Izquierdo, A.; Gironella, M.; Massaguer, A.; May, F.E.; Salas, A.; Sans, M.; Poulsom, R.; Thim, L.; Piqué, J.M.; Panés, J. Trefoil peptide TFF2 treatment reduces VCAM-1 expression and leukocyte recruitment in experimental intestinal inflammation. *J. Leukoc. Biol.* **2004**, *75*, 214–223. [CrossRef] [PubMed]
32. Giraud, A.S.; Pereira, P.M.; Thim, L.; Parker, L.M.; Judd, L.M. TFF-2 inhibits iNOS/NO in monocytes, and nitrated protein in healing colon after colitis. *Peptides* **2004**, *25*, 803–809. [CrossRef] [PubMed]
33. Dhar, D.K.; Wang, T.C.; Maruyama, R.; Udagawa, J.; Kubota, H.; Fuji, T.; Tachibana, M.; Ono, T.; Otani, H.; Nagasue, N. Expression of Cytoplasmic TFF2 Is a Marker of Tumor Metastasis and Negative Prognostic Factor in Gastric Cancer. *Lab. Investig.* **2003**, *83*, 1343–1352. [CrossRef]
34. Schmidt, P.H.; Lee, J.R.; Joshi, V.; Playford, R.J.; Poulsom, R.; Wright, N.A.; Goldenring, J.R. Identification of a metaplastic cell lineage associated with human gastric adenocarcinoma. *Lab. Investig.* **1999**, *79*, 639–646.
35. Cai, Y.; Yi, M.; Chen, D.; Liu, J.; Guleng, B.; Ren, J.; Shi, H. Trefoil factor family 2 expression inhibits gastric cancer cell growth and invasion in vitro via interactions with the transcription factor Sp3. *Int. J. Mol. Med.* **2016**, *38*, 1474–1480. [CrossRef]
36. Longman, R.J.; Douthwaite, J.; Sylvester, P.A.; Poulsom, R.; Corfield, A.P.; Thomas, M.G.; Wright, N.A. Coordinated localisation of mucins and trefoil peptides in the ulcer associated cell lineage and the gastrointestinal mucosa. *Gut* **2000**, *47*, 792–800. [CrossRef] [PubMed]
37. Khoder, G.; Al-Yassir, F.; Al Menhali, A.; Saseedharan, P.; Sugathan, S.; Tomasetto, C.; Karam, S.M. Probiotics Upregulate Trefoil Factors and Downregulate Pepsinogen in the Mouse Stomach. *Int. J. Mol. Sci.* **2019**, *20*, 3901. [CrossRef] [PubMed]
38. Lukic, J.; Chen, V.; Strahinic, I.; Begovic, J.; Lev-Tov, H.; Davis, S.C.; Tomic-Canic, M.; Pastar, I. Probiotics or pro-healers: The role of beneficial bacteria in tissue repair. *Wound Repair Regen.* **2017**, *25*, 912–922. [CrossRef]
39. Plaza-Díaz, J.; Ruiz-Ojeda, F.J.; Vilchez-Padial, L.M.; Gil, A. Evidence of the Anti-Inflammatory Effects of Probiotics and Synbiotics in Intestinal Chronic Diseases. *Nutrients* **2017**, *9*, 555. [CrossRef]
40. Liu, Y.; Alookaran, J.J.; Rhoads, J.M. Probiotics in Autoimmune and Inflammatory Disorders. *Nutrients* **2018**, *10*, 1537. [CrossRef]
41. Yoshioka, M.; Bolduc, C.; Raymond, V.; St-Amand, J. High-fat meal-induced changes in the duodenum mucosa transcriptome. *Obesity (Silver Spring)* **2008**, *16*, 2302–2307. [CrossRef] [PubMed]
42. De Giorgio, M.R.; Yoshioka, M.; Riedl, I.; Moreault, O.; Cherizol, R.G.; Shah, A.A.; Blin, N.; Richard, D.; St-Amand, J. Trefoil factor family member 2 (Tff2) KO mice are protected from high-fat diet-induced obesity. *Obesity (Silver Spring)* **2013**, *21*, 1389–1395. [CrossRef] [PubMed]
43. Ghanemi, A.; St-Amand, J. Interleukin-6 as a "metabolic hormone". *Cytokine* **2018**, *112*, 132–136. [CrossRef] [PubMed]
44. Hong, J.T.; Son, D.J.; Lee, C.K.; Yoon, D.Y.; Lee, D.H.; Park, M.H. Interleukin 32, inflammation and cancer. *Pharmacol. Ther.* **2017**, *174*, 127–137. [CrossRef]

45. Petruzzelli, M.; Wagner, E.F. Mechanisms of metabolic dysfunction in cancer-associated cachexia. *Genes Dev.* **2016**, *30*, 489–501. [CrossRef]
46. Tanaka, T.; Narazaki, M.; Kishimoto, T. IL-6 in inflammation, immunity, and disease. *Cold Spring Harb. Perspect. Biol.* **2014**, *6*, a016295. [CrossRef]
47. Judd, L.M.; Alderman, B.M.; Howlett, M.; Shulkes, A.; Dow, C.; Moverley, J.; Grail, D.; Jenkins, B.J.; Ernst, M.; Giraud, A.S. Gastric cancer development in mice lacking the SHP2 binding site on the IL-6 family co-receptor gp130. *Gastroenterology* **2004**, *126*, 196–207. [CrossRef]
48. Peritore, A.F.; Siracusa, R.; Crupi, R.; Cuzzocrea, S. Therapeutic Efficacy of Palmitoylethanolamide and Its New Formulations in Synergy with Different Antioxidant Molecules Present in Diets. *Nutrients* **2019**, *11*, 2175. [CrossRef]
49. Lasker, S.; Rahman, M.M.; Parvez, F.; Zamila, M.; Miah, P.; Nahar, K.; Kabir, F.; Sharmin, S.B.; Subhan, N.; Ahsan, G.U.; et al. High-fat diet-induced metabolic syndrome and oxidative stress in obese rats are ameliorated by yogurt supplementation. *Sci. Rep.* **2019**, *9*, 20026. [CrossRef]
50. Ghanemi, A.; Yoshioka, M.; St-Amand, J. Broken Energy Homeostasis and Obesity Pathogenesis: The Surrounding Concepts. *J. Clin. Med.* **2018**, *7*, 453. [CrossRef]
51. Ghanemi, A.; Melouane, A.; Yoshioka, M.; St-Amand, J. Exercise and High-Fat Diet in Obesity: Functional Genomics Perspectives of Two Energy Homeostasis Pillars. *Genes (Basel)* **2020**, *11*, 875. [CrossRef] [PubMed]
52. Sindhu, S.; Akhter, N.; Kochumon, S.; Thomas, R.; Wilson, A.; Shenouda, S.; Tuomilehto, J.; Ahmad, R. Increased Expression of the Innate Immune Receptor TLR10 in Obesity and Type-2 Diabetes: Association with ROS-Mediated Oxidative Stress. *Cell. Physiol. Biochem.* **2018**, *45*, 572–590. [CrossRef] [PubMed]
53. Karczewski, J.; Śledzińska, E.; Baturo, A.; Jończyk, I.; Maleszko, A.; Samborski, P.; Begier-Krasińska, B.; Dobrowolska, A. Obesity and inflammation. *Eur. Cytokine Netw.* **2018**, *29*, 83–94. [CrossRef] [PubMed]
54. Ghanemi, A.; St-Amand, J. Redefining obesity toward classifying as a disease. *Eur. J. Intern. Med.* **2018**, *55*, 20–22. [CrossRef]
55. Taupin, D.; Wu, D.-C.; Jeon, W.-K.; Devaney, K.; Wang, T.C.; Podolsky, D.K. The trefoil gene family are coordinately expressed immediate-early genes: EGF receptor– and MAP kinase–dependent interregulation. *J. Clin. Investig.* **1999**, *103*, R31–R38. [CrossRef]
56. Lefebvre, O.; Chenard, M.-P.; Masson, R.; Linares, J.; Dierich, A.; LeMeur, M.; Wendling, C.; Tomasetto, C.; Chambon, P.; Rio, M.-C. Gastric Mucosa Abnormalities and Tumorigenesis in Mice Lacking the pS2 Trefoil Protein. *Science* **1996**, *274*, 259–262. [CrossRef]
57. Hoffmann, W. Trefoil Factor Family (TFF) Peptides and Their Diverse Molecular Functions in Mucus Barrier Protection and More: Changing the Paradigm. *Int. J. Mol. Sci.* **2020**, *21*, 4535. [CrossRef]
58. Kirikoshi, H.; Katoh, M. Expression of TFF1, TFF2 and TFF3 in gastric cancer. *Int. J. Oncol.* **2002**, *21*, 655–659. [CrossRef]
59. Ghanemi, A.; Yoshioka, M.; St-Amand, J. Secreted protein acidic and rich in cysteine and inflammation: Another homeostatic property? *Cytokine* **2020**, *133*, 155179. [CrossRef]
60. Ghanemi, A.; Yoshioka, M.; St-Amand, J. Secreted protein acidic and rich in cysteine and cancer: A homeostatic hormone? *Cytokine* **2020**, *127*, 154996. [CrossRef]
61. Ghanemi, A.; Yoshioka, M.; St-Amand, J. Secreted Protein Acidic and Rich in Cysteine: Metabolic and Homeostatic Properties beyond the Extracellular Matrix Structure. *Appl. Sci.* **2020**, *10*, 2388. [CrossRef]
62. Ghanemi, A.; Melouane, A.; Yoshioka, M.; St-Amand, J. Secreted protein acidic and rich in cysteine and bioenergetics: Extracellular matrix, adipocytes remodeling and skeletal muscle metabolism. *Int. J. Biochem. Cell Biol.* **2019**, *117*, 105627. [CrossRef] [PubMed]

animals

MDPI

Article

Descriptive Pathological Study of Avian Schistosomes Infection in Whooper Swans (*Cygnus cygnus*) in Japan

Mohamed S. Ahmed [1,2], Reda E. Khalafalla [3], Ashraf Al-Brakati [4], Tokuma Yanai [5] and Ehab Kotb Elmahallawy [6,*]

1 Department of Pathology, Faculty of Veterinary Medicine, Kafrelsheikh University, Kafrelsheikh 33516, Egypt; aosayedahmed@yahoo.com
2 Department of Veterinary Pathology, Gifu University, 1-1 Yanagido, Gifu 501-1193, Japan
3 Department of Parasitology, Faculty of Veterinary Medicine, Kafrelsheikh University, Kafrelsheikh 33516, Egypt; redabast@hotmail.de
4 Department of Human Anatomy, College of Medicine, Taif University, P.O. Box 11099, Taif 21944, Saudi Arabia; a.albrakati@tu.edu.sa
5 Laboratory of Wildlife and Forensic Pathology, Biomedical Science Examination and Research Center, Department of Veterinary Medicine, Faculty of Veterinary Medicine, Okayama University of Science, Okayama 700-0005, Japan; tokumayanai@gmail.com
6 Department of Zoonoses, Faculty of Veterinary Medicine, Sohag University, Sohag 82524, Egypt
* Correspondence: eehaa@unileon.es

Received: 24 November 2020; Accepted: 7 December 2020; Published: 10 December 2020

check for updates

Simple Summary: Avian schistosomes are a group of parasites responsible for most of the reported cases of cercarial dermatitis outbreaks. Among others, *Trichobilharzia* is considered the largest genus of avian Schistosomatidae, and it infects more than 40 avian species. The present study involves a descriptive pathological study of avian schistosome in 54 whooper swans (*Cygnus cygnus*) from various rescue/rehabilitation centers in Honshu, Japan. Interestingly, adult schistosomes were detected in the lumen of mesenteric, serosal, portal, and testicular veins, in the capillaries of the intestinal lamina propria, and in the sinusoids of the adrenal gland, spleen, and liver of 23 (42.59%) swans. Schistosomes were assumed to be *Allobilharzia visceralis* based on the morphological characteristics of the worm and eggs found at histopathological examination of internal organs, along with suggestive pathological findings as well as the pathological findings. Collectively, the present study provides novel descriptive pathological data about schistosome infection in whooper swans with new insights on their role in the transmission and spreading of avian schistosomes in Japan.

Abstract: Cercarial dermatitis, or Swimmer's itch, is one of the emerging diseases caused by the cercariae of water-borne schistosomes, mainly *Trichobilharzia* spp. Since the zoonotic potential of *Allobilharzia visceralis* is still unknown, studies on this schistosome would be helpful to add knowledge on its possible role in causing human infections. In the present study, 54 whooper swans (*Cygnus cygnus*) from rescue/rehabilitation centers in Honshu, Japan, were necropsied to identify the cause of death. Grossly, 33 (61.11%) swans were severely emaciated and 23 (42.59%) had multiple reddened areas throughout the length of the intestine with no worms detected in the internal organs. Microscopically, adult schistosomes were found in the lumen of the mesenteric, serosal, portal, and testicular veins, in the capillaries of the intestinal lamina propria, and in the sinusoids of the adrenal gland, spleen, and liver of 23 (42.59%) swans. Hypertrophy of veins containing adult worms was identified in 15 (27.77%) swans, and vascular lumen obliteration was observed in 8 (14.81%) swans. Mild to severe villous atrophy and superficial enteritis were observed in 8 birds (14.81%), whereas bile pigments and hemosiderin were detected in the livers of 14 (25.92%) and 18 (33.33%) swans, respectively. In three swans (5.55%), schistosome parasites were found in the subcapsular veins of the testes. The schistosomes in the present study were assumed to be *A. visceralis* based on the microscopical and histological evidence of adult schistosomes found in the lumen of veins as well as the infection pathology, which was very similar to the schistosome-induced pathology previously reported in swans infected by *A. visceralis* in Europe and Australia. The swans examined herein most likely died from obstructive phlebitis associated with *A. visceralis*, but further molecular confirmation is required for identification of this species. However, the present study does not provide new data on the zoonotic potential, but only on the pathogenic potential of this schistosome in swans. Furthermore, our study provides a novel contribution to the description of the pathological effects of avian schistosomes infection in whooper swans in Japan.

Keywords: schistosome; *Allobilharzia visceralis*; whooper swans; obstructive phlebitis

1. Introduction

Avian schistosomes are a specialized group of parasites and have a particular importance due to their zoonotic potential [1–3]. These schistosomes inhabit the circulatory system of the definitive avian hosts and are commonly known as "blood flukes." Various species of birds can be infected with schistosomes, but infection is most prevalent in waterfowl [1,4–7]. Among others, *Trichobilharzia* is the largest genus of avian Schistosomatidae, covering more than 40 avian species [8], and they can be divided into visceral and nasal species based on their predilection sites. Visceral species migrate through the viscera and are typically found in mesenteric, renal, cloacal, and portal blood vessels [9,10].

Most of these digenean trematodes have an indirect lifecycle involving a gastropod intermediate host. Fresh-water snails are required for the development of schistosomes belonging to the genera *Bilharziella, Ornithobilharzia, Jilinobilharzia, Macrobilhazia,* and *Trichobilharzia* and salt or brackish mollusks are instead required for genera *Dendritobilharzia, Gigantobilharzia,* and *Austrobilharzia* [3,8,10,11]. Infected aquatic bird excrete schistosome eggs, that hatch and release miracidia that penetrate inside the intermediate hosts where they develop to cercaria [11,12]. Thereafter, cercaria is released from the snail intermediate hosts and invade the warm-blooded vertebrate host via skin penetration, in whose circulatory system they develop to adults [1,4,7].

Avian schistosomiasis is characterized by lesions similar to those present in mammals infected with schistosomes, e.g., obliterative endophlebitis, venous hypertrophy, necrosis, granulomatous reaction combined with a mixed inflammatory response, thrombosis of mesenteric veins, fibrinohemorrhagic colitis, and portal fibroplasia, due to the presence of adults and/or eggs in blood vessels [5,9,13–21]. However, extensive anatomopathological studies on avian schistosomiasis are lacking. In humans, the repeated penetration of the skin causes the human cercarial dermatitis (HCD), an allergic reaction also known as "swimmer's itch" [1,15,22]. Cercarial dermatitis can be caused by several species of avian schistosomes, e.g., those belonging to the genera *Trichobilharzia, Gigantobilharzia,* and *Austrobilharzia* [3,8,10,11,23]. The zoonotic potential of other species, such as the swan schistosome *Allobilharzia visceralis* remains unknown [6,24,25], despite it cannot be excluded that it can produce HCD. Human cercarial dermatitis is considered endemic in Japan and rice farmers are among the occupational groups at high risk of infection [1,15,26]. In many cases, an etiological diagnosis of HCD at species level can be difficult to achieve, and it cannot be excluded that some cases could be due to *A. visceralis.* Swans are present in Japan and can transport their schistosomes during their migrations [15,23,27]. Indeed, *A. visceralis* has been already reported in swans either in Japan other than in North America and Iceland [13,28–30]. Therefore, in the light of the scarce knowledge on the pathology of avian schistosomiasis and of the potential zoonotic implications of blood flukes infecting swans [1,15,31,32], this study evaluated the occurrence of blood flukes in swans from Japan, discussing anatomopathological findings.

2. Materials and Methods

2.1. Ethical Statement

This study was approved by the Animal Care and Use Committee of Gifu University (approval I: EA07-05) and the Department of Veterinary Pathology, Kafrelsheikh University. Appropriate Institutional Animal Care Guidelines were followed during all handling and procedures.

2.2. Animals and Sample Collection

Fifty-four swans were received from rescue/rehabilitation centers in Honshu, Japan, between May 2005 and June 2007. Of these 54 birds, 38 were found dead, 12 swans died shortly after their arrival, whereas 4 swans were severely or moderately emaciated and dehydrated and were euthanized to avoid them unnecessary suffering. To determine the cause of death, the swans were submitted to the veterinary pathology department of the Gifu University for postmortem examination. Thirty-one swans were young (24–36 months), and the remaining were adults (48–72 months). Birds were categorized as immature if they still had brown feathers in their plumage, a pink-gray beak, and gray feet, whereas birds with fully white plumage, an orange beak, and black feet were categorized as mature [19,33]. This study followed the guidelines and measures of the Department of Veterinary Pathology, Gifu University, Japan, for the care and use of animals. In addition, before proceeding with euthanasia, appropriate veterinary care consistent with international, national, and institutional guidelines was guaranteed to the swans.

2.3. Gross and Histopathological Examination

Necropsies were performed on all swans in accordance with a standardized protocol. This procedure began with a review of the relevant history followed a full examination to detect anatomopathological alterations. To identify small foreign fragments or any lesions, the contents of the gizzard and intestine were carefully washed. Tissue samples were collected from all organs and from any noticeable lesions. The specimens were fixed in 10% phosphate-buffered formalin, embedded in paraffin, sectioned at a thickness of 4 µm, and then stained with hematoxylin and eosin [34]. Liver sections were also stained with Hall's bilirubin stain for bile pigment, and specimens of the liver and spleen were stained with Berlin blue stain for iron [34,35].

2.4. Parasitological Examination

It is difficult to describe the morphological features of the worms in this study, because the adult worms were very small and typically present only in the lumen of the affected veins. The different stages of the parasites observed in the various histopathological sections were incidentally reported during the measurement of lead (Pb) content in the soft tissues (liver and kidney). The morphology of the different stages of the adult worm in the blood vessels of different damaged internal organs and the effect of eggs in the intestinal mucosa of the affected birds were used for localization of the parasite during histopathological examination, as reported elsewhere [36].

3. Results

3.1. Gross Examination

Thirty-three out of 54 necropsied whooper swans were severely emaciated and lean, with atrophied pectoral muscles, serious atrophy of pericardial fat, and an absence of fat depots. Twenty-three birds showed multiple reddened areas throughout the entire length of the intestine, which were most prominent in the ileum, cecum, and colon. The main histological lesions were found in the intestinal tract, liver, adrenal gland, spleen, and testis; these lesions were caused by both worms and eggs (Table 1).

Table 1. Summary of histopathological lesions and worm findings in 23 infected whooper swans.

No. of Swans	**1**	**2**	**3**	**4**	**5**	**6**	**7**	**8**	**9**	**10**	**11**	**12**	**13**	**14**	**15**	**16**	**17**	**18**	**19**	**20**	**21**	**22**	**23**
Sex/Age	**F/A**	**F/A**	**F/A**	**M/Y**	**M/Y**	**M/Y**	**M/Y**	**F/A**	**F/A**	**F/Y**	**M/A**	**M/Y**	**M/Y**	**F/A**	**M/Y**	**F/Y**	**ND/Y**	**F/A**	**F/Y**	**F/ND**	**M/Y**	**F/A**	**M/Y**
Emaciation	++	+++	+	+	+	++	+	+++	+	+	++	+	+	+	++	+	+	++	+++	++	+	+	+
Parasites in serosal vein	+	++	+	++	+	++	+	++	+	+	++	+	+	++	+	+	+	++	+	+	+	++	++
Parasites in mesenteric V	++	++	+	+	++	++	++	+	+	+	+	+	++	+	+	+	+	+	+	+	+	+	+
Parasites in portal vein	+	+	+	-	-	+	+	++	-	-	+	-	-	-	+	-	+	+	+	+	-	+	+
Parasites in hepatic sinusoids	+	+	-	+	-	+	+	+	-	-	++	-	-	-	++	-	+	+	+	+	-	+	+
Parasites in adrenal sinusoids	+	+++	+	-	-	-	++	-	-	+	-	-	+	-	-	+	-	++	+++	-	-	++	-
Parasites *in splenic veins*	-	-	+	+	-	-	+	+	+++	-	+	+	-	-	-	-	+	+	-	-	+	-	-
Parasites *in subcapsular veins*	++−	++	-	-	-	-	-	++	-	-	-	-	-	-	-	-	-	-	-	-	-	-	-
Bile pigment deposition	++	++	-	+	-	+++	-	+++	+	-	++	-	+	-	++	-	-	+	+	+	-	+	+
Hemosiderin pigment	+++	++	-	++	+	++	-	+++	++	-	++	-	+	-	++	+	+	++	++	+	+	+	+
Venous hypertrophy	++	++	-	-	++	-	++	++	-	-	++	-	+	-	++	-	+	++	++	-	-	++	-
Obliterative endophlebitis	+	+	-	-	+	-	-	+	-	-	+	-	-	-	++	-	-	++	+	-	-	-	-
Villous atrophy		+	-	-	+	+	-	+	++	-	+	-	-	+	-	-	-	++	-	-	-	-	-

F: female M: male A: adult Y: young NA: not analyzed ND: not determined N: negative + mild ++ moderate +++ severe.

3.2. Histopathological Examination

Adult schistosomes were found in 43% (23/54) of the swans. In these cases, one or more adult worms were detected in the veins but not in the arteries. Adult worms were found in the lumen of the mesenteric veins, serosal veins, portal veins, testicular veins, capillaries of the intestinal lamina propria, and sinusoids of the adrenal gland, spleen and liver. Macrophages containing brownish pigment were occasionally seen in the parenchyma surrounding the worms, most commonly in the splenic veins and the hepatic sinusoids. Some affected veins, mainly the serosal and mesenteric veins, showed endophlebitis, irregular intimal thickening due to the infiltration of inflammatory cells, and hypertrophy of the muscular fibers in the tunica media.

3.2.1. Intestine

Numerous sections of adult schistosomes were found in the mesenteric and serosal veins throughout the intestine in all 23 infected birds, being the ileum, caecum, and colon the most affected areas. Vessels containing adult schistosomes showed endophlebitis characterized by myointimal hyperplasia, with infiltration of plasma cells, heterophils, and eosinophils in the surrounding tissues (Figure 1A,B). In 12 swans, the mesenteric and serosal veins, along with the veins between the muscular layers of the intestine, exhibited nodular hypertrophy of the tunica media. Eight swans suffered from obliterative endophlebitis with complete occlusion of the venous lumen (Figure 1C). Superficial enteritis was present in eight birds, and mild to severe villous atrophy was observed in association with numerous parasitic eggs in the lamina propria (in both the small and large intestine) have been observed by microscopical or histological evidence. The eggs were surrounded by venous congestion and diffuse infiltration of the lamina propria, with a variable number of lymphocytes and a few plasma cells, heterophils, and eosinophils (Figure 1D).

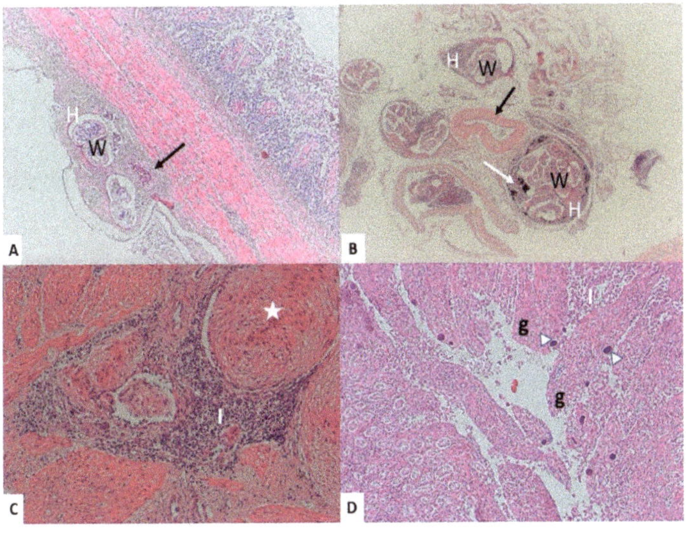

Figure 1. Effect of the parasite in the intestine. (**A**) Adult worms (W) are seen in the thickened walls of the serosal vein (H). Note the normal thickness of the artery (black arrow). (**B**) Brownish pigment–laden macrophages (white arrow) around the worm (W) in the thickened wall of the mesenteric veins (H). (**C**) The vein lumen was almost occluded due to marked myointimal hyperplasia in the veins of the muscular layer of the intestine (white star), with perivascular inflammatory reaction (I). (**D**) Several schistosome eggs (white arrowheads) present in the intestinal lamina propria and surrounded by an inflammatory reaction of lymphocytes and plasma cells (I); the intestinal villi are markedly blunted (g). Hematoxylin and eosin stain (100×).

3.2.2. Liver

Adult worms were found in the portal veins and hepatic sinusoids of 14 birds. In five cases, mild to severe inflammatory reactions were observed around the parasites or eggs in the hepatic parenchyma, with degeneration of the hepatic cells and infiltration of a large number of inflammatory cells in the hepatic sinusoids and the portal triads (Figure 2A,B). Fourteen swans had areas of *bile pigment deposition* (biliverdin) in the liver parenchyma, which stained positively with Hall's stain (Figure 2C). In addition, mild to marked deposition of hemosiderin pigment, positive on Berlin blue staining, was apparent in the liver of 18 swans (Figure 2D).

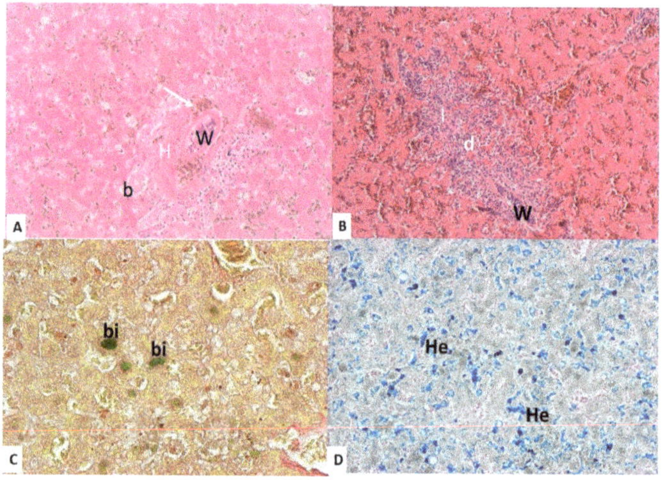

Figure 2. Effect of the parasite in the liver. (**A**) Adult worms (W) present in the thickened walled of the portal vein (H) with hemosiderin pigment deposition (white arrow) and bile duct hyperplasia (b). (**B**) Schistosome parasite (W) found in the hepatic sinusoids surrounded by degenerated hepatocyte (d) and massive inflammatory reaction (I). Hematoxylin and eosin stain (100×). (**C**) Emerald green–colored clumps of bile pigment (bi), Hall stain (400×). (**D**) Macrophages laden with bluish pigment (He), Berlin blue stain (100×).

3.2.3. Adrenal Glands

Numerous sections of adult schistosomes were observed within the adrenal sinusoids of 10 swans, and some sinusoids were completely occluded, resulting in pressure on the surrounding cells (Figure 3A). An inflammatory reaction was seen around the worms in six birds, with infiltration of lymphocytes and plasma cells and degeneration of the adrenal gland cells (Figure 3B).

3.2.4. Spleen

Adult worms were present in the subcapsular sinusoids and splenic veins of 10 swans (Figure 3C). Furthermore, mild to marked deposition of hemosiderin pigment was reported in the spleen of 18 swans (Figure 2D).

3.2.5. Testes

Multiple adult worms were found in the superficial subcapsular veins underneath the tunica albuginea in three swans. In these cases, infiltration of inflammatory cells, predominantly lymphocytes, macrophages, and a few heterophils, was seen in the surrounding parenchyma (Figure 3D).

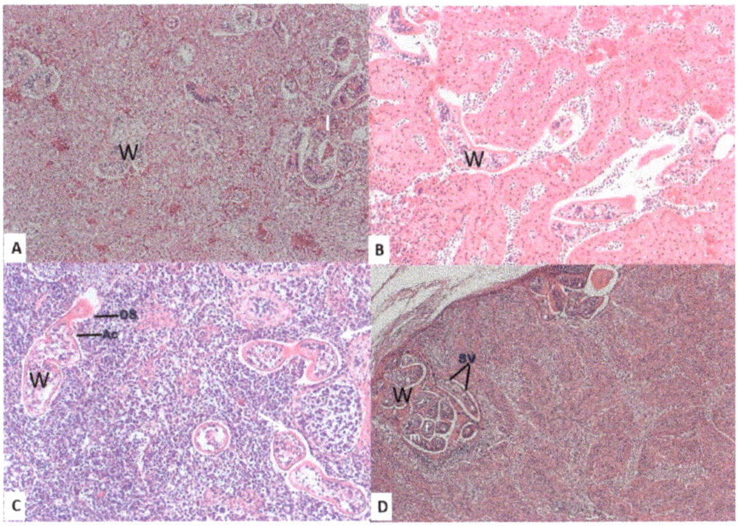

Figure 3. Effect of the parasite in the adrenal gland, spleen, and testis. (**A**, **B**) Multiple cross-sections of adult worms (W) found in the sinusoids of the adrenal gland surrounded by infiltration of mononuclear inflammatory cells (I). (**C**) Adult worms (W) found in the splenic veins. Note the oral sucker (Os) and acetabulum (Ac) of the parasite. (**D**) Multiple cross-sections of adult schistosomes (W) completely occlude the subcapsular veins of the testis and were surrounded by the infiltration of mononuclear inflammatory cells (I). Note the seminal vesicles of the parasite (Sv) and the presence of female (f) in the ventral groove of the male (m) parasite. Hematoxylin and eosin stain (100×).

3.3. Parasitological Findings

Based on the available information, including the species of the affected bird and its location, the morphological characteristics of the schistosome worm and eggs in the intestinal lamina propria, and pathological findings, the schistosomes of the present study were assumed to be *A. visceralis*. The death of the investigated swans was suspected to be due to obstructive phlebitis associated with the suspected parasite. Eggs were found abundantly in the intestinal lamina propria and were mostly ovoid to asymmetrical in shape (Figure 1D); however, confirmation at the species level requires further molecular investigation. Moreover, the schistosome flukes occurred in abundance in the veins of different internal organs with varying morphological characteristics, i.e., oral sucker, posterior sucker, or acetabulum), seminal vesicles, and testis (Figure 3C). Some adult schistosome parasites were found in pairs, with the male carrying the female in its ventral groove or gynecophoric canal (Figure 3D).

4. Discussion

Schistosomes are considered to be highly pathogenic in migratory waterfowl [37]. Because the worm is very small and located in the blood vessels, schistosomes in whooper swans can be overlooked on gross necropsy [9,36]. It should be stressed that Swimmer's itch is considered an emerging disease in various parts of the world, resulting in various nervous or pulmonary symptoms on the basis of the infecting species [38]. Furthermore, avian schistosomes have been considered the most neglected parasitic zoonosis among aquatic birds worldwide [23]. To the best of our knowledge, there are no published studies describing the pathological effects of schistosome infection in whooper swans in Japan. Thus, this study provides a novel contribution to this research topic and adds knowledge on a potentially zoonotic parasite.

We detected adult schistosomes in 43% (23/54) of whooper swans on necropsy; the worms were mostly present in the veins of the large and small intestine, liver, adrenal gland, spleen, and testis.

These findings are consistent with previous studies reporting that vascular lesions caused by avian schistosome infection in birds are comparable with lesions observed in visceral schistosomiasis in mammals [9,13,20]. Given the fact that this study was carried out during the period 2005–2007, we planned to perform molecular characterization of the parasite but there were no available samples to do perform this step. In Japan, Hayashi et al. (2017) [13] detected for the first time *A. visceralis* in the capillaries of several organs of whooper swans using molecular methods, without microscopical or histological evidence of eggs or worm. Meanwhile, studies performed in Iceland [28,29] and North America [30] identified vascular lesions caused by schistosomes in whooper swans and tundra swans, respectively. We believe that emaciation and weakness in all 23 infected swans may have resulted from the severe vascular effects associated with schistosome infection, namely, the obstruction of venous return in the mesenteric, intestinal, splenic, and portal veins as well as enteropathy. Both adult schistosomes and eggs contributed to the enteropathy: the adults caused obliterative vascular lesions, whereas the migration of the eggs led to enteritis with villous atrophy [19]. However, in cases such as these, it is not clear whether the parasites are the cause of emaciation [31,39], as important data, such as bodyweight and parasitic load of healthy birds for comparison, are missing [15]. We did not have data on the body weight and parasitic load of apparently healthy whooper swans from this region for comparison. In the current study, the blood flukes infecting the whooper swan were assumed to likely be *A. visceralis*, on the basis on the species of the affected bird, morphological characteristics of the worm and eggs found in the internal organs, and pathological findings associated with their presence in the blood vessels of different organs in both adult and juvenile birds. This method of identification was previously accepted and is in agreement with the findings of Kolářová et al. (2010) [36]. However, further accurate identification methods (i.e., molecular characterization methods are still needed. We were unable to describe the morphological features of adult worms in this study because of the difficulty in obtaining intact specimens: adult worms are very small and are usually present only in the lumen of affected veins, which is consistent with some previous reports [11,19]. Furthermore, these findings are supported by the results from Hayashi et al. (2017) [13], who did not detect egg-like structures of the schistosome in the swans but there was no any gross abnormality or necrosis in the organs of affected swans and assumed that schistosomes did not cause severe damage to the swans examined. Similarly, a recent study reported unidentified schistosomes and their eggs only by histopathological examination [18]. In this study, flukes were found inside the lumen of blood vessels of the muscular layer and in the mucosa of the esophagus, intestine, and caeca but with a slight inflammatory response in only three cases, represented by hemorrhage and infiltration of some inflammatory cells, such as lymphocytes and heterophiles [18]. In contrast, Brant (2007) [24] detected adult worms and egg-tissue debris in a nodule of the inferior mesenteric vein and suggested that, to identify the species of parasite, it is important to investigate the correlation between the pathological lesions and the general condition of the swans, as well as to determine the presence or absence of eggs. The disease features were similar to those described in several reports of schistosome infection in swans from Europe and Australia, including the black swan (*Cygnus atratus*) and the mute swan (*Cygnus olor*) in Australia [27,40] and the whooper swan in Europe [27]. Our results indicated that the number of young birds affected was higher than the numbers of adults, i.e., 61% (14/23) of affected swans were immature. The higher prevalence of infection in the young birds might be due to lower immunity, as compared with the increased immunity in adults that results from repeated exposure to schistosome parasites [41]. In the present study, most infected swans 78% (18/23) showed endophlebitis of the veins containing adult worms, with infiltration of leukocytes into the surrounding tissues. This may have resulted from the irritation of the vessel walls caused by the worms, which led to myointimal hyperplasia and, in some instances, to occlusion of the affected blood vessels. This concept and previous findings are consistent with the reports of Warren (1977) [42], Bolhuis et al. (2004) [19], and Kolářová et al. (2001) [43], all of whom suggested that viable adult schistosomes cause proliferation of the vascular intima either via mechanical injury to the intima or via the secretion of antigens as an immune (allergic) reaction against the schistosomes. Bolhuis et al. (2004) [19] revealed the occurrence of *Trichobilharzia* sp. in five of eight mute swans, whereas pathological lesions including moderate to severe, diffuse, hyperplastic endophlebitis were reported in the intestinal veins together with splenic and hepatic hemosiderosis [19]. In the current study, we did not find any fibrosis in the portal triad in the birds examined. This is consistent with the findings of Kolářová et al. (2006) [15] but in contrast to those of Bolhuis et al. (2004) [19], who reported mild to extensive fibroplasia of the portal triads in mute swans and attributed this finding to the aberrant localization of female schistosomes in the bile ducts. Similarly, Wojcinski et al. (1987) [44] reported the same lesions in ducks infected with schistosomes but found no evidence of parasites in bile ducts, and Robinson and Maxie (1993) [20] reported that in mammals, severe cases of schistosomiasis might result in occlusion of the lumen of the veins, and lesions may extend to the intrahepatic branches of the portal vein, leading to prominent portal fibrosis. Bolhuis et al. (2004) [19] also reported the development of granulomas due to the severe perivascular inflammatory reaction around the veins harboring the adult parasite in the liver of juvenile and adult birds; in contrast, Brant (2007) [24] did not find any granulomas in the portal triads of infected swans.

In the present work, worm eggs were found multifocally in the lamina propria of the small and/or large intestine, and 35% (8/23) of swans showed mild to severe villous atrophy (villous blunting, fusion, and edema) and superficial enteritis, which might have resulted from the migration of schistosome eggs through the intestinal wall. This explanation is supported by a previous study conducted by Wojcinski et al. (1987) [44]. In addition, in their study, Bolhuis et al. (2004) [19] reported lymphocytic and granulocytic enteritis associated with the presence of eggs of schistosomes in the intestinal mucosa of examined swans. However, Horák et al. (2002) reported that in human schistosomiasis, some eggs fail to reach the intestinal lumen and are instead disseminated through the circulatory system to the liver, lungs, and other organs, where they cause reactions ranging from very mild to marked granulomatous inflammation. Robinson and Maxie (1993) [20] stated that schistosome eggs release antigens that induce a delayed hypersensitivity response and cause the formation of small granulomas, which are characterized by the infiltration of eosinophils, mononuclear leukocytes, and giant cells as well as reactive fibrosis. In the present study, we observed bile pigments and hemosiderin in the liver of 61% (14/23) and 78% (18/23) of whooper swans infected with avian schistosomes, respectively, whereas adult worms and/or eggs were detected in the liver of 61% (14/23) of infected swans. This indicates that cholestatic jaundice may be caused by avian schistosomiasis, as found by Akagami et al. (2010) [16]. Schistosomes were detected in the sinusoids of the adrenal gland in 44% (10/23) of swans in the present study; this finding has not previously been reported, except in one study by Hayashi et al. (2017) [13]. A unique finding of this study is the detection of worms in the sinusoids of the testes in 13% (3/23) of infected swans. We believe that the presence of parasites in the adrenal glands and in the testes was due to the migration of parasites through the vascular system of heavily infected birds.

5. Conclusions

In conclusion, our study provides interesting data that describe the pathological effects of schistosome infection, assumed to be *A. visceralis*, in whooper swans in Japan, which provides a novel contribution to this field of research. It could be suggested that these parasites were the cause of death in the infected swans in this study, because they were found in the blood vessels of all infected swans and caused obstructive phlebitis. Additional molecular studies on schistosome infection in whooper swans and in their snail intermediate hosts are required to better characterize the parasite species.

Author Contributions: M.S.A. and T.Y. involved in the conception of the research idea and methodology design and performed data analysis and interpretation. R.E.K., A.A.-B. and E.K.E. participated of the methodology, sampling, the laboratory work and data analysis and prepared the manuscript for publication. M.S.A., R.E.K., A.A.-B., T.Y. and E.K.E. contributed their scientific advice, prepared the manuscript for publication, and performed the revision. All authors have read and agreed to the published version of the manuscript.

Funding: This work was supported by the Taif University Researchers Supporting Program (Project number: TURSP-2020/151), Taif University, Saudi Arabia.

Acknowledgments: The authors sincerely thank the staff members of the rescue/rehabilitation centers for their efforts in the collection of swans. They also thank the members of the Department of Veterinary Pathology, Faculty of Applied Biological Science, Gifu University, and Biomedical Science Examination and Research Center, Okayama University of Science, Japan, for their support. The authors thank Taif University Researchers Supporting Program (Project number: TURSP-2020/151), Taif University, Saudi Arabia for their support.

Conflicts of Interest: The authors declare no conflict of interest.

References

1. Horak, P.; Mikes, L.; Lichtenbergova, L.; Skala, V.; Soldanova, M.; Brant, S.V. Avian schistosomes and outbreaks of cercarial dermatitis. *Clin. Microbiol. Rev.* **2015**, *28*, 165–190. [CrossRef] [PubMed]
2. Turjanicová, L.; Mikeš, L.; Pecková, M.; Horák, P. Antibody response of definitive hosts against antigens of two life stages of the neuropathogenic schistosome Trichobilharzia regenti. *Parasites Vectors* **2015**, *8*, 1–11. [CrossRef] [PubMed]
3. Azimov, D. *Schistosomes of Animals and Man*; Izdatel'stvo 'FAN': Taskhent, Uzbekistan, 1975.
4. Webster, B.L.; Southgate, V.R.; Littlewood, D.T. A revision of the interrelationships of Schistosoma including the recently described Schistosoma guineensis. *Int. J. Parasitol.* **2006**, *36*, 947–955. [CrossRef]
5. Atkinson, C.T.; Thomas, N.J.; Hunter, D.B. *Parasitic Diseases of Wild Birds*; John Wiley & Sons: Hoboken, NJ, USA, 2009.
6. Brant, S.V.; Loker, E.S. Molecular systematics of the avian schistosome genus Trichobilharzia (Trematoda: Schistosomatidae) in North America. *J. Parasitol.* **2009**, *95*, 941–963. [CrossRef] [PubMed]
7. Rudolfová, J. New findings of schistosomes in wildfowl and snails. *Helminthologia* **2001**, *38*, 248–249.
8. Skrjabin, K. Family Schistosomatidae Looss, 1899. *Trematodes Anim. Man* **1951**, *5*, 225–414.
9. Horak, P.; Kolarova, L.; Adema, C.M. Biology of the schistosome genus Trichobilharzia. *Adv. Parasitol.* **2002**, *52*, 155–233.
10. Farley, J. A review of the family Schistosomatidae: Excluding the genus Schistosoma from mammals. *J. Helminthol.* **1971**, *45*, 289–320. [CrossRef]
11. Khalil, L. Family Schistosomatidae Stiles & Hassall, 1898. *Keys Trematoda* **2002**, *1*, 419–432.
12. McLaren, D.J.; Hockley, D.J. Blood flukes have a double outer membrane. *Nature* **1977**, *269*, 147–149. [CrossRef]
13. Hayashi, K.; Ichikawa-Seki, M.; Ohari, Y.; Mohanta, U.K.; Aita, J.; Satoh, H.; Ehara, S.; Tokashiki, M.; Shiroma, T.; Azuta, A.; et al. First detection of Allobilharzia visceralis (Schistosomatidae, Trematoda) from Cygnus cygnus in Japan. *Parasitol. Int.* **2017**, *66*, 925–929. [CrossRef]
14. Randall, C.; Reece, R.L. *Color Atlas of Avian Histopathology*; Mosby-Wolfe: London, UK; Baltimore, MD, USA, 1996.
15. Kolarova, L.; Rudolfova, J.; Hampl, V.; Skirnisson, K. Allobilharzia visceralis gen. nov., sp. nov. (Schistosomatidae-Trematoda) from Cygnus cygnus (L.) (Anatidae). *Parasitol. Int.* **2006**, *55*, 179–186. [PubMed]
16. Akagami, M.; Nakamura, K.; Nishino, H.; Seki, S.; Shimizu, H.; Yamamoto, Y. Pathogenesis of venous hypertrophy associated with schistosomiasis in whooper swans (Cygnus cygnus) in Japan. *Avian Dis.* **2010**, *54*, 146–150. [CrossRef] [PubMed]
17. Paré, J.A.; Black, S.R. Schistosomiasis in a collection of captive Chilean flamingos (Phoenicopterus chilensis). *J. Avian Med. Surg.* **1999**, 187–191.
18. Oyarzún-Ruiz, P.; Muñoz, P.; Paredes, E.; Valenzuela, G.; Ruiz, J. Gastrointestinal helminths and related histopathological lesions in black-necked swans Cygnus melancoryphus from the Carlos Anwandter Nature Sanctuary, Southern Chile. *Rev. Bras. De Parasitol. Vet.* **2019**, *28*, 613–624. [CrossRef] [PubMed]
19. van Bolhuis, G.H.; Rijks, J.M.; Dorrestein, G.M.; Rudolfova, J.; van Dijk, M.; Kuiken, T. Obliterative endophlebitis in mute swans (Cygnus olor) caused by Trichobilharzia sp. (Digenea: Schistosomatidae) infection. *Vet. Pathol.* **2004**, *41*, 658–665. [PubMed]
20. Robinson, W.F.; Maxie, M.G. The cardiovascular system. In *Pathology of Domestic Animals*, 4th ed.; Jubb, K.V.F., Kennedy, P.C., Palmer, N., Eds.; Academic Press: San Diego, CA, USA, 1993; Volume 3, pp. 1–100.
21. Pence, D.B.; RHODES, M.J. Trichobilharzia physellae (Digenea: Schistosomatidae) from endemic waterfowl on the high plains of Texas. *J. Wildl. Dis.* **1982**, *18*, 69–74. [CrossRef]
22. Leedom, W.S.; Short, R.B. Cercaria pomaceae sp. n., a dermatitis-producing schistosome cercaria from Pomacea paludosa, the Florida apple snail. *J. Parasitol.* **1981**, 257–261. [CrossRef]

23. Lashaki, E.K.; Teshnizi, S.H.; Gholami, S.; Fakhar, M.; Brant, S.V.; Dodangeh, S. Global prevalence status of avian schistosomes: A systematic review with meta-analysis. *Parasite Epidemiol. Control* **2020**, *9*, e00142. [CrossRef]
24. Brant, S.V. The occurrence of the avian schistosome Allobilharzia visceralis Kolakrova, Rudolfova, Hampl et Skirnisson, 2006 (Schistosomatidae) in the tundra swan, Cygnus columbianus (Anatidae), from North America. *Folia Parasitol (Praha)* **2007**, *54*, 99–104. [CrossRef]
25. Jouet, D.; Ferte, H.; Hologne, C.; Kaltenbach, M.L.; Depaquit, J. Avian schistosomes in French aquatic birds: A molecular approach. *J. Helminthol.* **2009**, *83*, 181–189. [CrossRef] [PubMed]
26. Chamot, E.; Toscani, L.; Rougemont, A. Public health importance and risk factors for cercarial dermatitis associated with swimming in Lake Leman at Geneva, Switzerland. *Epidemiol. Infect.* **1998**, *120*, 305–314. [CrossRef] [PubMed]
27. Kolárová, L. Avian schistosomes of the genus Trichobilharzia in final hosts in Europe. *Bull. Scand. Soc. Parasitol.* **2005**, *14*, 85–86.
28. Kolarova, L.; Skirnisson, K.; Horak, P. Schistosome cercariae as the causative agent of swimmer's itch in Iceland. *J. Helminthol.* **1999**, *73*, 215–220. [CrossRef] [PubMed]
29. Huelsenbeck, J.P.; Ronquist, F. MRBAYES: Bayesian inference of phylogenetic trees. *Bioinformatics* **2001**, *17*, 754–755. [CrossRef]
30. Petersen, A. *Íslenskir Fuglar (Icelandic Birds.)*; Vaka-Helgafell: Reykjavík, Iceland, 1998.
31. Wobeser, G.A. *Diseases of Wild Waterfowl*; Springer Science & Business Media: New York, NY, USA, 2012.
32. Blankespoor, H.; Reimink, R. The Control of Swimmer's Itch in Michigan: Past, Present, and Future. *Mich. Acad.* **1991**, *24*, 7–23.
33. Cramp, S.; Perrins, C. *The Birds of the Western Palearctic*; Oxford University Press: Oxford, UK, 1977; Volumes 1–9.
34. Bancroft, J.D.; Gamble, M. *Theory and Practice of Histological Techniques*; Elsevier Health Sciences: Amsterdam, The Netherlands, 2008.
35. Watanaba, Y.; Sakaguchi, H.; Hosoda, Y. *The Methods of Preparing Histologic Sections*, 6th ed.; Igaku Shoin Company Ltd.: Tokyo, Japan, 1992; pp. 81–140.
36. Kolarova, L.; Horak, P.; Skirnisson, K. Methodical approaches in the identification of areas with a potential risk of infection by bird schistosomes causing cercarial dermatitis. *J. Helminthol.* **2010**, *84*, 327–335. [CrossRef]
37. Soulsby, E. *Helminths Arthropods and Protozoa of Domesticated Animals*; Baillière Tindall: London, UK, 1982.
38. Picot, H.; Bourdeau, P.; Bardet, R.; Kerjan, A.; Piriou, M.; Le, A.G.; Bayssade-Dufour, C.; Chabasse, D.; Mott, K. Cercarial dermatitis in Europe: A new public health problem? *Bull. World Health Organ.* **1996**, *74*, 159–163.
39. Pennycott, T.W. Lead poisoning and parasitism in a flock of mute swans (Cygnus olor) in Scotland. *Vet. Rec.* **1998**, *142*, 13–17. [CrossRef] [PubMed]
40. Palmer, D.; Ossent, P. Nasal schistosomiasis in mute swans in Switzerland. *Rev. Suisse De Zool.* **1984**, *91*, 709–715. [CrossRef]
41. Guth, B.; Blankespoor, H.; Reimink, R.; Johnson, W. Prevalence of dermatitis-producing schistosomes in natural bird populations of lower Michigan. *Proc. Helminthol. Soc. Wash.* **1979**, *46*, 58–63.
42. Warren, K.S. Modulation of immunopathology and disease in schistosomiasis. *Am. J. Trop. Med. Hyg.* **1977**, *26*, 113–119. [CrossRef] [PubMed]
43. Kolarova, L.; Horak, P.; Cada, F. Histopathology of CNS and nasal infections caused by Trichobilharzia regenti in vertebrates. *Parasitol. Res.* **2001**, *87*, 644–650. [PubMed]
44. Wojcinski, Z.W.; Barker, I.K.; Hunter, D.B.; Lumsden, H. An outbreak of schistosomiasis in Atlantic brant geese, Branta bernicla hrota. *J. Wildl. Dis.* **1987**, *23*, 248–255. [CrossRef]

animals

MDPI

Article

Genomic Characterization of *Salmonella* Minnesota Clonal Lineages Associated with Poultry Production in Brazil

Diéssy Kipper [1], Laura M. Carroll [2], Andrea K. Mascitti [1], André F. Streck [3], André S. K. Fonseca [4], Nilo Ikuta [4] and Vagner R. Lunge [1,4,*]

1 Laboratório de Diagnóstico Molecular, Universidade Luterana do Brasil (ULBRA), Canoas, Rio Grande do Sul 92425-020, Brazil; diessykipper@hotmail.com (D.K.); andreakaroline88@hotmail.com (A.K.M.)
2 Department of Food Science, Cornell University, Ithaca, New York, NY 14850, USA; laura.carroll@embl.de
3 Laboratório de Diagnóstico em Medicina Veterinária, Universidade de Caxias do Sul (UCS), Caxias do Sul, Rio Grande do Sul 95070-560, Brazil; afstreck@ucs.br
4 Simbios Biotecnologia, Cachoeirinha, Rio Grande do Sul 94940-030, Brazil; fonseca@simbios.com.br (A.S.K.F.); ikuta@simbios.com.br (N.I.)
* Correspondence: vagner.lunge@gmail.com; Tel.: +55-5199984-1770

Received: 29 September 2020; Accepted: 3 November 2020; Published: 5 November 2020

check for updates

Simple Summary: *Salmonella* is a leading cause of foodborne illnesses and a global public health concern. *Salmonella enterica* serotype Minnesota has been increasingly isolated from Brazilian poultry farms. The present study investigated the phylogenetic relationships, evolution and genetic characteristics of *S.* Minnesota isolates from Brazilian poultry farms. The results demonstrated two main *S.* Minnesota lineages in the poultry production chain from Brazil, both presenting genes for antibiotic resistance and virulence. The present study also provides insights into the temporal evolution, population structure, and genetic characteristics of the two *S.* Minnesota lineages disseminated in Brazilian poultry farms.

Abstract: *Salmonella* serotype Minnesota has been increasingly detected in Brazilian poultry farms and food products (chicken meat, eggs) in recent years. In addition, *S.* Minnesota isolates from poultry are generally resistant to several antibiotics and persistent in farm environments. The present study aimed to assess phylogenomic diversity of *S.* Minnesota isolates from the poultry production chain in Brazil. In total, 107 worldwide *S.* Minnesota whole genomes (including 12 from Brazil) were analyzed using a comparative approach. Phylogenetic analysis demonstrated two clades more related to poultry production in Brazil: *S.* Minnesota poultry lineages I and II (SM-PLI and SM-PLII). Phylodynamic analysis demonstrated that SM-PLI had a common ancestor in 1915, while SM–PLII originated circa 1971. SM-PLII encompassed a higher number of isolates and presented a recent increase in effective population size (mainly from 2009 to 2012). Plasmids IncA/C2 and ColRNA, antimicrobial resistance genes (*aph(3′)-Ia*, *blaCMY-2*, *qnrB19*, *sul2*, and *tet(A)*) and mainly a virulence genetic cluster (including the yersiniabactin operon) were detected in isolates from SM-PLI and/or SM-PLII. This study demonstrates the dissemination of two distinct *S.* Minnesota lineages with high resistance to antibiotics and important virulence genetic clusters in Brazilian poultry farms.

Keywords: phylodynamic; whole-genome sequencing (WGS); chicken; antimicrobial resistance genes; virulence genetic cluster

1. Introduction

Salmonella is a leading cause of foodborne illnesses and a global public health concern [1]. It is a Gram-negative, rod-shaped facultative anaerobic bacterium belonging to the family Enterobacteriaceae. The genus *Salmonella* is divided into two species (*Salmonella enterica* and *Salmonella bongori*), but it is also classified into several serotypes by immunological assays. So far, more than 2600 serotypes have already been identified within the *Salmonella* genus worldwide, many of them associated with enteric and systemic diseases in domestic animals and humans [2].

In poultry production, *Salmonella* is disseminated into the flocks and farm environments via the avian feces. Other animals may become infected through contaminated poultry litter or close contact with an infected bird. High *Salmonella* bacterial content in the enteric tract of broilers and layers can result in the contamination of chicken meat, eggs, and other poultry products in slaughterhouses [3].

Salmonella enterica serotype Minnesota was first isolated in a turkey farm from Minnesota (United States) in 1936 [4]. Since then, this serotype has been detected in different sources, including the natural environment, plants, animal-producing farms, and foods [5–7]. Poultry products seem to be an important source of human infection with this bacterial foodborne pathogen. In addition, bacteriological analyses have demonstrated that *S.* Minnesota isolates are resistant to antibiotics, including extended-spectrum cephalosporins [8].

In Brazil, *S.* Minnesota has been frequently detected on poultry farms (10% to 30%) since the beginning of this century [9,10]. In addition to the farm environment, *S.* Minnesota has also been detected in slaughterhouses and foods [10]. A very high frequency (reaching 86.6%) was observed in several poultry farms from the Brazilian Center West Region around 2010 [6]. *S.* Minnesota was even detected in chicken carcasses in Brazilian markets, as well as in poultry products exported to Portugal [8,11]. The present study aimed to evaluate the population structure, phylogenetic relationships, temporal evolution, and genetic characteristics (e.g., plasmids and antibiotic resistance and virulence genes) of the *S.* Minnesota strains isolated from Brazilian poultry production chain.

2. Material and Methods

2.1. Bacterial Isolates and Molecular Biology Assays

Three *S.* Minnesota isolates were obtained from poultry farms in the state of Mato Grosso do Sul, Center West Region from Brazil, in 2018 (Table S1). Single colonies of each isolate were removed from xylose lysine desoxycholate (XLD) agar plates and placed in brain heart infusion (BHI) broth, following overnight incubation at 35 °C. DNA was extracted using a commercial method according to the manufacturer's instructions (NewGene, Simbios Biotecnologia, Cachoeirinha, RS, Brazil) and was further characterized by PCR/sequencing to confirm the genus *Salmonella* and serotype Minnesota with the following experimental approaches: (i) *invA* real-time PCR for *Salmonella* detection (reagents NewGene SALAmp, Simbios Biotecnologia, Cachoeirinha, RS, Brazil), and (ii) *rrn*H operon intergenic sequence ribotyping (ISR) analysis for serotype assignment [12].

2.2. Whole-Genome Sequencing

The PureLink® Genomic DNA Mini Kit was used to extract DNA following the manufacturer's instructions (Thermo Fisher Scientific, Waltham, MA, USA), and DNA was visualized on a 2% agarose gel stained with ethidium bromide. Sequencing libraries were prepared using the Nextera XT kit (Illumina, Inc., San Diego, CA, USA). DNA concentration was adjusted to 0.2 ng/µL, and sequencing was performed on an Illumina NextSeq platform, using 150 bp paired-end reads (Wadsworth Center, New York State Department of Health (NYSDOH), Albany, NY, USA).

2.3. Acquisition of Genomic Data and in Silico Identification of Genetic Elements

Trimmomatic version 0.33 [13] was used to trim raw Illumina sequence reads and remove low-quality bases. The quality of the resulting trimmed reads was assessed using FastQC version

0.11.2 [14] prior to de novo assembly using SPAdes version 3.6.0 [15]. The quality of draft genomes was evaluated using QUAST version 5.0.2 [16], and per-base average coverage was estimated by mapping each isolate's trimmed reads to its respective assembled contigs using BBmap version 38.26 [17] and Samtools version 1.9 [18]. Assemblies were annotated using Prokka version 1.12 [19]. SISTR version 0.3.1 [20] was used to perform in silico serotyping, and each isolate was also assigned to a sequence type (ST) using seven-gene multi-locus sequence typing (MLST; https://github.com/tseemann/mlst).

The isolates sequenced here were analyzed together with publicly available *S.* Minnesota genomes. Among the genome sequences available in the National Center for Biotechnology Information's (NCBI's) Sequence Read Archive (SRA) database [21], 104 were selected to represent as many countries, sources, and years as possible and were downloaded. These whole-genome sequences (WGS), plus the three new Brazilian *S.* Minnesota sequenced here, were used in all analyses (Table S1).

ABRicate version 0.8 (https://github.com/tseemann/abricate) was used to detect antimicrobial resistance genes, virulence factors, and plasmid replicons in each assembled genome, using the ResFinder database [22], Virulence Factor Database (VFDB) [23], and PlasmidFinder [24] database, respectively (accessed 11 June 2018). *Salmonella* pathogenicity islands (SPIs) were additionally detected in each genome using the nucleotide Basic Local Alignment Search Tool (BLASTN) [25]. For all searches, minimum nucleotide identity and coverage thresholds of 75% and 50% were used, respectively.

2.4. Identification of Single-Nucleotide Polymorphisms (SNPs) and Construction of Maximum Likelihood Phylogenies

Single-nucleotide polymorphisms (SNPs) were identified among all 107 *S.* Minnesota assemblies (i.e., the three isolates sequenced here, plus 104 genomes downloaded from NCBI; Table S1) using kSNP3 version 3.1 [26] and the optimal *k*-mer size determined by Kchooser ($k = 19$). The maximum parsimony tree produced by kSNP3 was used to cluster the genomes on the basis of the core SNPs identified.

The CFSAN SNP Pipeline was used to identify high-quality SNPs (hqSNPs) using trimmed Illumina reads associated with two different clusters, the first with the 28 SM-LI (*Salmonella* Minnesota lineage I) isolates and the second with the 44 SM-LII (*Salmonella* Minnesota lineage II) isolates. The genome assembly of isolate SRR1646144_UK_2012 was used as reference (i.e., assembly with N50 > 100,000 nt and <50 contigs). The resulting SNP matrix of preserved sites was used to build a phylogeny using the maximum likelihood (ML) method implemented in W-IQ-TREE (the IQ-TREE web server; accessed 11 December 2019) [27], using ModelFinder to select the optimal substitution model [28] and 1000 replicates of the UltraFast bootstrap approximation [29].

2.5. Tip-Dated Evolutionary Analysis

The linear regression approach implemented in TempEst version 1.5 [30] was used to evaluate the temporal signal and clock-likeness of the ML phylogenies constructed using hqSNPs detected among the SM-LI and SM-LII genomes. The resulting R^2 value produced by TempEst was 0.45 for SM-LI and 0.53 for SM-LII. Thus, these two separate datasets were queried individually in subsequent temporal analyses.

A tip-dated phylogeny was constructed using BEAUti version 1.8.2 and BEAST version 1.8.2 [31], using combinations of the general time reversible (GTR) model [32] and one of (i) a strict clock and coalescent constant size population model, (ii) a strict clock and coalescent Bayesian skyline model, (iii) a lognormal relaxed clock and coalescent constant size population model, and (iv) a lognormal relaxed clock and coalescent Bayesian skyline model, for multiple datasets including SM-LI and SM-LII. For all models, the initial clock rate was set to 2.1×10^{-7} substitutions/site/year.

The Markov chain Monte Carlo (MCMC) algorithm implemented in BEAST was run for 1×10^9 generations, and parameters were logged every 1×10^5 generations. The optimal model (i.e., the strict clock and coalescent Bayesian skyline model) was identified using marginal likelihood estimates obtained via path-sampling using 10 steps of at least 1×10^9 generations, and by assessing effective sample size (ESS) values and mixing of parameters in Tracer version 1.6.0 [33]. Five independent

MCMC runs using the optimal model were performed, using chain lengths of 1×10^9 generations, sampling every 1×10^5 generations. The resulting log files were viewed in Tracer to ensure that ESS values were sufficiently high (i.e., >200 for all parameters) and that all parameters had mixed adequately with 10% burn-in. LogCombiner version 1.8.3 was used to combine the log and tree files of five independent runs, and TreeAnnotator version 1.8.2 [34] was used to construct a maximum clade credibility (MCC) tree, using 10% burn-in and common ancestor node heights. FigTree version 1.4.2 (http://tree.bio.ed.ac.uk/software/figtree/) was used to annotate the resulting phylogeny, using bars to denote 95% highest posterior density (HPD) intervals for node heights and branch labels to denote posterior probabilities.

2.6. Identification of Clade-Associated Genes within S. Minnesota

Roary version 3.12.0 [35] was used to identify orthologous genes present in the *S.* Minnesota core and pan genome, using a minimum protein BLAST (BLASTP) identity value of 90% (-i 90). Scoary version 1.6.14 [36] was used to identify genes associated with each of two clades (i.e., SM-PLI (*Salmonella* Minnesota poultry lineage I) and SM-PLII (*Salmonella* Minnesota poultry lineage II)) within the *S.* Minnesota lineages, using a *p*-value cutoff of 0.05.

3. Results

3.1. WGS Data of S. Minnesota and Sequence Types (STs)

Raw sequencing reads obtained in this study and downloaded from NCBI (Table S1) were assembled with a median of 67 contigs larger than 1 kb (ranging from 28 to 457 kb), a median N50 of 227,625 bp (ranging from 21,874 to 429,939 bp), and median average coverage of 70× (ranging from 20× to 345×). The median length of the 107 assembled *S.* Minnesota genomes (made of contigs > 1000 bp) was 4.81 Mbp (ranging from 4.49 to 5.18 Mbp). In silico analysis showed that 102 sequences matched to ST 548 and five sequences to ST 285 (Table S1). The difference between ST 548 and ST 285 was in one single-nucleotide polymorphism of the *hisD* gene.

3.2. S. Minnesota Isolates of Brazilian Origin Are Confined to Two Lineages

A maximum parsimony phylogeny constructed using core SNPs (n = 39,752) identified among all 107 *S.* Minnesota genomes revealed the distribution of all sequences in several clusters with no strong relationship to specific countries and sources (poultry, human, environment, food, animal feed, and livestock). According to this phylogeny, Brazilian isolates were grouped into two major specific clusters, here called *Salmonella* Minnesota lineages I and II (SM-LI and SM-LII) (Figure 1).

Phylogenomic relationships among the two clusters (SM-LI and SM-LII) were, thus, further investigated. Using the high-quality SNP (hqSNP) calling approach implemented in the CFSAN SNP Pipeline, the maximum likelihood (ML) phylogeny clearly demonstrated that Brazilian genomes clustered into SM-LI and SM-LII. SM-LI included a total of 28 isolates: 11 from the United States, five from Brazil, five from Mexico, three from the United Kingdom, three from Haiti, and one from the Netherlands. This lineage differed by 0–322 pairwise hqSNPs (median 160) and included *S.* Minnesota isolates from four different sources: poultry, food, human, and the environment. A subclade within this lineage, referred to here as SM-PLI, contained eight genomes, including five from Brazil, two from the United States, and one from the Netherlands, and differed by 0–74 pairwise hqSNPs (median 50). These isolates were derived from different sources, including five from poultry, two from foods, and one from human feces (Figure 2A). SM-LII included 44 isolates: 23 from the United Kingdom, 11 from the Portugal, seven from Brazil, and three from Chile. This second lineage differed by 0–202 pairwise hqSNPs (median 37) and included isolates from three different sources: 21 from poultry, 20 from food, and three from humans. This whole clade is referred to hereafter as SM-PLII, since it included mainly poultry isolates (Figure 2B).

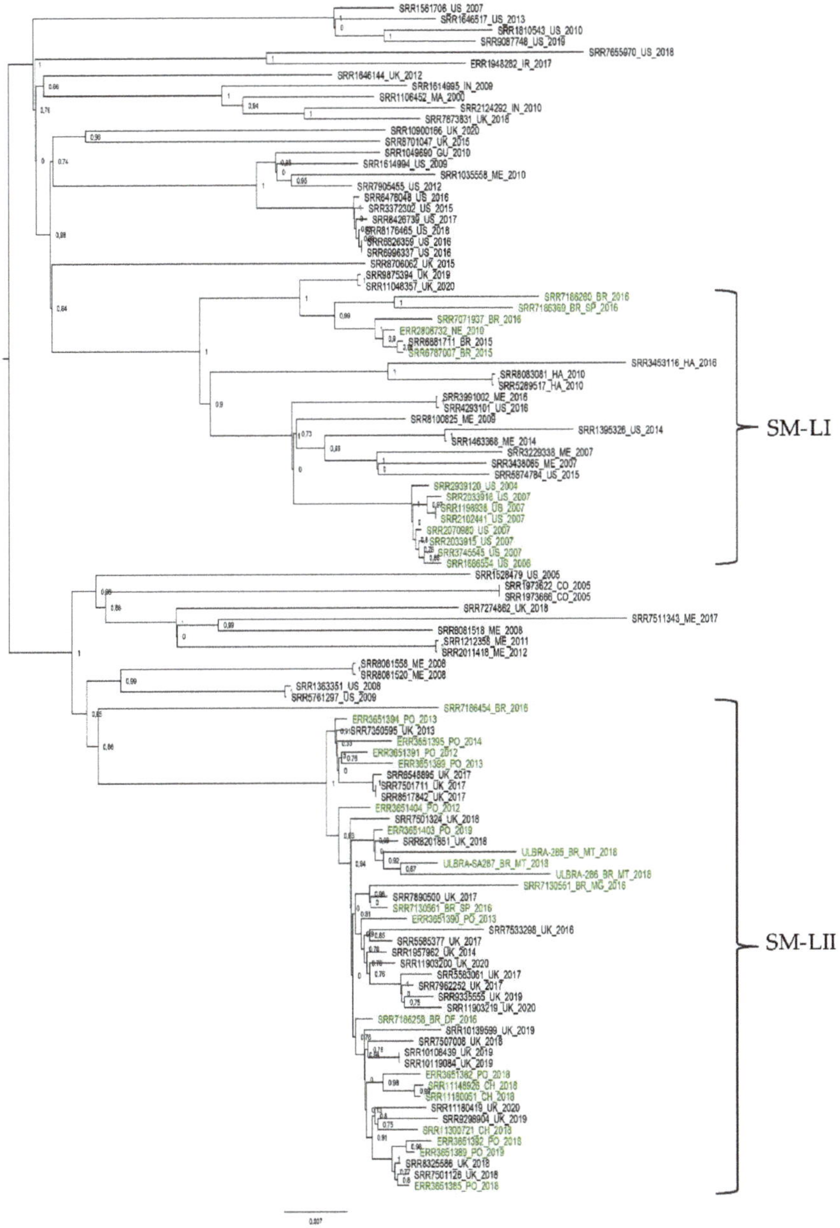

Figure 1. Maximum parsimony phylogeny construct using core single-nucleotide polymorphisms (SNPs) identified among 107 *Salmonella* Minnesota genomes using kSNP3. All Brazilian *S.* Minnesota isolates were grouped into two clades (*Salmonella* Minnesota lineages I and II (SM-LI and SM-LII)), denoted using Roman numerals. The label colors denote the source of isolates (green for poultry genomes). The phylogeny constructed using the maximum parsimony method implemented in kSNP3 is midpoint rooted, and branches withbootstrap values are labeled.

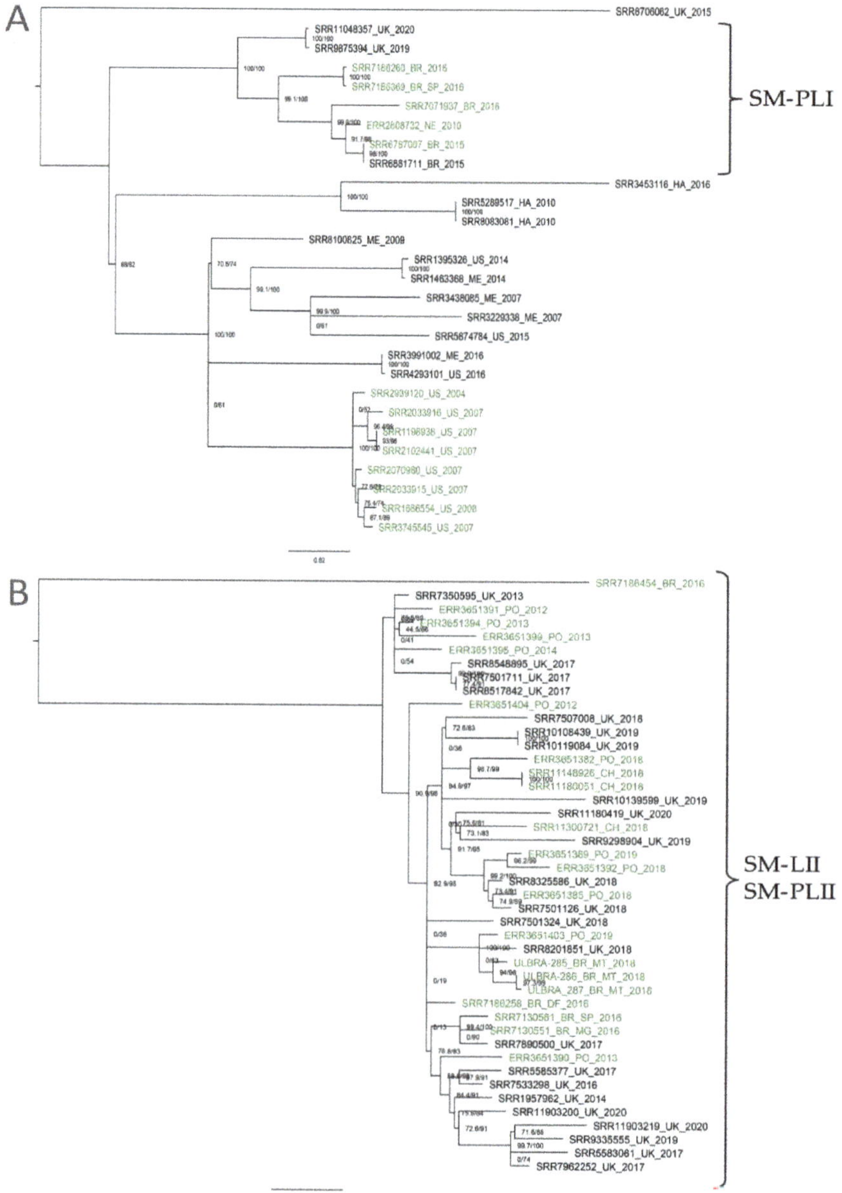

Figure 2. Maximum likelihood phylogeny constructed using high-quality SNPs (hqSNPs) identified among 28 SM-LI and 44 SM-LII genomes using the CFSAN SNP Pipeline. The label colors denote the source of isolates (green for poultry). The phylogeny was constructed using IQ-TREE and is midpoint rooted, with branch lengths representing the number of substitutions per site, and the bootstrap values are labeled. (**A**) 28 SM-LI genomes. In clade SM-PLI ($n = 8$) are five Brazilian isolates, two from the United Kingdom, and one from Netherlands, deposited in the National Center for Biotechnology Information (NCBI). (**B**) 44 SM-LII genomes. In clade SM-PLII ($n = 44$) are the three isolates sequenced in this study, four Brazilian isolates, three isolates from Chile, 11 isolates from Portugal, and 23 isolates from the United Kingdom, deposited in the NCBI.

3.3. Bayesian Phylogenetic Analysis of *S.* Minnesota

The evolutionary rate for the SM-LI isolates was predicted to be 1.27×10^{-7} substitutions/site/year (95% HPD 1.96×10^{-8}–2.39×10^{-7}) and shared a common ancestor emerging in the year 1676 (95% HPD 928–1765). SM-PLI shared a common ancestor that existed circa 1915 (95% HPD 1375–1982) (Figure 3A). The evolutionary rate for the clade SM-PLII was predicted to be 4.29×10^{-7} substitutions/site/year (95% HPD 3.06×10^{-7}–5.49×10^{-7}) and shared a common ancestor emerging in 1971 (95% HPD 1908–2006). Most SM-PLII isolates (97%; 43/44) shared a common ancestor emerging even more recently in 2004 (95% HPD 1986–2016), suggesting the high dissemination of this lineage in the beginning of the 2000s (Figure 3B).

Historical demographic trends of the median estimate of the *S.* Minnesota effective population sizes of SM-LI and SM-PLII over time were reconstructed using a Bayesian skyline approach. The SM-LI effective population size remained constant from 1985 to 2000 (Figure 4A). The SM-PLII effective population size remained constant from 1985 until 2009, when there was an increase until 2012, after which the effective population size remained constant through 2020 (Figure 4B).

3.4. Genes That Confer Resistance to Tetracyclines and Sulfonamides Are Prevalent among the *S.* Minnesota Poultry Lineages

Of the 107 *S.* Minnesota genomes queried here, 11.2% (12/107) did not have plasmid replicons, while 88.8% (95/107) possessed one to six replicons. The following replicons were detected (in order of frequency): ColRNAI ($n = 61$; 57.1%), IncA/C2 ($n = 47$; 43.9%), IncFIC(FII) ($n = 23$; 21.5%), ColpVC ($n = 15$; 14.1%), and IncFII(S) ($n = 11$; 10.2%). Plasmid replicons Col(MGD2), Col(Ye449), Col156, Col8282, IncFIB(AP001918), IncFIB(pB171), IncFIB(pECLA), IncFIB(pHCM2), IncFIB(29), IncFII(SARC14), IncFII(p14), IncFII(p96A), IncFII(pECLA), IncFII(pHN7A8), IncFII(pKPX1), IncFII(pRSB107), IncFII, IncFII_1_pSFO, IncI1, IncY, and pSL483 were each detected among 107 genomes, but in fewer than 10 isolates each (i.e., with frequencies less than 10%).

A separate analysis of the eight SM-PLI genomes demonstrated the occurrence of six different plasmid replicons. One SM-PLI sequence (12.5%) did not have plasmid replicons, while the remaining seven (87.5%) possessed one to three of them. The following replicons were detected most frequently: IncA/C2 ($n = 4$; 50%) and ColRNAI ($n = 3$; 37.5%) (Figure S1). Among the 44 SM-PLII genomes, 13 different plasmid replicons were detected, and each isolate genome harbored one to six of these replicons. The following replicons were detected most frequently: IncA/C2 ($n = 43$; 97.7%) and ColRNAI ($n = 40$; 90.1%) (Figure S1).

Twenty-eight different antimicrobial resistance genes were detected among 107 isolates, with each genome harboring 2–11 genes and/or integrons. The *aac(6′)-Iaa* and *mdf(A)* genes, which confer resistance to amynoglicosides (*aac(6′)-Iaa*), benzalkonium chloride (*mdf(A)*), and rhodamine (*mdf(A)*), were detected in all 107 genomes (100%). The *sul2*, *tet(A)*, *blaCMY-2*, *aph(3′)-Ia_1*, *qnrB19*, and *ant(3′′)*-Ia genes, which confer resistance to sulfonamides, tetracyclines, cephamycins, cephalosporins, aminoglycoside phosphotransferases, fluoroquinolones, and streptomycins, respectively, were less frequent ($n = 55$ (51.4%), $n = 48$ (44.6%), $n = 42$ (39.2%), $n = 39$ (36.5%), $n = 38$ (35.5%), $n = 25$ (23.3%), respectively). The remaining 20 genes, which confer resistance to aminoglycosides, cephalosporins, diaminopyrimidines, penams, penems, phosphomycins, phenicols, tetracycline, and sulfonamides, were detected in fewer than 8% of the isolates.

Among the eight SM-PLI genomes, 12 different antimicrobial resistance genes and/or integrons were detected. Apart from genes detected in 100% of the isolates (i.e., *aac(6′)-Iaa* and *mdf(A)*), the following other antimicrobial resistance genes were present: *sul2* and *tet(A)* in four isolates (50%) each (Figure S1, Supplementary Materials). In addition, 13 different antimicrobial resistance genes and/or integrons were detected among the 44 SM-PLII genomes. Apart from genes detected in 100% of the isolates (i.e., *aac(6′)-Iaa* and *mdf(A)*), other antimicrobial resistance genes included *sul2* and *tet(A)* in 43 isolates (97.7%), *blaCMY-2* in 42 isolates (95.4%), *aph(3′)-Ia* and *qnrB19* in 28 isolates (86.3%), and *ant(3′′)-Ia* in 23 isolates (52.7%) (Figure S1).

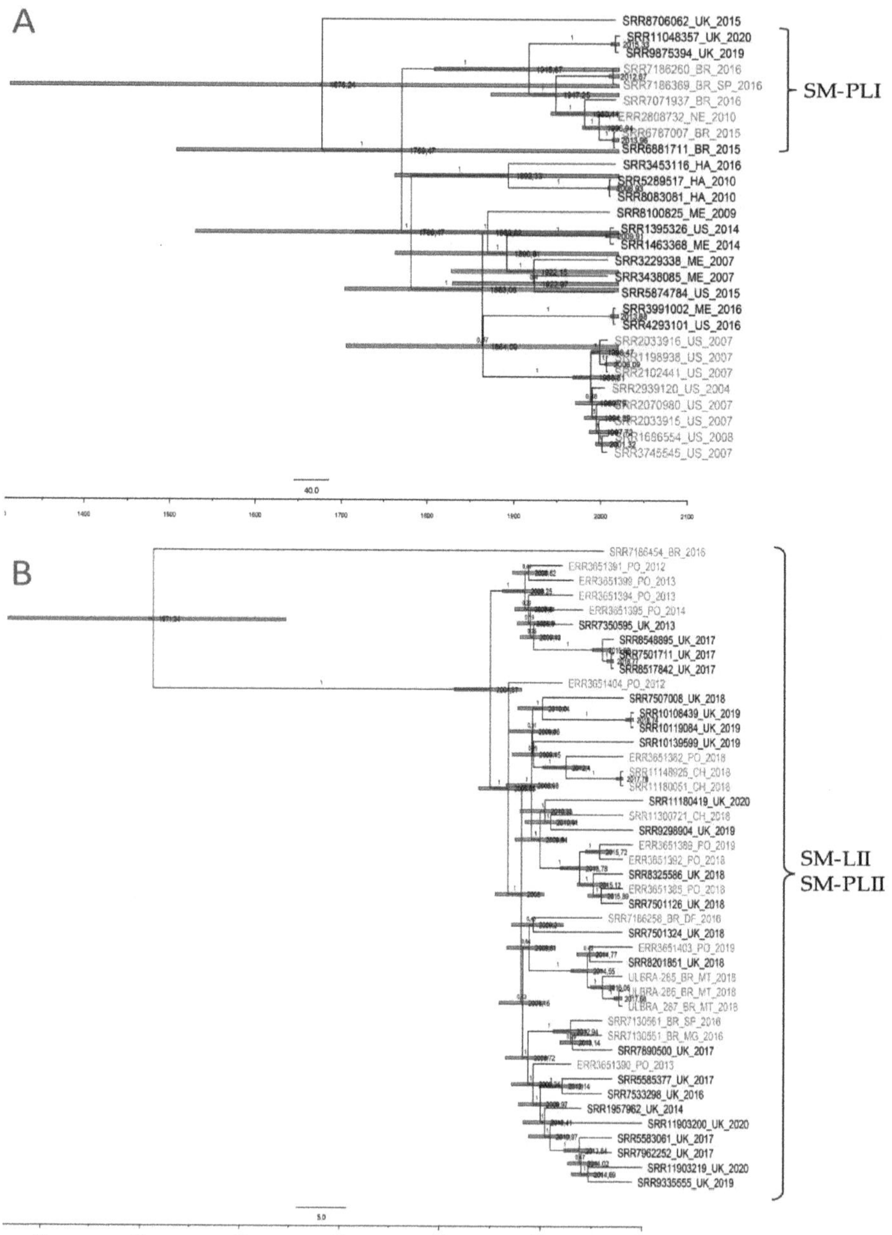

Figure 3. Maximum clade credibility tree constructed using high-quality SNPs (hqSNPs) identified among two *S.* Minnesota lineages using the CFSAN SNP Pipeline, rooted using BEAST. Time in years is plotted along the *x*-axis. Branch labels denote posterior probabilities of branch support, and node bars correspond to 95% highest posterior density (HPD) intervals for node heights. The label colors denote the source of isolates (green for poultry genomes). (**A**) 28 SM-LI genomes shared a common ancestor emerging in the year 1676. Clade SM-PLI shared a common ancestor that existed circa 1915. (**B**) 44 SM-PLII genomes shared a common ancestor emerging in the year 1971.

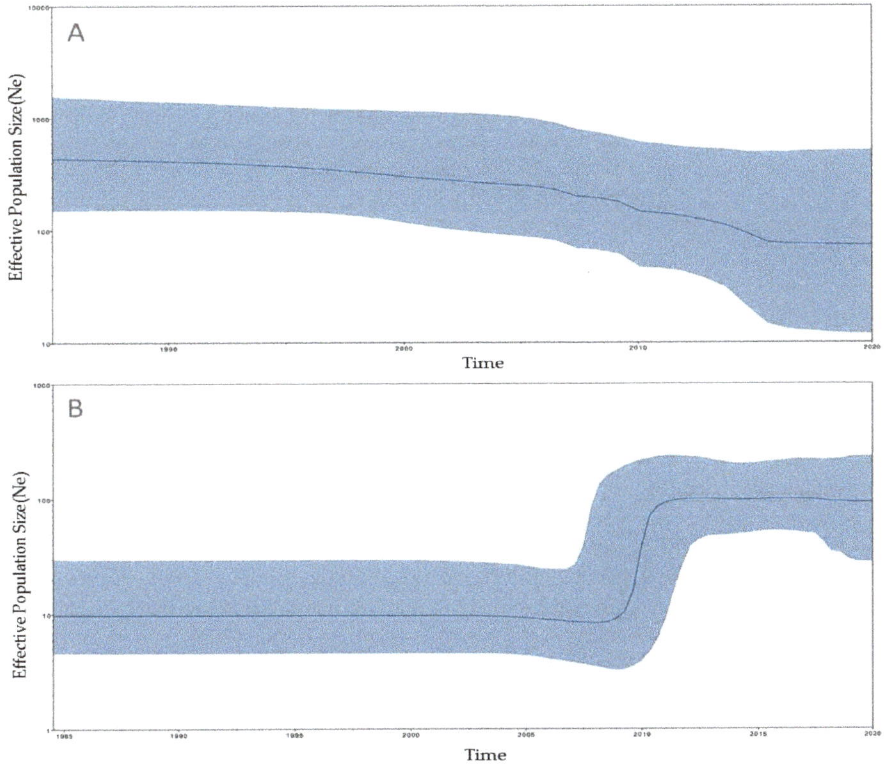

Figure 4. Bayesian skyline plot constructed via BEAST and Tracer, using high-quality SNPs (hqSNPs) detected among SM-LI and SM-LII/SM-PLII. The x-axis represents time in years, while the y-axis denotes the effective population size. The dark-blue line represents the median, while light-blue shading represents the 95% highest posterior density (HPD) interval. (**A**) Bayesian skyline plot detected among 28 SM-LI genomes. (**B**) Bayesian skyline plot detected among 44 SM-LII/SM-PLII genomes.

3.5. Virulence Mapping and Pan-Genome of S. Minnesota

To understand the pathogenicity repertoire of *S.* Minnesota isolates, genetic virulence factors were queried in the 107 genomes. Four pathogenicity islands (SPI2, SPI5, SPI13, and SPI14) were detected in all isolates, two (SPI3 and SPI9) were detected in 106 isolates (99.1%), two (SPI4 and SPI1) were detected in 103 isolates (96.2%), and C63PI was detected in 99 isolates (92.5%). A separate analysis of the eight SM-PLI genomes demonstrated that seven pathogenicity islands (SPI2, SPI3, SPI4, SPI5, SPI9, SPI13, and SPI14) were detected in all isolates, C63PI was detected in seven isolates (87.5%), and SPI1 was detected in five isolates (62.5%). Among the 44 SM-PLII genomes, seven pathogenicity islands (SPI1, SPI2, SPI5, SPI9, SPI13, SPI14, and C63PI) were detected in all isolates, SPI3 was detected in 43 isolates (97.2%), and SPI4 was detected in 40 isolates (90.9%). Overall, 160 *Salmonella* virulence genes were detected, with 113 genes present in all isolates. Noteworthy, there was the additional occurrence of some specific virulence genes in Brazilian lineages; 50% SM-PLI genomes (4/8) and 93.1% SM-PLII (41/44) genomes carried *fyuA*, *irp1*, *irp2* and the operon *ybtABPQSTUX* (Figure S2) with a median of 100% identity and 97% coverage.

Of the 15,320 genes identified among the 107 *S.* Minnesota genomes, 3873 (25.2%) were core genes (i.e., present among all 107 genomes), while the remaining 11,447 (74.8%) comprised the pan-genome (Figure S3).

4. Discussion

S. Minnesota is a foodborne pathogen recently associated with the Brazilian poultry production chain. This serotype has been increasingly detected in avian farms from the Center West, one of the fastest growing poultry-producing regions in Brazil [6]. In this study, three *S.* Minnesota strains from this region were isolated and sequenced and compared to other genomes submitted to NCBI's SRA database as *S.* Minnesota (n = 104), including nine more from Brazil.

In order to study the phylogenetic relationships of Brazilian *S.* Minnesota isolates of poultry origin, all 107 complete genomes were first assigned to STs using seven-gene MLST. Only STs 548 and 285 were detected, and the former was more frequent, as previously reported [7,37]. In the phylogeny (Figure 1), ST 285 was nested within ST 548. ST 285 is rare and normally detected in Mexico, although some strains have been detected in the United Kingdom and the United States from environment, livestock, human and avian sources (http://enterobase.warwick.ac.uk/species/senterica/search_strains?query=st_search).

Despite encompassing two STs, the *S.* Minnesota genomes queried here displayed considerable genomic diversity, and Brazilian isolates clustered within two specific clades (SM-LI and SM-LII). Additionally, it could be observed that some European *S.* Minnesota genomes also clustered with SM-PLI and SM-PLII. Noteworthy, the occurrence of *S.* Minnesota isolates in Europe has already been previously described, including in poultry meat imported from Brazil [8,11]. A more recent study also associated some *S.* Minnesota isolates (n = 3) with poultry production in Brazil [37]. These previously sequenced *S.* Minnesota genomes from Brazil clustered in one unique clade together with isolates from the United Kingdom, all being predominantly found in humans and food, according to a core genome phylogeny [37]. Furthermore, a temporal study of *Salmonella enterica* serotypes from broiler farms in Brazil showed that *S.* Minnesota was the most frequent serotype in broiler flocks, and the transmission on the surveyed farms was predominantly horizontal and through different contamination sources [6].

The Bayesian temporal phylogenetic evaluation showed that the common ancestor of the SM-PLI and SM-PLII presented tMRCAs in the 20th century (around 1915 and 1971, respectively). Interestingly, 97.7% (43/44) SM-PLII isolates shared a common ancestor that existed circa 2004, and a recent increase in effective population size was also estimated (mainly from 2009 to 2012; Figure 4B). There are too few isolates from this lineage associated with poultry production in the specific Brazilian producing regions to conclusively say that *S.* Minnesota is spreading due to SM-PLII in Brazil. Further studies should be carried out with more *S.* Minnesota genomes from poultry sources to reach at more detailed information about the main lineages and their temporal evolution in this specific animal production chain. However, the three isolates sequenced here, and other information obtained from field reports demonstrated the high recent dissemination of this serotype, probably related to the recent expansion of poultry production in Brazil in the last two decades [38,39]. The increased global trade of poultry meat and recent major changes in international microbiological food regulations have further evidenced the occurrence of this *Salmonella* serotype in chicken meat and other poultry products [11,40,41].

S. Minnesota isolates sequenced here and others from poultry were predicted to be resistant to multiple antibiotics and to carry genes *ant(3'')-Ia*, *aph(3')-Ia*, *blaCMY-2*, *mdf(A)*, *qnrB19*, *sul2*, and *tet(A)*, which confer resistance to the class of aminoglycosides, betalactams, fluoroquinolones, sulfonamides, and tetracyclines. These genes and even a multidrug resistance (MDR) profile have already been described in other studies of *S.* Minnesota [11,37,40]. This gene set was probably selected as a result of management practices in the Brazilian poultry production chain. A recent study reported several places in Brazil as hotspots of antimicrobial resistance emergence [41].

Most SM-PLI and SM-PLII isolates also possessed some recognized virulence genes, such as *fyuA*, *irp1*, *irp2*, and the operon *ybtAPQSTUX* (i.e., median of 100% identity and 97% coverage). This last gene cluster is usually located in a chromosomal region called the highly pathogenic island (HPI). HPI encodes a yersiniabactin-mediated iron acquisition system previously demonstrated in pathogenic strains of *Yersinia* and several members of the Enterobacteriaceae, including *Salmonella* [42]. HPI has been reported in other *Salmonella* serotypes, such as Infantis [43] and Seftenberg [42]; however, to our knowledge, this is the first study identifying HPI in *S.* Minnesota. The HPI presence in *S.* Minnesota could provide a more concerning metabolic profile in different ways: (i) improving the environmental fitness and persistence of the bacteria [44], (ii) suppressing the host immune response [45], and (iii) influencing the expression of virulence determinants or additional genes not associated with this specific island, which may increase their ability to initiate infection [44]. These additional genetic properties may therefore, be, determinants for the dissemination and persistence of *S.* Minnesota in Brazilian poultry farms [6]. New studies would be necessary to experimentally confirm this genomic evidence.

5. Conclusions

The present study provided insights into the evolution and genomic content of *S.* Minnesota, particularly the lineages currently circulating in the poultry production chain in Brazil. Two specific lineages (SM-PLI and SM-PLII) were identified, as well as numerous isolates that possessed genes conferring antibiotic resistance and high genetic virulence potential. There are still few studies in the literature evaluating this important *Salmonella* serotype, and there were no data on the evolutionary analysis of *S.* Minnesota lineages. This information can contribute to the improvement of the management of all production systems affected by this serotype, particularly avian flocks in the poultry production chain from Brazil.

Supplementary Materials: The following are available online at http://www.mdpi.com/2076-2615/10/11/2043/s1: Table S1. Metadata of *S.* Minnesota isolates from NCBI and three isolates sequenced in this study; Figure S1. Presence and absence of 28 antimicrobial resistance genes and 26 plasmids replicons among 107 *S.* Minnesota genomes; Figure S2. Presence and absence of 47 virulence genes among 107 *S.* Minnesota genomes; Figure S3. Pie plots of gene content in core, soft core, shell, and cloud genomes describing the pan genome for *S.* Minnesota.

Author Contributions: A.S.K.F. and V.R.L. obtained and maintained the bacterial isolates. D.K., A.K.M., and N.I. performed the molecular biology analysis. D.K. performed the genomic analyses. D.K. and V.R.L. reviewed the literature and wrote the original draft preparation; D.K., L.M.C., A.F.S., and V.R.L. reviewed and edited the manuscript. All authors read and agreed to the final published version of the manuscript.

Funding: This study was financed in part by the Coordenação de Aperfeiçoamento de Pessoal de Nível Superior–Brasil (CAPES)—Finance Code 001. This study was also financed by Simbios Biotecnologia. V.R.L. was financially supported by the National Council for Scientific and Technological Development from Brazil (CNPq—Conselho Nacional de Desenvolvimento Científico e Tecnológico; process number 311010/2017-2).

Acknowledgments: The authors wish to thank the FDA GenomeTrakr network for support through the collaborative research agreement U18 FD006229 and the Wadsworth Center Advanced Genomic Technologies Cluster for sequencing three of the isolates. The authors also thank Renato Hohl Orsi and Martin Wiedmann for their guidance and support.

Conflicts of Interest: The authors declare no conflict of interest.

References

1. Lee, K.M.; Runyon, M.; Herrman, T.J.; Phillips, R.; Hsieh, J. Review of Salmonella detection and identification methods: Aspects of rapid emergency response and food safety. *Food Control* **2015**, *47*, 264–276. [CrossRef]
2. Mezal, E.H.; Sabol, A.; Khan, M.A.; Ali, N.; Stefanova, R.; Khan, A.A. Isolation and molecular characterization of Salmonella enteric serovar Enteritidis from poultry house and clinical samples during 2010. *Food Microbiol.* **2014**, *38*, 67–74. [CrossRef]
3. Silva, C.; Calva, E.; Maloy, S. One health and food-borne disease: Salmonella transmission between humans, animals, and plants. *Microbiol. Spectr.* **2014**, *2*, OH-0020-2013. [CrossRef] [PubMed]
4. Edwards, P.R.; Bruner, D.W. Two new Salmonella types isolated from fowls. *J. Hyg.* **1938**, *38*, 716–720. [CrossRef]
5. Jiménez, M.; Martinez-Urtaza, J.; Rodriguez-Alvarez, M.X.; Leon-Felix, J.; Chaidez, C. Prevalence and genetic diversity of Salmonella spp. in a river in a tropical environment in Mexico. *J. Water Health* **2014**, *12*, 874–884. [CrossRef]
6. Voss-Rech, D.; Vaz, C.S.; Alves, L.; Coldebella, A.; Leao, J.A.; Rodrigues, D.P.; Back, A. A temporal study of Salmonella enterica serotypes from broiler farms in Brazil. *Poult. Sci.* **2015**, *94*, 433–441. [CrossRef] [PubMed]
7. Wang, H.; Hoffmann, M.; Laasri, A.; Jacobson, A.P.; Melka, D.; Curry, P.E.; Hammack, T.S.; Zheng, J. Complete Genome Sequence of Salmonella enterica subsp. enterica serovar Minnesota Strain. *Genome Biol. Evol.* **2017**, *9*, 2727–2731. [CrossRef]

8. Campos, J.; Mourão, J.; Silveira, L.; Saraiva, M.; Correia, C.B.; Maçãs, A.P.; Peixe, L.; Antunes, P. Imported poultry meat as a source of extended-spectrum cephalosporin-resistant CMY-2-producing Salmonella Heidelberg and Salmonella Minnesota in the European Union, 2014–2015. *Int. J. Antimicrob. Agents* **2018**, *51*, 151–154. [CrossRef] [PubMed]
9. Costa, R.G.; Festivo, M.L.; Araujo, M.S.; Reis, E.M.; Lázaro, N.S.; Rodrigues, D.P. Antimicrobial susceptibility and serovars of Salmonella circulating in commercial poultry carcasses and poultry products in Brazil. *J. Food Prot.* **2013**, *76*, 2011–2017. [CrossRef] [PubMed]
10. Mendonça, E.P.; de Melo, R.T.; Nalevaiko, P.C.; Monteiro, G.P.; Fonseca, B.B.; Galvão, N.N.; Giombelli, A.; Rossi, D.A. Spread of the serotypes and antimicrobial resistance in strains of Salmonella spp. isolated from broiler. *Braz. J. Microbiol.* **2019**, *50*, 515–522. [CrossRef]
11. Silveira, L.; Nunes, A.; Pista, Â.; Isidro, J.; Belo Correia, C.; Saraiva, M.; Batista, R.; Castanheira, I.; Machado, J.; Gomes, J.P. Characterization of Multidrug-Resistant Isolates of Salmonella entérica Serovars Heidelberg and Minnesota from Fresh Poultry Meat Imported to Portugal. *Microbial. Drug Resist.* 2020. [CrossRef]
12. Kipper, D.; Hellfeldt, R.M.; De Carli, S.; Lehmann, F.K.M.; Fonseca, A.S.K.; Ikuta, N.; Lunge, V.R. Salmonella serotype assignment by sequencing analysis of intergenic regions of ribosomal RNA operons. *Poult. Sci.* **2019**, *98*, 5989–5998. [CrossRef] [PubMed]
13. Bolger, A.M.; Lohse, M.; Usadel, B. Trimmomatic: A flexible trimmer for Illumina sequence data. *Bioinformatics* **2014**, *30*, 2114–2120. [CrossRef] [PubMed]
14. Babraham Bioinformatics. FastQC v. 0.11.2. 2014. Available online: http://www.bioinformatics.babraham.ac.uk/projects/fastqc/ (accessed on 10 January 2020).
15. Bankevich, A.; Nurk, S.; Antipov, D.; Gurevich, A.A.; Dvorkin, M.; Kulikov, A.S.; Lesin, V.M.; Nikolenko, S.I.; Pham, S.; Prjibelski, A.D.; et al. SPAdes: A new genome assembly algorithm and its applications to single-cell sequencing. *J. Comp. Biol.* **2012**, *19*, 455–477. [CrossRef]
16. Gurevich, A.; Saveliev, V.; Vyahhi, N.; Tesler, G. QUAST: Quality assessment tool for genome assemblies. *Bioinformatics* **2013**, *29*, 1072–1075. [CrossRef]
17. Bushnell, B. BBMap v. 38.26. 2015. Available online: https://sourceforge.net/projects/bbmap/ (accessed on 25 January 2020).
18. Li, H.; Handsaker, B.; Wysoker, A.; Fennell, T.; Ruan, J.; Homer, N.; Marth, G.; Abecasis, G.; Durbin, R. 1000 Genome Project Data Processing Subgroup. The Sequence Alignment/Map format and SAMtools. *Bioinformatics* **2009**, *25*, 2078–2079. [CrossRef]
19. Seemann, T. Prokka: Rapid prokaryotic genome annotation. *Bioinformatics* **2014**, *30*, 2068–2069. [CrossRef]
20. Yoshida, C.E.; Kruczkiewicz, P.; Laing, C.R.; Lingohr, E.J.; Gannon, V.P.; Nash, J.H.; Taboada, E.N. The Salmonella In Silico Typing Resource (SISTR): An Open Web-Accessible Tool for Rapidly Typing and Subtyping Draft Salmonella Genome Assemblies. *PLoS ONE* **2016**, *11*, e0147101. [CrossRef]
21. Leinonen, R.; Sugawara, H.; Shumway, M. International Nucleotide Sequence Database Collaboration. The sequence read archive. *Nucleic Acids Res.* **2011**, *39*, D19–D21. [CrossRef]
22. Zankari, E.; Hasman, H.; Cosentino, S.; Vestergaard, M.; Rasmussen, S.; Lund, O.; Aarestrup, F.M.; Larsen, M.V. Identification of acquired antimicrobial resistance genes. *J. Antimicrob. Chemother.* **2012**, *67*, 2640–2644. [CrossRef]
23. Chen, L.; Yang, J.; Yu, J.; Yao, Z.; Sun, L.; Shen, Y.; Jin, Q. VFDB: A reference database for bacterial virulence factors. *Nucleic Acids Res.* **2005**, *33*, D325–D328. [CrossRef]
24. Carattoli, A.; Zankari, E.; García-Fernández, A.; Voldby, L.M.; Lund, O.; Villa, L.; Møller, A.F.; Hasman, H. In silico detection and typing of plasmids using PlasmidFinder and plasmid multilocus sequence typing. *Antimicrob. Agents Chemother.* **2014**, *58*, 3895–3903. [CrossRef] [PubMed]
25. Camacho, C.; Coulouris, G.; Avagyan, V.; Ma, N.; Papadopoulos, J.; Bealer, K.; Madden, T.L. BLAST+: Architecture and applications. *BMC Bioinform.* **2009**, *10*, 421. [CrossRef]
26. Gardner, S.N.; Hall, B.G. When whole-genome alignments just won't work: kSNP v2 software for alignment-free SNP discovery and phylogenetics of hundreds of microbial genomes. *PLoS ONE* **2013**, *8*, e81760. [CrossRef]
27. Trifinopoulos, J.; Nguyen, L.T.; von Haeseler, A.; Minh, B.Q. W-IQ-TREE: A fast online phylogenetic tool for maximum likelihood analysis. *Nucleic Acids Res.* **2016**, *44*, W232–W235. [CrossRef]
28. Kalyaanamoorthy, S.; Minh, B.Q.; Wong, T.; von Haeseler, A.; Jermiin, L.S. ModelFinder: Fast model selection for accurate phylogenetic estimates. *Nat. Methods* **2017**, *14*, 587–589. [CrossRef]

29. Hoang, D.T.; Chernomor, O.; von Haeseler, A.; Minh, B.Q.; Vinh, L.S. UFBoot2: Improving the Ultrafast Bootstrap Approximation. *Mol. Biol. Evol.* **2018**, *35*, 518–522. [CrossRef] [PubMed]
30. Rambaut, A.; Lam, T.T.; Max Carvalho, L.; Pybus, O.G. Exploring the temporal structure of heterochronous sequences using TempEst (formerly Path-O-Gen). *Virus Evol.* **2016**, *2*, vew007. [CrossRef]
31. Drummond, A.J.; Suchard, M.A.; Xie, D.; Rambaut, A. Bayesian phylogenetics with BEAUti and the BEAST 1.7. *Mol. Biol. Evol.* **2012**, *29*, 1969–1973. [CrossRef]
32. Tavaré, S. Some probabilistic and statistical problems in the analysis of DNA sequences. *Lect. Math. Life Sci.* **1986**, *17*, 57–86.
33. Rambaut, A.; Drummond, A.J.; Xie, D.; Baele, G.; Suchard, M.A. Posterior Summarization in Bayesian Phylogenetics Using Tracer 1.7. *Syst. Biol.* **2018**, *67*, 901–904. [CrossRef] [PubMed]
34. Heled, J.; Bouckaert, R.R. Looking for trees in the forest: Summary tree from posterior samples. *BMC Evol. Biol.* **2013**, *13*, 221. [CrossRef] [PubMed]
35. Page, A.J.; Cummins, C.A.; Hunt, M.; Wong, V.K.; Reuter, S.; Holden, M.T.; Fookes, M.; Falush, D.; Keane, J.A.; Parkhill, J. Roary: Rapid large-scale prokaryote pan genome analysis. *Bioinformatics* **2015**, *31*, 3691–3693. [CrossRef]
36. Brynildsrud, O.; Bohlin, J.; Scheffer, L.; Eldholm, V. Rapid scoring of genes in microbial pan-genome-wide association studies with Scoary. *Genome Biol.* **2016**, *17*, 238; [CrossRef] [PubMed]
37. Monte, D.F.; Lincopan, N.; Berman, H.; Cerdeira, L.; Keelara, S.; Thakur, S.; Fedorka-Cray, P.J.; Landgraf, M. Genomic Features of High-Priority Salmonella enterica Serovars Circulating in the Food Production Chain, Brazil, 2000–2016. *Sci. Rep.* **2019**, *9*, 11058. [CrossRef]
38. Gonçalves, V.S.; de Moraes, G.M. The application of epidemiology in national veterinary services: Challenges and threats in Brazil. *Prev. Vet. Med.* **2017**, *137*, 140–146. [CrossRef]
39. De Carli, S.; Gräf, T.; Kipper, D.; Lehmann, F.K.M.; Zanetti, N.; Siqueira, F.M.; Cibulski, S.; Fonseca, A.S.K.; Ikuta, N.; Lunge, V.R. *Molecular and phylogenetic analyses of Salmonella Gallinarum trace the origin and diversification of recent outbreaks of fowl typhoid in poultry farms. Vet. Microbiol.* **2017**, *212*, 80–86. [CrossRef] [PubMed]
40. Moura, Q.; Fernandes, M.R.; Cerdeira, L.; Ienne, S.; Souza, T.A.; Negrão, F.J.; Lincopan, N. Draft genome sequence of a multidrug-resistant CMY-2-producing Salmonella enterica subsp. enterica serovar Minnesota ST3088 isolated from chicken meat. *J. Glob. Antimicrob. Resist.* **2017**, *100*, 67–69. [CrossRef]
41. Van Boeckel, T.P.; Pires, J.; Silvester, R.; Zhao, C.; Song, J.; Criscuolo, N.G.; Gilbert, M.; Bonhoeffer, S.; Laxminarayan, R. Global trends in antimicrobial resistance in animals in low- and middle-income countries. *Science* **2019**, *365*, eaaw1944. [CrossRef]
42. Petermann, S.R.; Sherwood, J.S.; Logue, C.M. The Yersinia high pathogenicity island is present in Salmonella enterica Subspecies I isolated from turkeys. *Microb. Pathog.* **2008**, *45*, 110–114. [CrossRef]
43. Aviv, G.; Tsyba, K.; Steck, N.; Salmon-Divon, M.; Cornelius, A.; Rahav, G.; Grassl, G.A.; Gal-Mor, O. A unique megaplasmid contributes to stress tolerance and pathogenicity of an emergent Salmonella enterica serovar Infantis strain. *Environ. Microbiol.* **2014**, *16*, 977–994; [CrossRef]
44. Oelschlaeger, T.A.; Zhang, D.; Schubert, S.; Carniel, E.; Rabsch, W.; Karch, H.; Hacker, J. The high-pathogenicity island is absent in human pathogens of Salmonella enterica subspecies I but present in isolates of subspecies III and VI. *J. Bacteriol.* **2003**, *185*, 1107–1111. [CrossRef]
45. Autenrieth, I.; Hantke, K.; Heesemann, J. Immunosuppression of the host and delivery of iron to the pathogen: A possible dual role of siderophores in the pathogenesis of microbial infections? *Med. Microbiol. Immunol.* **1991**, *180*, 135–141; [CrossRef]

animals

Article

Comparison of the Effectiveness of Two Different Vaccination Regimes for Avian Influenza H9N2 in Broiler Chicken

Shaimaa Talat [1], Reham R. Abouelmaatti [2], Rafa Almeer [3], Mohamed M. Abdel-Daim [3,4] and Wael K. Elfeil [5,*]

1 Department of Birds and Rabbits Medicine, Faculty of Veterinary Medicine, Sadat City University, Menoufiya 32958, Egypt; shaimaa610@gmail.com
2 Department of Animal Epidemiology and Zoonosis, Sharkia Veterinary Directorate, General Organization of Veterinary Services (GOVS), Ministry of Agriculture, Sharkia 44511, Egypt; r.abouelmaatti@yahoo.com
3 Department of Zoology, College of Science, King Saud University, Riyadh 11451, Saudi Arabia; ralmeer@ksu.edu.sa (R.A.); abdeldaim.m@vet.suez.edu.eg (M.M.A.-D.)
4 Pharmacology Department, Faculty of Veterinary Medicine, Suez Canal University, Ismailia 41522, Egypt
5 Avian and Rabbit Medicine Department, Faculty of Veterinary Medicine, Suez Canal University, Ismailia 41522, Egypt
* Correspondence: elfeil@vet.suez.edu.eg; Tel.: +20-64-320-7052

Received: 29 August 2020; Accepted: 9 October 2020; Published: 14 October 2020

Simple Summary: The low pathogenic avian influenza H9N2 virus has been associated with severe economic losses in broiler chicken flocks. Problems associated with its control strategy are potential early infection and level of immune response that may be high in one-day-old chicks due to maternally derived antibodies. Herein, two vaccination regimes were evaluated in commercial broilers kept under either field or laboratory conditions. Two different vaccine types and concentrations were used, and the results highlighted a significantly higher protection against early infection when a homologous vaccine of high antigenic mass was applied at 7 days of life. Shedding was significantly reduced in this regime.

Abstract: Low pathogenic avian influenza virus is one of the major threats that has been affecting the poultry industry in the Middle East region for decades. Attempts to eradicate this disease have failed. Currently, there are commercial vaccines that are either imported or produced locally from recently circulating isolates of H9N2 in Egypt and Middle Eastern countries. This present work focused on comparing the effectiveness of two vaccines belonging to these categories in Egypt. Two commercial broiler flocks (Cobb-500 Broiler) with maternally derived immunity (MDA) against H9N2 virus were employed and placed under normal commercial field conditions or laboratory conditions. Immunity was evaluated on the basis of detectable humoral antibodies against influenza H9N2 virus, and challenge was conducted at 28 days of life using a recent wild H9N2 virus. The results showed that vaccination on the 7th day of life provided significantly higher immune response in both vaccine types, with significantly lower virus shedding compared to vaccination at day 1 of life, regardless of field or laboratory conditions. In addition, the vaccine produced from a recent local H9N2 isolate (MEFLUVAC-H9-16) provided a significantly higher humoral immune response under both field and laboratory conditions, as measured by serology and virus shedding (number of shedders and amount of shedding virus), being significantly lower following challenge on the 28th day of life, contrary to the imported H9 vaccine. In conclusion, use of H9N2 vaccine at 7 days of life provided a significantly higher protection than vaccination at day 1 of life in birds with MDA, suggesting vaccination regimes between 5–8-days of life for broiler chicks with MDA. Moreover, use of a vaccine prepared from a recently circulating H9N2 virus showed significantly higher protection and was more suitable for birds in the Middle East.

Keywords: avian influenza; homologous vaccine; heterologous vaccine; broiler; early infection

1. Introduction

The poultry industry has been suffering from several pathogens in Egypt during recent decades, including avian influenza viruses (AIV) that may be either highly pathogenic avian influenza (HPAIV; H5N1, H5N2, H5N8) or low-pathogenic avian influenza (LPAIV; H9N2) viruses, velogenic Newcastle disease virus (vNDV), infectious bronchitis virus (IBV; variant 1, variant 2, and classic wild virus), infectious bursal disease (either variant or virulent virus), multidrug-resistant bacteria (MDR; *Escherichia coli*, *Salmonella*, *Pasteurella*, etc.), in addition to coccidia species. All these pathogens have caused severe economic losses and have badly affected the veterinary care strategies [1–10]. Avian influenza (AI) is a contagious viral disease, belonging to the Orthomyxoviridae family, and is a segmented, single-stranded, negative sense RNA virus [11,12]. Avian influenza viruses (AIV) belong to type-A and are divided into subtypes on the basis of antigenic relationships of the surface glycoproteins (hemagglutinin and neuraminidase) into 18 hemagglutinins (HA) and 11 neuraminidases (NA), with variable combinations. These glycoproteins are considered the main antigenic components of the virus and act as immune modulators for pattern recognition receptors of the immune system. Structural variations within these pathogen surface glycoproteins were shown to affect the different host responses, whether they be avian, fish, or mammalian [13–16]. On the basis of the pathogenicity of the avian virus, it is further classified into two types known as a highly pathogenic avian influenza virus "H5/H7" (HPAIV) and a low pathogenic avian influenza virus (LPAIV) [12,17,18]. The H9N2 avian influenza virus is associated with one of the major viral problems affecting the poultry industry in Egypt since it was officially reported for the first time in 2011 until now [19]. Virus infection leads to high economic losses in both layers and for breeders due to a drop in egg production. Broilers may also show severe losses during co-infection with other pathogens, especially Infectious Bronchitis Virus (IBV),Newcastle disease virus (NDV), bacteria such as *E. coli* and *Mycoplasma*, or even live virus vaccines [5,9,20,21]. Recently several reports have highlighted the immunosuppressive effect associated with LPAI-H9N2 in poultry flocks either by altering the differentiation of lymphocytes or inflammatory cytokines or the depletion and apoptosis of some immune cells [22–29]. Moreover, some reports have discussed the effect of H9N2 on the alteration of blood biochemical and hematological parameters [30]. Regarding the potency and efficacy of the H9N2 inactivated vaccine in Egypt, there is a paucity of knowledge addressing this issue.

This work focuses on evaluating the value of applying the H9N2 vaccine at 1 day or 7 days of life on the developed immune response under both farm commercial conditions and laboratory standard conditions in broiler chicks with maternally derived immunity (MDA). Two commercially available vaccines were compared: one imported that is based on an old Middle East isolate (1998) and another produced in Egypt from a recent Middle East isolate (2016). Protection following challenge was assessed against live H9N2 virus in birds kept under standard laboratory conditions only.

2. Materials and Methods

2.1. Ethical Approval

Animal studies were approved by the Animal Welfare and Research Ethics Committee of Suez Canal University and all procedures were conducted strictly in accordance with the Guide for the Care and Use of Laboratory Animals. Every effort was made to minimize animal suffering.

2.2. Birds and Vaccines

A total of 108,120 one-day-old commercial Cobb-500 broilers from vaccinated broiler breeders with H9N2 vaccine was used in this experiment. All birds were given vaccines for infectious bursal disease

(IBD), AIV-H5, and Newcastle disease (ND) as is routine for commercial broilers in Egypt. Two commercial inactivated H9N2 vaccines were used in this trial (vaccines A and B). Vaccine A (MEFLUVAC-H9ND-16) is produced by MEVAC Co. Egypt and prepared from the A/ck/Egypt/ME/543V/2016(H9N2) virus. Vaccine B (Gallimune 208 H9ND) is produced by Merial Incorporation, France, and was brought from a local agency in Egypt. Vaccine B is prepared from A/chicken/Iran/Av1221/1998. Both were used according to the manufacturer's recommendations.

2.3. Experiment Design

2.3.1. Laboratory Groups

A total of 120 one-day-old commercial Cobb-500 broiler chicks with maternally derived antibodies for H9N2 virus (MDA) were divided into 6 different experimental groups: group 1 was vaccinated with MEFLUVAC-H9ND-16 (vaccine A) and group-2 received an imported H9ND vaccine (vaccine B)—both were administered at day 1 of life. Group 3 took vaccine A and group 4 took vaccine B, but at the 7th day of life. Group 5 served as a positive control (non-vaccinated, challenged group) and group 6 served as a negative control (non-vaccinated, non-challenged group). All vaccines were provided as per the manufacturer's recommendations, as shown in Table 1. Challenge was conducted in G1-5 (10 birds from each group) at the 28th day of life using a previously identified AIV-H9N2 virus [31].

Table 1. Experimental design for different groups (G-1-10).

	Group No.	Bird No.	Vaccine Regime			Challenge at 28 Day of Age	Assessment of Protection
			Vaccine Type	Age/Days	Dose/mL		
Experiment 1 lab experiment	G-1	20	A	1	0.3	+++	Follow up of immune response of vaccinated birds at weeks post vaccination to H9, H5, ND, IBD, and IB vaccines using HI and ELISA tests. Viral shedding detected by real-time PCR.
	G-2	20	B	1	0.3	+++	
	G-3	20	A	7	0.3	+++	
	G-4	20	B	7	0.3	+++	
	G-5	20	-	——	—	+++	
	G-6	20	-	——	—	——	
Experiment 2 field group	G-7	27K	A	1	0.3	-	Follow up of immune response of vaccinated birds on weekly basis. Measure of performance parameters and field exposure. Natural exposure monitoring by RT-PCR.
	G-8	27K	B	1	0.3	-	
	G-9	27K	A	6	0.3	-	
	G-10	27K	B	6	0.3	-	

2.3.2. Field-monitored Groups

A total of 108,000 broiler chickens (Cobb-500) produced from vaccinated broiler breeders with H9N2 vaccine and showing maternally derived antibodies for H9N2 virus (MDA) were placed equally in 4 pens, each with 27,000 birds (G-7-10). Group 7 took a commercial local H9ND vaccine (A), while group 8 took a commercial imported H9ND vaccine (B); both products were administered at the 1st day of life by subcutaneous (S/C) injection using the manufacturer's recommended dose. Group 9 took vaccine A while group 10 took vaccine B at the 7th day of life. Birds in groups 7–10 were brought from the same broiler breeder flock and the same hatchery and kept under commercial field conditions with proper biosecurity measures and took the same ratio and management standers.

2.4. Hemagglutination Inhibition (HI) Test

The HI test was used to monitor post-vaccination humoral immune response for each vaccine using avian influenza H9N2 antigens (one representative of the circulating virus in Egypt and another imported antigen). Chicken sera were examined for HA-specific antibodies against H9N2 virus by HI test according to the Office International des Epizooties (OIE) manual (OIE, 2015). Serial twofold serum dilutions in phosphate buffer saline (PBS) were subsequently mixed with equal volumes (25 μL) of the virus containing 4 hemagglutinating units (HAU), then 25 μL of washed chicken red blood cells were added. After we incubated the HI titers for 40 min at room temperature, we determined them as reciprocals of highest serum dilutions in which inhibition of hemagglutination was observed.

2.5. Challenge Virus

Vaccinated birds grown in isolated rooms were challenged at 4 weeks of age by intranasal inoculation of 6 $\log_{10}$ embryo infective dose$_{50}$ (EID_{50}) of the previously isolated wild type AI-H9N2 virus [31].

2.6. qRT-PCR for Virus Shedding

Tracheal swabs were collected from the challenged birds for detection of virus shedding by RT-PCR at 3 and 7 days post challenge, as per the OIE manual [32], using specific primers and probes, as previously described [31]. qRT-PCR titers were converted into $\log_{10}$ $EID_{50}/_{mL}$, as described previously [33]. Briefly, a triplicate of 6 10-fold dilutions of challenge AIV-H9N2 (AIV-H9N2; 10^6 $EID_{50}/_{mL}$) were used to generate a standard curve using stock virus dilutions from 10^{-1} to 10^{-6}. Since Ct is defined as the point at which the curve crosses the horizontal threshold line, we plotted virus $\log_{10}$ titers of a specimen against the Ct value, and the best fit line was constructed. The linear range of the assay ranged from 1 to 10^6 $EID_{50}/_{mL}$, with a correlation coefficient of 0.99. System detection limit was 0.5 $EID_{50}/_{mL}$, as has been standardized and described previously [31]. AIV-H9N2 quantity in unknown samples were derived by plotting the Ct of an unknown against the standard curve and were expressed in $\log_{10}$ $EID_{50}/_{mL}$ equivalents.

2.7. Statistical Analysis

Where necessary, data were analyzed by Student's *t*-test or by ANOVA followed by application of Duncan's new multiple range test to determine the significance of differences between individual treatments and corresponding control [34].

3. Results

3.1. Different AIV-H9N2 Virus Hemagglutinin Segment Amino Acid Identity Degrees

The hemagglutination segment (HA) amino acids identity degree showed higher similarities with vaccine A seed, ranging from 93.8 to 98.8% with different isolated viruses from Middle Eastern countries while with vaccine B, the degree of similarity was lower as it ranged from 89.5 to 92.8%, as shown in Table 2.

Table 2. Different avian influenza (AIV)-H9N2 virus hemagglutinin segment amino acid identity degrees.

Items	Alg. 2017	Egypt 2018	Iraq 2017	KSA 2018	Leb. 2017	Libya 2015	Mor. 2018	Pak. 2018	Tun. 2015	UEA 2017	Vaccine A	Vaccine B
Alg./2017		94.59	94.78	96.39	94.59	96.39	99.28	91.88	91.76	98.10	93.68	92.24
Egypt/2018	94.59		94.79	93.68	94.64	95.54	94.64	92.54	94.58	96.46	98.86	91.79
Iraq/2017	94.78	94.79		94.34	93.32	93.93	93.21	94.46	93.11	93.04	94.43	90.71
KSA/2018	96.39	93.68	91.34		94.22	95.49	96.57	90.43	92.31	96.39	94.78	91.88
Leb./2017	94.59	94.64	92.32	94.22		96.79	94.82	90.89	93.41	94.64	94.75	92.86
Libya/2015	96.39	95.54	93.93	95.49	96.79		96.25	92.86	95.33	96.07	94.64	93.93
Mor./2018	99.28	94.64	93.21	96.57	94.82	96.25		91.96	92.31	99.82	94.75	92.14
Pak./2018	91.88	90.54	94.46	90.43	90.89	92.86	91.96		89.84	91.79	94.18	89.11
Tun./2015	91.76	92.58	90.11	92.31	93.41	95.33	92.31	89.84		92.31	95.48	89.56
UEA/2017	98.10	94.46	93.04	96.39	94.64	96.07	99.82	91.79	92.31		96.57	91.96
Vaccine A	94.68	98.86	94.43	94.78	93.75	94.64	94.75	94.18	95.48	96.57		90.61
Vaccine B	92.24	91.79	90.71	91.88	92.86	93.93	92.14	89.11	89.56	91.96	91.61	

Alg.: Algeria; **Leb.:** Lebanon; **Mor.:** Morocco; **Pak.:** Pakitsan.

3.2. Immune Response to Other Vaccines at 28th Day of Life

Birds in all groups showed immune responses for vaccinations with infectious bursal disease vaccine, avian Influenza-H5 vaccine, and Newcastle disease vaccines. No significant differences were found among the different groups, as is shown in Table 3.

Table 3. Serological response of broiler chickens to infectious bursal disease virus (IBDV), Newcastle disease (ND), and avian influenza-H5N1 (AI-H5) vaccines at 28 days of age.

Group No.	Bird No.	Vaccine Regime			ELISA Mean Titers	HI Titer Log_2	
		Vaccine Type	Age/days	Dose/mL	IBD 28 Days	AI-H5 28 Days	ND 28 Days
G-1	20	A	1	0.3	17,553 ± 1105	3.7 ± 0.51	4.8 ± 0.72
G-2	20	B	1	0.3	17,703 ± 1120	3.8 ± 0.61	4.9 ± 0.61
G-3	20	A	7	0.3	17,612 ± 1090	3.6 ± 0.42	4.7 ± 0.66
G-4	20	B	7	0.3	16,217 ± 1220	3.6 ± 0.52	4.8 ± 0.62
G-5	20	-	-	-	17,533 ± 1140	3.7 ± 0.65	4.9 ± 0.56
G-6	20	-	-	-	17,533 ± 1170	3.7 ± 0.72	4.8 ± 0.81

ELISA = enzyme-linked immunosorbent assay; HI = hemagglutination inhibition test; IBDV = infectious bursal disease virus; ND = Newcastle disease virus; AI-H5 = avian influenza-H5N1.

3.3. Immune Response in Groups Kept under Laboratory Conditions

HI assay using antigen A (representing recently circulating H9N2 virus in the Middle East), not H9N2 virus challenge, revealed that birds in groups 3–4 (vaccinated at 7 days of life) had significantly higher ($p \leq 0.05$) immune responses at 28 and 35 days of life, compared to groups 1 and 2 that were vaccinated at day 1 of life. Moreover, group 1 (vaccine A) showed a significantly higher immune response ($p \leq 0.05$) at 21, 28, and 35 days of life compared to birds in group 2 (vaccine B). At 7 and 14 days of life, birds in group 1 showed a higher but not significantly different (p value ≥ 0.05) immune response compared to group 2, as shown in Figure 1 and Table 3. Birds in group 3 (vaccine A at D-7) showed a significantly higher immune response ($p \leq 0.05$) at 28 and 35 days of life in comparison with birds in group 4 (vaccine B). Yet, at 7, 14, and 21 days of life, birds in group 3 showed a higher but non-significant difference in the immune response ($p \geq 0.05$) compared to group 4, as shown in Figure 1 and Table 3. Birds in groups 5 and 6 showed non-detectable (nt) HI titer at 21 and 28 days of life, which reflected complete weaning from the maternally derived antibodies at 21 days of age. Birds in group 6 showed an undetectable immune response at 35 days of life, which ensured a negative control condition. Birds in group 6 developed seroconversion at 35 days of life (7 days post-challenge), which reflected the positive effect of the challenge virus. Performing HI assay using antigen B (representing the imported vaccine, not the recently circulating virus in the Middle East) without challenge showed that birds in groups 3–4 (vaccinated at the 7th day of life) developed a significantly higher ($p \leq 0.05$) immune response at 28 and 35 days of life versus groups 1-2 that were vaccinated at day 1 of life. There was no significant difference between the HI titers of the different groups vaccinated at the same age. Birds in group 5 showed significantly lower HI titers using antigen B as compared with antigen A at 7 days post-challenge, as shown in Table 4.

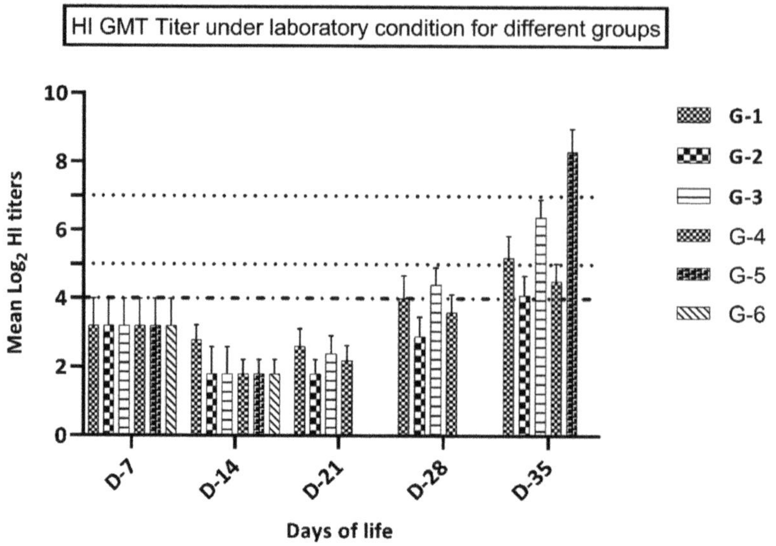

Figure 1. GMT of HI titers in groups 1-6 (kept under laboratory conditions).

Table 4. Hemagglutination inhibition (HI) test results in bird groups (G-1-6) using two-antigens.

Days of Life	Antigen Type	Experimental Groups					
		G-1	G-2	G-3	G-4	G-5	G-6
D-7	Antigen A	3.2 ± 0.79	3.2 ± 0.79	3.2 ± 0.79	3.2 ± 0.79	3.2 ± 0.79	3.2 ± 0.79
	Antigen B	2.6 ± 0.69	2.6 ± 0.69	2.6 ± 0.69	2.6 ± 0.69	2.6 ± 0.69	2.6 ± 0.69
D-14	Antigen A	2.8 ± 0.54	1.8 ± 0.42	1.8 ± 0.49	1.8 ± 0.56	1.8 ± 0.48	1.8 ± 0.32
	Antigen B	2.1 ± 0.44	2.2 ± 0.54	1.6 ± 0.74	1.6 ± 0.64	1.6 ± 0.74	1.6 ± 0.64
D-21	Antigen A	2.6 ± 0.55	1.8 ± 0.67	2.4 ± 0.52	2.2 ± 0.42	nd	nd
	Antigen B	2.2 ± 0.54	2.3 ± 0.64	2.1 ± 0.54	2.1 ± 0.54	nd	nd
D-28	Antigen A	4.1 ± 0.71	2.9 ± 0.59	4.4 ± 0.57	3.6 ± 0.46	nd	nd
	Antigen B	3.1 ± 0.44	3.1 ± 0.54	3.4 ± 0.64	3.2 ± 0.64	nd	nd
D-35	Antigen A	5.4 ± 0.61	4.0 ± 0.57	6.4 ± 0.52	4.5 ± 0.67	8.3 ± 0.65	nd
	Antigen B	4.2 ± 0.54	4.1 ± 0.48	5.1 ± 0.45	4.9 ± 0.64	7.4 ± 0.82	nd

Antigen A: antigen prepared from recently circulating H9N2 virus similar to vaccine A seed virus; antigen B: imported antigen representing vaccine B seed virus; D-7: 7 days of life; D-14: 14 days of life; D-21: 21 days of life; D-28: 28 days of life; D-35: 35 days of life; nd: non-detectable level; G-1: vaccine A at D-1; G-2: vaccine B at D-1; G-3: vaccine A at D-7; G-4: vaccine B at D-7; G-5: non-vaccinated, challenged (positive control); G-6: non-vaccinated, non-challenged (negative control).

3.4. Protection Following Challenge with a Wild Type H9N2 at the 28th Day of Life

3.4.1. Seroconversion 7-DPC with Recent Middle Eastern H9N2

At 7-DPC (days post-challenge), birds in group 5 (non-vaccinated, challenged) showed seroconversion with an average Geometric mean titer (GMT) HI titer of 8.3 ± 0.65 using antigen representing the recently circulating H9N2 virus in Egypt. At the same time, the titer was 7.4 ± 0.82 using the standard imported H9N2 antigen. Birds in group 2 and group 4 showed a significant increase in immune response (HI titer) at 7-DPC in comparison with birds of the same group and age, but unchallenged. Birds in group 1 and group 3 at 7-DPC demonstrated a declined immune response compared to those unchallenged in the same group and age, as shown in Table 5.

Table 5. The seroconversion at 7-DPC (days post-challenge) with recent Middle East H9N2 virus with two types of AIV-H9 antigen.

Group No.	Bird No.	Vaccine Regime			GMT Log_2 HI Titer (n = 10)	
					7 Days Post-Challenge	
		Vaccine Type	Age/days	Dose/mL	Local Antigen	Imported Antigen
1	10	A	1	0.3	4.1 ± 1.2 *	3.2 ± 1.21 *
2	10	B	1	0.3	7.0 ± 2.57 *	5.9 ± 2.57 *
3	10	A	7	0.3	5.1 ± 0.92 *	4.8 ± 0.89 *
4	10	B	7	0.3	6.5 ± 1.67 *	5.5 ± 1.87 *
5	10	-	-	-	8.3 ± 0.65 *	7.4 ± 0.82 *
6	10	-	-	-	-	-

*: mean there is a significant difference between means when $p > 0.05$.

3.4.2. Virus Shedding Following Challenge with H9N2 at 28 Days of Life

Birds in groups 3 and 4 (vaccinated at 7 days of life) showed a significantly lower number of shedders at 3-DPC in comparison with groups 1 and 2 (vaccinated at day 1 of life). Of groups vaccinated on the first day of life, group 1 (vaccine A) showed a significant reduction in virus shedding; number of shedders and amount of shed virus at 3/7-DPC compared to group 2 (vaccine B) (Table 6). Birds in group 3 (vaccine A at D-7) showed a significant reduction in virus shedding in terms of number of shedders and amount of shed virus at 3/7-DPC compared to group 2 (vaccine B), as shown in Table 6. Birds in group 2 (vaccine B) showed a reduction in the number of shedders compared to birds in group 5 (non-vaccinated, challenged), while there was no significant difference in the amount of virus shedding via the cloacal route at 3-DPC between birds in group 2 (vaccine B at day 1 of life) and group 5 (non-vaccinated, challenged). Moreover, birds in both groups (group 2 and group 5) showed the same virus shedding amount via tracheal route at 7-DPC, while birds in group 6 showed non-detectable (nd) virus shedding at 3- and 7-DPC in both tracheal and cloacal swaps.

Table 6. Virus shedding at 3- and 7-days post-challenge.

Group No.	Vaccinal Regime		Assessment of Protection							
			3-DPC				7-DPC			
	Vaccine Type	Vaccine Age	Tracheal Swabs No./EID50	%	Cloacal Swabs No./EID50	%	Tracheal Swabs No./EID50	%	Cloacal Swabs No./EID50	%
G-1	A	1	4/10 (2.1 ± 0.9) [b]	40%	3/10 (1.5 ± 0.3) [c]	30%	3/10 (1.8 ± 0.7) [b]	30%	3/10 (1.8 ± 0.8) [b]	30%
G-2	B	1	6/10 (2.8 ± 0.8) [c]	60%	4/10 (2.1 ± 0.4) [c]	40%	3/10 (2.3 ± 1.1) [c]	30%	4/10 (2.5 ± 0.8) [c]	40%
G-3	A	7	2/10 (1.6 ± 0.6) [a]	20%	2/10 (1.1 ± 0.3) [a]	20%	1/10 (1.3 ± 0.0) [a]	10%	2/10 (1.8 ± 0.5) [a]	20%
G-4	B	7	4/10 (2.4 ± 0.7) [c]	40%	3/10 (1.9 ± 0.3) [c]	30%	2/10 (1.9 ± 0.7) [c]	20%	3/10 (2.1 ± 0.6) [c]	30%
G-5	-	-	10/10 (3.1 ± 0.9) [d]	100%	6/10 (2.1 ± 0.3) [c]	60%	7/10 (2.3 ± 1.9) [c]	70%	10/10 (3.1 ± 1.8) [d]	100%
G-6	-	-	nd	-	nd	-	nd	-	nd	-

[abcd] means different superscripts differ significantly ($p \leq 0.05$); DPC: days post-challenge; EID_{50}: egg infectious $dose_{50}$; nd: non-detectable level; G-1: vaccine A at day 1; G-2: vaccine B at day 1; G-3: vaccine A at day 7; G-4: vaccine B at day 7; G-5: non-vaccinated, challenged (+ control); G-6: non-vaccinated, non-challenged (control).

3.5. Immune Response in Groups Kept under Field Condition

Birds in groups 9–10 (vaccinated at 7 days of life) showed a significantly higher immune response at 28 and 35 days of life in comparison with groups 7 and 8 that were vaccinated at day 1 of life. In groups vaccinated at the first day of life, group 7 (vaccine A) showed a significantly higher immune response ($p \leq 0.05$) at 28 and 35 days of life compared to birds in group 8 (vaccine B), while at 7, 14, and 21 days of life, birds in this group showed a non-significant increase ($p \geq 0.05$) in the immune response versus group 8 (Figure 2). Birds in group 9 (vaccine A at 7 days of life) showed a significantly higher immune response ($p \leq 0.05$) at 28 and 35 days of life in comparison with birds in group 10 (vaccine B), while at 14 and 21 days of life, birds in group 9 showed a non-significant increase ($p \geq 0.05$) in the immune response compared to group 10 (Figure 2).

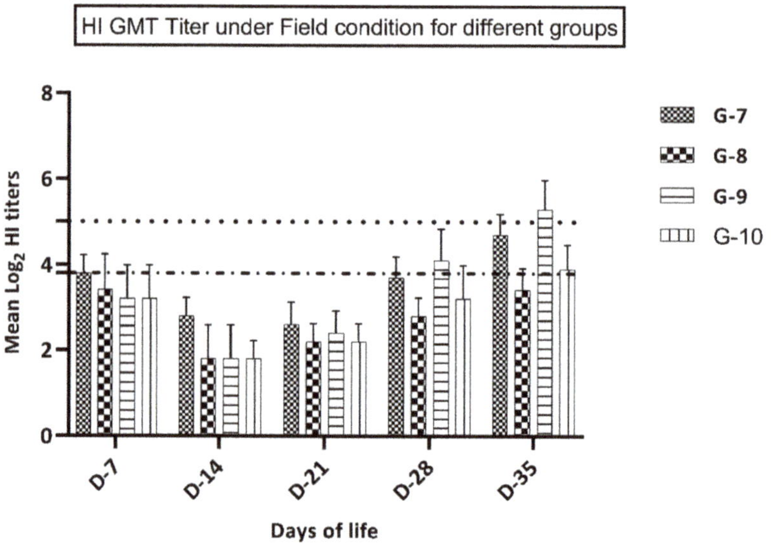

Figure 2. GMT HI titer in groups 7–10 (kept under field conditions).

4. Discussion

Broiler chicks in Egypt and the Middle East almost always arise from broiler-breeders' flocks vaccinated against H9N2. Accordingly, the vast majority of one-day-old broiler chicks produced in the region carry MDA against H9N2, which compromises the use of the inactivated H9N2 vaccines [29,31]. However, the immune response to other applied vaccines (IBD, NDV, H5) among all bird groups showed detectable antibody levels, with no significant differences after receiving one of the two vaccines employed either at day 1 of life or 7 days of life, or among non-vaccinated controls, which agrees with the previous reports of Kilany et al., Sultan et al., and Khalil et al., who claimed that applying vaccines does not interfere with the immune response of other different vaccines [30,35,36].

Commercial broilers with MDA against AIV-H9N2 face difficulties in developing an immune response following vaccination with inactivated H9N2 vaccines at day 1 of life due to interference. However, the most common regime for H9N2 vaccination in Egypt is to administer a single-dose between days 1–5 of life in broiler sectors, resulting in frequent vaccine failure. Results from the present study show that commercial broilers with MDA against H9N2 develop significantly higher immune response when applied at 7 days of life rather than day 1 of life, regardless the vaccine type used (either A or B). This result explains in part the repeated H9N2 vaccination failure in commercial boiler flocks with MDA (vaccinated at day 1 of life). Interference of the vaccine with the high titer of MDA against H9N2 (average = 6–8 $\log_2$) leads to this failure, as previously reported [37–39]. Under standard laboratory conditions, birds receiving vaccine A developed significantly higher immune response compared to vaccine B when administered at the same age (day 1 of life and 7 days of life). This may be referred to the amount of antigen in each vaccine, with vaccine A containing a higher amount of antigen (350 HAU unit/dose), while vaccine B contained around 200 HAU unit/dose [38]. As previously reported by Kilany et al. (2016), increasing the dose from 200 to 250 or 350 HAU can improve the immune response and protection against H9N2 [6].

Virus shedding is an important factor in the epidemiology of avian influenza; the lower the amount of virus shedding (amount of virus shedding and number of shedders' birds), the better we can control avian influenza. Results from the current study showed that use of the inactivated H9N2 vaccine at 7 days of life significantly reduced the virus shedding at 3- and 7-DPC compared to the inoculation at day 1 of life. Birds receiving vaccine A at day 1 of life significantly showed lower virus shedding in amount and number of shedders compared to those receiving vaccine B at the same age. However, birds receiving vaccine B at day 1 of life showed a significant reduction in virus shedding compared to the non-vaccinated challenge group, with tracheal shedding at 3-DPC and cloacal shedding at 7-DPC. No significant virus shedding was observed in the tracheal and cloacal swabs at 7-DPC between group 5 (non-vaccinated challenged) and group 2 (vaccine B at day 1 of life), which may have been due to the lower antigenic mass in the vaccine dose and higher level of MDA at day 1 of life. This negatively impacts the development of immune response, in agreement with the previous reports by Kilany et al. (2016), who demonstrated that lower antigenic masses (less than 128–200 HAU/dose) do not significantly reduce virus shedding compared to non-vaccinated challenged birds [40].

Applying vaccine-A at 7 days of life showed a significant reduction in virus shedding at 3- and 7-DPC compared to administering it at day 1 of life. This is contrary to the findings from vaccine B at 1 or 7 days of life, which may be explained by the higher antigenic mass in vaccine A along with the decline of MDA at 7 days of life, consent with Sun et al. (2012) and Khalil et al. (2015), who reported a significantly higher protection in chickens with H9N2 vaccines containing a higher antigenic mass than 250 HAU/dose. Moreover, Elfeil et al. (2019) reported a significant reduction in virus shedding in turkey following vaccination with H9N2 vaccine (350 HAU/dose) [36,40,41].

Commercial farm conditions always differ from laboratory conditions. In this study, birds kept under farm conditions and vaccinated at 7 days of life showed a significantly higher immune response than those vaccinated at day 1 of life. This matches with the results of laboratory groups and confirms the observation that vaccination at 7 days of life provides a significantly higher immune response and expected protection [36,42]. In addition, groups kept under farm commercial conditions of mass production (25,000 birds/pen) showed 1–3 $\log_2$ lower HI titers than those kept under laboratory conditions, indicating that there is around 7–25% difference in expected immune response between farm and laboratory conditions. This finding highlights the need to perform more research trials under commercial farm conditions, including virus challenge under Biosafety level-3 (BSL-3) isolators, bearing in mind that the negative pressure inside the isolators may affect virus spreading, as mentioned previously in the case of AIV-H9N2 in turkey poults, as well as in Newcastle disease virus and infectious bronchitis virus in chicken [40–44].

5. Conclusions

Application of AIV-H9N2 inactivated vaccine at 7 days of life provides a significantly higher protection on the basis of antibody level and reduction of virus shedding, number of shedders, and amount of virus shed per bird versus vaccines given at day 1 of life. Use of a homologous vaccine with high antigenic mass could also help in the reduction virus shedding and provide a significantly higher immunity and protection. Application of such a regime could help the control strategies of AIV-H9N2 in commercial broiler flocks in endemic areas and reduce the epidemiological load of AIV-H9N2 virus in the environment.

Author Contributions: Conceptualization, S.T., W.K.E.; methodology, S.T., W.K.E.; software, S.T., R.R.A., W.K.E.; validation, S.T., R.R.A., W.K.E.; formal analysis, S.T., R.R.A., W.K.E.; investigation, S.T., R.R.A., R.A., M.M.A.-D.,W.K.E.; resources, S.T., R.R.A., R.A., M.M.A.-D., W.K.E.; data curation, S.T., R.R.A., R.A., M.M.A.-D., W.K.E.; writing—original draft preparation, S.T., R.R.A., R.A., M.M.A.-D., W.K.E.; writing—review and editing, S.T., R.R.A., R.A., M.M.A.-D., W.K.E.; visualization S.T., R.R.A., W.K.E.; supervision S.T., R.R.A., W.K.E.; project administration, S.T., R.R.A., W.K.E.; funding acquisition, S.T., R.R.A., R.A., M.M.A.-D., W.K.E. All authors have read and agreed to the published version of the manuscript.

Funding: This research was funded by the Researchers Supporting Project number (RSP-2020/96), King Saud University, Riyadh, Saudi Arabia.

Acknowledgments: The author would like to extend their sincere appreciation to Professor Hesham Sultan, Sadat City University, Egypt, for technical support and advice. The authors would like to extend their sincere appreciation to the Researchers Supporting Project number (RSP-2020/96), King Saud University, Riyadh, Saudi Arabia.

Conflicts of Interest: The authors declare no conflict of interest and the funders had no role in the design of the study; in the collection, analyses, or interpretation of data; in the writing of the manuscript; or in the decision to publish the results.

References

1. Dia, M.S.; Hafez, M.S.A.E.; Ashry, M.A.; Elfeil, W.K. Occurrence of avian influenza h5n1 among chicken, duck farms and human in Egypt. *Am. J. Anim. Vet. Sci.* **2019**, *14*, 26–32. [CrossRef]
2. Eid, H.M.; Algammal, A.M.; Elfeil, W.K.; Youssef, F.M.; Harb, S.M.; Abd-Allah, E.M. Prevalence, molecular typing, and antimicrobial resistance of bacterial pathogens isolated from ducks. *Vet. World* **2019**, *12*, 677–683. [CrossRef]
3. Sedeik, M.E.; Awad, A.M.; Rashed, H.; Elfeil, W.K. Variations in Pathogenicity and Molecular Characterization of Infectious Bursal Disease Virus (IBDV) in Egypt. *Am. J. Anim. Vet. Sci.* **2018**, *13*, 76–86. [CrossRef]
4. Eid, H.I.; Algammal, A.M.; Nasef, S.A.; Elfeil, W.K.; Mansour, G.H. Genetic variation among avian pathogenic *E. coli* strains isolated from broiler chickens. *Asian J. Anim. Vet. Adv.* **2016**, *11*, 350–356. [CrossRef]
5. Ayoub, M.A.; Elfeil, W.K.; El Boraey, D.; Hammam, H.; Nossair, M.A. Evaluation of some vaccination programs in protection of experimentally challenged broiler chicken against newcastle disease virus. *Am. J. Anim. Vet. Sci.* **2019**, *14*, 197–206. [CrossRef]
6. Sultan, H.A.; Talaat, S.; Elfeil, W.K.; Selim, K.; Kutkat, M.A.; Amer, S.A.; Choi, K.S. Protective efficacy of the Newcastle disease virus genotype VII–matched vaccine in commercial layers. *Poult. Sci.* **2020**, *99*, 1275–1286. [CrossRef] [PubMed]
7. Elfeil, W.K.; Ezzat, M.E.; Fathi, A.; Alkilany, M.-A.A.; Abouelmaatti, R.R. Prevalence and Genotypic Analysis and Antibiotic Resistance of Salmonella Species Isolated from Imported and Freshly Slaughtered Chicken. *Am. J. Anim. Vet. Sci.* **2020**, *15*, 134–144. [CrossRef]
8. Fawzy, M.; Ali, R.; Elfeil, W.; Saleh, A.; Eltarabilli, M. Efficacy of inactivated velogenic Newcastle disease virus genotype VII vaccine in broiler chickens. *Vet. Res. Forum* **2020**, *11*, 113–120. [CrossRef] [PubMed]
9. Sultan, H.A.; Ali, A.; El Feil, W.K.; Bazid, A.H.I.; Zain El-Abideen, M.A.; Kilany, W.H. Protective Efficacy of Different Live Attenuated Infectious Bronchitis Virus Vaccination Regimes against Challenge with IBV Variant-2 Circulating in the Middle East. *Front. Vet. Sci.* **2019**, *6*, 341. [CrossRef] [PubMed]
10. Rady, M.; Ezz-El-Din, N.; Mohamed, K.F.; Nasef, S.; Samir, A.; Elfeil, W.K. Correlation between ESβL Salmonella Serovars Isolated from Broilers and their Virulence Genes. *J. Hell. Vet. Med Soc.* **2020**, *71*, 2163–2170. [CrossRef]
11. Capua, I. *Avian Influenza and Newcastle Disease: A Field and Laboratory Manual*; Springer: Milan, Italy, 2009.
12. Swayne, D.E.; Glisson, J.R. *Diseases of Poultry*; Wiley-Blackwell: Ames, Iowa, 2013.
13. Abouelmaatti, R.R.; Algammal, A.M.; Li, X.; Ma, J.; Abdelnaby, E.A.; Elfeil, W.M.K. Cloning and analysis of Nile tilapia Toll-like receptors type-3 mRNA. *Cent. Eur. J. Immunol.* **2013**, *38*, 277–282. [CrossRef]
14. Elfeil, W.K.; Abouelmaatti, R.R.; Sun, C.; Han, W.; Li, X.; Ma, J.; Lei, L.; Liu, S.; Yang, Y.; Wang, Y.; et al. Identification, cloning, expression of a novel functional anasplatyrhynchos mRNA TLR4. *J. Anim. Vet. Adv.* **2012**, *11*, 1727–1733. [CrossRef]
15. Elfeil, W.M.K.; Algammal, A.M.; Abouelmaatti, R.R.; Gerdouh, A.; Abdel-Daim, M.M. Molecular characterization and analysis of TLR-1 in rabbit tissues. *Cent. Eur. J. Immunol.* **2016**, *41*, 236–242. [CrossRef] [PubMed]
16. Abouelmaatti, R.R.; Algammal, A.M.; Elfeil, W.M.K.; Elshaffy, N.M.; Li, X.; Ma, J.; Fawzy, M.; Wahdan, A.; El-Tarabili, R.; Shabana, I.I. Genetic characterization, cloning, and expression of Toll-like Receptor 1 mRNA Oreochromis niloticus. *Vet. Arh.* **2020**, *90*, 193–204. [CrossRef]
17. Capua, I.; Alexander, D.J. Avian influenza: Recent developments. *Avian Pathol.* **2004**, *33*, 393–404. [CrossRef]
18. Spackman, E. *Avian Influenza Virus*; Humana Press: Totowa, NJ, USA, 2008; Volume 436.
19. El-Zoghby, E.F.; Arafa, A.S.; Hassan, M.K.; Aly, M.M.; Selim, A.; Kilany, W.H.; Selim, U.; Nasef, S.; Aggor, M.G.; Abdelwhab, E.M.; et al. Isolation of H9N2 avian influenza virus from bobwhite quail (*Colinus virginianus*) in Egypt. *Arch. Virol.* **2012**, *157*, 1167–1172. [CrossRef]
20. Monne, I.; Hussein, H.A.; Fusaro, A.; Valastro, V.; Hamoud, M.M.; Khalefa, R.A.; Dardir, S.N.; Radwan, M.I.; Capua, I.; Cattoli, G. H9N2 influenza A virus circulates in H5N1 endemically infected poultry population in Egypt. *Influenza Other Respir. Viruses* **2013**, *7*, 240–243. [CrossRef]

21. El Sayed, M.; Alyousef, Y.; Al Sayed, A.; Elfeil, W. Evaluation of the antibody response of two local Saudi lines and commercial chickens vaccinated against newcastle diseases virus and infectious bursal disease virus. *Sci. J. King Faisal Univ.* **2019**, *20*, 105–113.
22. Gharaibeh, S. Pathogenicity of an Avian Influenza Virus Serotype H9N2 in Chickens. *Avian Dis.* **2008**, *52*, 106–110. [CrossRef]
23. Hsu, S.M.; Chen, T.H.H.; Wang, C.H. Efficacy of Avian Influenza Vaccine in Poultry: A Meta-analysis. *Avian Dis.* **2010**, *54*, 1197–1209. [CrossRef]
24. Ahad, A.; Thornton, R.N.; Rabbani, M.; Yaqub, T.; Younus, M.; Muhammad, K.; Mahmood, A.; Shabbir, M.Z.; Kashem, M.A.; Islam, M.Z. Risk factors for H7 and H9 infection in commercial poultry farm workers in provinces within Pakistan. *Prev. Vet. Med.* **2014**, *117*, 610–614. [CrossRef] [PubMed]
25. Qiang, F.; Youxiang, D. The effects of H9N2 influenza A on the immune system of broiler chickens in the Shandong Province. *Transbound. Emerg. Dis.* **2011**, *58*, 145–151. [CrossRef] [PubMed]
26. Farzin, H.; Toroghi, R.; Haghparast, A. Up-regulation of pro-inflammatory cytokines and chemokine production in avian influenza H9N2 virus-infected human lung epithelial cell line (A549). *Immunol. Investig.* **2016**, *45*, 116–129. [CrossRef] [PubMed]
27. Arafat, N.; Eladl, A.H.; Marghani, B.H.; Saif, M.A.; El-shafei, R.A. Enhanced infection of avian influenza virus H9N2 with infectious laryngeotracheitis vaccination in chickens. *Vet. Microbiol.* **2018**, *219*, 8–16. [CrossRef]
28. Bonfante, F.; Cattoli, G.; Leardini, S.; Salomoni, A.; Mazzetto, E.; Davidson, I.; Haddas, R.; Terregino, C. Synergy or interference of a H9N2 avian influenza virus with a velogenic Newcastle disease virus in chickens is dose dependent. *Avian Pathol.* **2017**, *46*, 488–496. [CrossRef]
29. Nagy, A.; Mettenleiter, T.C.; Abdelwhab, E.M. A brief summary of the epidemiology and genetic relatedness of avian influenza H9N2 virus in birds and mammals in the Middle East and North Africa. *Epidemiol. Infect.* **2017**, *145*, 3320–3333. [CrossRef]
30. Sultan, A.H.; Abd El-Razik, G.A.; Allam, S.T.; El-Deeb, A.H. Inactivated oil emulsion H9N2 vaccine in broiler chickens: Pathogenesis and Clinicopathological studies. *Am. J. Res. Commun.* **2015**, *3*, 38–53.
31. Elfeil, W.; Abouelmaatti, R.; Diab, M.; Mandour, M.; Rady, M. Experimental Infection of Chickens by Avian Influenza H9N2 Virus: Monitoring of Tissue Tropism and Pathogenicity. *J. Egypt. Vet. Med. Assoc* **2018**, *78*, 369–383.
32. OIE. Manual of Diagnostic Tests and Vaccines for Terrestrial Animals-Avian Influenza. In *OIE Terrestrial Manual 2015*; OIE: Rome, Italy, 2015.
33. Nolan, T.; Hands, R.E.; Bustin, S.A. Quantification of mRNA using real-time RT-PCR. *Nat. Protoc.* **2006**, *1*, 1559. [CrossRef]
34. Steel, R.G.D.; Torrie, J.H. *Principles and Procedures of Statics*; Mcgraw Hill Book Comp. Inc.: London, UK, 1960.
35. Kilany, W.; Bazid, A.-H.; Ali, A.; El-Deeb, A.; Zain El Abideen, M.; Sayed, M.; El-Kady, M. Comparative Effectiveness of Two Oil Adjuvant–Inactivated Avian Influenza H9N2 Vaccines. *Avian Dis.* **2016**, *60*, 226–231. [CrossRef]
36. Khalil, A.; Hussein, H.; Tolba, S.; El-Sanousi, A. Preparation and Evaluation of H9n2 Vaccine Adjuvated with Montanide ISA71 VG. *Glob. Vet.* **2015**, *15*, 670–674. [CrossRef]
37. Elfeil, W.K.; Abouelmaatti, R.R.; Ibrahim, H.H.; Ali, A.; Kilany, W.H.; Rady, A.; El-Sayed, M. Comparison of the effectiveness of two local and imported inactivated combined H9N2-ND vaccines in broiler flocks in Egypt. In Proceedings of the IX International Veterinary Conference: One World, One Health, Sharm El Sheikh City, Egypt, 9–13 March 2009.
38. El-Deeb, A.H.; Kilany, W.; Hanafie, A.; Echeverry, F.; El-Kady, M. Comparative Field Evaluation of Protective Efficacy of Commercially Available H9N2 Vaccines in Breeders in Egypt. In Proceedings of the 19th World Veterinary Poultry Association Congress, Cape Town, South Africa, 7–11 September 2015.
39. Elfeil, W.; Hanfie, A.; Rady, M.; Kilany, W.; Ibrahim, H.; Elkady, M.; Elsayed, M. Evaluation of Different H9N2 vaccination regime in commercial Broiler breeders flocks. In Proceedings of the XX World Veterinary Poultry Association Congress, Edinburgh International Conference Centre (EICC), Edinburgh, UK, 2 May 2017.
40. Kilany, W.; Ali, A.; Bazid, A.-H.; El-Deeb, A.; Zain El Abideen, M.; Sayed, M.; El-Kady, M. A Dose-Response Study of Inactivated Low Pathogenic Avian Influenza H9N2 Virus in Specific-Pathogen-Free and Commercial Broiler Chickens. *Avian Dis.* **2016**, *60*, 256–261. [CrossRef] [PubMed]

41. Elfeil, W.; Yousef, H.; Fawzy, M.; Ali, A.; Kilany, W.; Ibrahim, H.; Elsayed, M. Protective efficacy of MEFLUVAC H9 in turkey poults in both lab and Field condition. In Proceedings of the XXIst World Veterinary Poultry Association Congress, Angkok International Trade and Exhibition Centre, Bangkok, Thailand, 16–20 September 2019.
42. Sun, Y.; Pu, J.; Fan, L.; Sun, H.; Wang, J.; Zhang, Y.; Liu, L.; Liu, J. Evaluation of the protective efficacy of a commercial vaccine against different antigenic groups of H9N2 influenza viruses in chickens. *Vet. Microbiol.* **2012**, *156*, 193–199. [CrossRef] [PubMed]
43. Shahar, E.; Haddas, R.; Goldenberg, D.; Lublin, A.; Bloch, I.; Bachner Hinenzon, N.; Pitcovski, J. Newcastle disease virus: Is an updated attenuated vaccine needed? *Avian Pathol.* **2018**, *47*, 467–478. [CrossRef]
44. Elhady, M.A.; Ali, A.; Kilany, W.H.; Elfeil, W.K.; Ibrahim, H.; Nabil, A.; Samir, A.; El Sayed, M. Field Efficacy of an Attenuated Infectious Bronchitis Variant 2 Virus Vaccine in Commercial Broiler Chickens. *Vet. Sci.* **2018**, *5*, 49. [CrossRef]

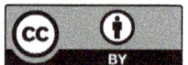

animals

MDPI

Article

Molecular Characterization and Developing a Point-of-Need Molecular Test for Diagnosis of Bovine Papillomavirus (BPV) Type 1 in Cattle from Egypt

Mohamed El-Tholoth [1,2,3], Michael G. Mauk [2], Yasser F. Elnaker [4], Samah M. Mosad [1], Amin Tahoun [5], Mohamed W. El-Sherif [6], Maha S. Lokman [7,8], Rami B. Kassab [8,9], Ahmed Abdelsadik [10], Ayman A. Saleh [11] and Ehab Kotb Elmahallawy [12,13,*]

1. Department of Virology, Faculty of Veterinary Medicine, Mansoura University, Mansoura 35516, Egypt; tholothvirol@mans.edu.eg (M.E.-T.); dr.sama786@yahoo.com (S.M.M.)
2. Department of Mechanical Engineering and Applied Mechanics, University of Pennsylvania, Philadelphia, PA 19104, USA; mmauk@seas.upenn.edu
3. Health Sciences Division, Veterinary Sciences Program, Al Ain Men's Campus, Higher Colleges of Technology, Al Ain 17155, UAE
4. Department of Animal Medicine (Infectious Diseases), Faculty of Veterinary Medicine, The New Valley University, El-Karga 72511, New Valley, Egypt; yasserelnaker@yahoo.com
5. Department of Animal Medicine, Faculty of Veterinary Medicine, Kafrelshkh University, Kafrelsheikh 33511, Egypt; amin12_veta@yahoo.com
6. Department of Surgery, Anesthesiology and Radiology, Faculty of Veterinary Medicine, The New Valley University, El-Karga 72511, New Valley, Egypt; drmwt@hotmail.com
7. Biology Department, College of Science and Humanities, Prince Sattam bin Abdul Aziz University, Alkharj 11942, Saudi Arabia; ms.hussein@psau.edu.sa
8. Department of Zoology and Entomology, Faculty of Science, Helwan University, 11795 Cairo, Egypt; rami.kassap@yahoo.com
9. Department of Biology, Faculty of Science and Arts, Al Baha University, Almakhwah, Al Baha 1988, Saudi Arabia
10. Zoology Department, Faculty of Science, Aswan University, Aswan 81528, Egypt; aabdelsadik@aswu.edu.eg
11. Department of Animal Wealth Development, Genetics and Genetic Engineering, Faculty of Veterinary Medicine, Zagazig University, Zagazig 44519, Egypt; lateefsaleh@yahoo.com
12. Department of Biomedical Sciences, University of Leon, 24071 León, Spain
13. Department of Zoonoses, Faculty of Veterinary Medicine, Sohag University, Sohag 82524, Egypt

* Correspondence: eehaa@unileon.es

Received: 17 September 2020; Accepted: 17 October 2020; Published: 21 October 2020

check for updates

Simple Summary: Bovine papillomatosis is a disease caused by bovine papillomavirus (BPV), which is a diverse group of oncogenic viruses that challenge cattle industry, resulting in significant economic losses. The present study investigated the occurrence of bovine papillomatosis among cattle (n = 308) with cutaneous warts on the head and neck from New valley Province, Egypt through molecular detection of BPV-1, -2, -4, -5, and -10. The work also involved a phylogenetic analysis of the positive samples for detection of the genetic relatedness of the virus. Interestingly, BPV-1 DNA was detected in 84.6% of the collected samples. Furthermore, the study included the development of an isothermal nucleic acid amplification test, which is a field test combining molecular and lateral flow immunoassays for point-of-need testing appropriate for veterinary use in resource-limited settings. Collectively, our study provided interesting data related to the combined use of molecular and immunoassays methods in the detection of the virus besides better understanding the genetic relatedness of the circulating genotypes of BPV-1 in Egypt. Our study suggested further research to explore more about the other genotypes of BPV in the Egyptian environment that could be helpful for the implementation of control strategies for combating this disease.

Abstract: Bovine papillomatosis is a viral disease of cattle causing cutaneous warts. A diagnosis of this viral infection is very mandatory for combating the resulting economic losses. Given the limited data available about bovine papillomavirus (BPV) in Egypt, the present study involved the molecular diagnosis of bovine papillomavirus type-1 (BPV-1), -2, -4, -5, and -10 in cattle presenting cutaneous warts on the head and neck from New Valley Province, Egypt. The phylogenetic analysis of the detected types of BPV was also performed, followed by developing a point-of-need molecular assay for the rapid identification of identified BPV types. In this regard, a total of 308 cattle from private farms in Egypt were clinically examined, of which 13 animals presented cutaneous warts due to suspected BPV infection. The symptomatic animals were treated surgically, and biopsies from skin lesions were collected for BPV-1, -2, -4, -5, and -10 molecular identification using polymerase chain reaction (PCR). The presence of BPV-1 DNA was confirmed in 11 collected samples (84.6%), while BPV-2, -4, -5, and -10 were not detected. Sequencing of the PCR products suggested the Egyptian virus is closely related to BPV found in India. An isothermal nucleic acid amplification test (NAAT) with labeled primers specific for the BPV-1 L1 gene sequence, and based on recombinase polymerase amplification (RPA), in combination with a lateral flow strip assay for the detection of RPA products, was developed and tested. The point-of-need molecular assay demonstrated a diagnostic utility comparable to PCR-based testing. Taken together, the present study provides interesting molecular data related to the occurrence of BPV-1 in Egypt and reveals the genetic relatedness of the Egyptian BPV-1 with BPV-1 found in buffalo in India. In addition, a simple, low-cost combined test was also validated for diagnosis of the infection. The present study suggests the necessity of future investigations about the circulating strains of the virus among the cattle in Egypt to assess their genetic relatedness and better understand the epidemiological pattern of the disease.

Keywords: bovine papillomavirus; cattle; Egypt; nucleic acid lateral flow immunoassay; PCR

---

1. Introduction

Papillomaviruses are small nonenveloped viruses within the *Papillomaviridae* family with icosahedral symmetry, 55 to 60 nm in diameter, with a double-stranded DNA (dsDNA) genome and approximately 8-kilobase pairs in length [1,2]. The replication of these viruses occurs in the nuclei of squamous epithelial cells, and these viruses exhibit tropism to skin and mucosal tissues, causing benign and malignant tumors that replicate in the nuclei of squamous epithelial cells [3–6]. This group of viruses constitutes a wide range of DNA viruses that are found in mammals, birds, reptiles, and human beings [7]. In accordance with its occurrence in animals, the virus was identified in many domestic species, including bovine, ovine, swine, felines, and canines [8]. The resulting virus got its name based on the species from which the virus was characterized, as in case of bovine-named bovine papillomaviruses (BPVs) [8]. To our knowledge, twenty-six types of BPV have been described; 23 of them are grouped into five genera, with three types still unclassified [9]. The Deltapapillomavirus has four types: BPV-1, BPV-2, BPV-13, and BPV-14. The Xipapillomavirus genus has two species: Xipapillomavirus 1 (BPV-3, BPV-4, BPV-6, BVP-9, BPV-10, BPV-11, and BPV-15) and Xipapillomavirus 2 (BPV-12). The other two genus are Epsilonpapillomavirus 1 (BPV-5 and BPV-8) and Dyoxypapillomavirus 1 (BPV-7) [1,10–13]. Lastly, two recently described types (BPV-17) and BPV-20) are still unclassified as species. Taken into account, BPVs are generally species-specific; however, BPV-1, BPV-2, and BPV-13 can infect both cattle and equids [14–16]. Bovine papillomatosis is the resulting viral disease characterized by cutaneous warts or papillomas that represent proliferative lesions ranging from small nodular lesions to large cauliflower warts that are often rough and spiny to the touch and gray to black in color [17]. The transmission of BPV between animals may occur due to contaminated milking, ear-marking, grooming equipment, and animals rubbing on contaminated objects, such as wire fences [17]. Venereal warts may be transmitted sexually [6,17]. The prevalence of

BPV is high in calves and yearlings, although all ages can be infected [17]. Steers are less frequently affected than heifers [6,18]. Regarding its occurrence in Egypt, some previous reports involved limited clinical and epidemiological studies on BPV in Egypt [18,19], but little yet is known about its occurrence in Egypt.

The accurate detection of the infected cases represents one of the main strategies for controlling the virus. In this regards, a tentative diagnosis is based on the clinical signs, while a confirmative diagnosis relies on histopathology, electron microscopy of the specimens, immunohistochemistry, and molecular or nucleic acid-based tests, e.g., polymerase chain reaction (PCR) [20,21]. To the authors' knowledge, there are no reports of in vitro cultivation of BPV [22,23]. Importantly, the development of a low-cost, minimally instrumented, simple-to-use method for the rapid (30 to 60 min) detection of BPV would facilitate and inform the implementation of control measures and help reduce its economic impact. This method would enable sample testing in the field (e.g., on the farm) or at remote testing sites close to the farmer. In addition, it would eliminate the need for sample transport to central laboratories and the consequent delay times of days or weeks between sample collections and test results. Taking into consideration molecular tests based on specific enzymatic amplification of part of the virus genome, combined with either real-time or subsequent (post-amplification) detection of the amplicon (amplification product), are many advantages that include the highest sensitivity and specificity among all diagnostics methods [21,24]. However, conventional implementations of such molecular tests require relatively expensive instruments, i.e., benchtop thermal cyclers that provide precise and rapid temperature cycling of the sample, and are typically limited to use in facilities with reliable electric power and trained technicians [25]. In the past decade, the advent of isothermal amplification methods that use constant temperature instead of thermal cycling have fostered dramatic simplifications in point-of-care molecular diagnostics systems [26]. In laboratory settings, the amplification process is assayed by real-time fluorescent monitoring or post-amplification gel or capillary electrophoresis. These are costly or inconvenient for use outside of the laboratory. Alternatively, lateral flow strips (also called LF immunoassays or immunochromatography) provide convenient and simple noninstrumented methods for the detection of amplicons and are especially amenable to field tests. They are of low cost, compact (palm size), do not require electricity, and have a long shelf life [27]. For the detection of nucleic acids, the amplification primers are conjugated with antigen labels that bind with capture and reporter antibodies on the strip. The amplification product is blotted on the strip, and the presence of the amplicon (positive test result) is indicated by a darkened test line (and control line), whereas a negative test should, in principle, be implied by changes in only the control line [28]. For isothermal amplification, recombinase polymerase amplification (RPA) has a lower incubation temperature (37 °C), requires only two primers, compared to four or six with Loop-mediated isothermal amplification (LAMP), and generally exhibits very rapid amplification (10 to 20 min). RPA has demonstrated a sensitivity comparable to PCR, and for this work, with regard to point-of-need testing, RPA would appear advantageous [26,29–31]. Furthermore, LF immunoassays have proven suitable for on-site detection and field use in developing countries [27]. Combined RPA and LF immunoassays have previously been described for veterinary use for infectious bronchitis virus and Newcastle disease virus, as well as influenza virus (H9 subtype) detection [28,32]. Given the above information, our study was focused on the molecular detection and phylogenetic analysis of BPV-1, -2, -4, -5, and -10 in cattle from New Valley Province, Egypt presenting cutaneous warts on the head and neck that indicate a likely BPV infection. Furthermore, the work involved development of a field test combining RPA and LF immunoassays for point-of-need molecular testing as appropriate for veterinary use in resource-limited settings.

2. Materials and Methods

2.1. Ethical Statement

The ethical approval was performed as described by the ethical standards of Veterinary Medicine, Mansoura University, Egypt, which complies with all relevant Egyptian legislations. Cattle owners gave consent orally, which is in harmony with ethical regulations of the nation.

2.2. Animals

The study was carried out during the summer of 2016. A total number of 308 cattle (*Bos Taurus*) from private farms in New Valley Province, Egypt were examined (Table 1). Of which, 13 animals (9 females and 4 males, all aged 1 to 2 years) showed clinical signs consistent with BPV infection. Cattle over 2 years of age did not present any such clinical manifestations, and the history of these cases did not reveal the appearance of external signs of infection at any point in their lives. The clinically diseased cattle exhibited small, firm nodules on the head and cauliflower growths on the neck (Figure 1A,B). The skin lesions were grayish to black in color. The body temperatures of the infected cattle were within the normal range, and their appetites were normal.

Table 1. Details of examined animals (n = 308) that showed clinical signs of bovine papillomatosis and positive result by bovine papillomavirus type-1-polymerase chain reaction (BPV-1-PCR).

Farm Number	Age Range (Year)	Total Number of Animals/Farm	Sex of Examined Animals		No, Sex, and Age of Animals Showed Clinical Signs and Positive Result by BPV-1-PCR
			Female	Male	
1	1–4	15	10	5	0
2	1–5	19	11	8	1 male (13 month)
3	1–3	13	9	4	0
4	1–5	21	13	8	1 Female (18 months) 1 male (24 month)
5	1–5	16	10	6	0
6	1–3	10	8	2	1 male (23 month)
7	1–4	15	11	4	0
8	1–3	18	12	6	0
9	1–3	12	8	4	0
10	1–5	14	10	4	1 Female (14 month)
11	1–4	16	11	5	1 Female (13 month)
12	1–5	15	10	5	0
13	1–3	20	12	8	0
14	1–4	14	10	4	1 Female (20 month)
15	1–4	17	11	6	1 Female (15 month)
16	1–5	10	8	2	0
17	1–4	19	12	7	1 Female (14 month)
18	1–5	19	13	6	0
19	1–3	12	9	3	1 Female (17 month)
20	1–5	13	9	4	1 Female (22 month)
Total (%)		308 (100%)	207 (67.2%)	101 (32.8%)	11 (3.6%) 8 females (2.6%) 3 males (1.0%)

2.3. Surgical Treatment of the Cutaneous Warts and Sampling

Diseased animals were sedated with 0.2 mg/kg xylazine 2% solution (Xyla-Ject, ADWIA Pharmaceuticals Co., Sharqia Governorate, Egypt) by intramuscular injection, and lidocaine HCL 2% (Hospira, Inc, 300 N Field Dr, Lake Forest, IL 60045, USA) was infiltrated around the cutaneous warts after preparation of the surgical site. Animals were restrained and typed before surgical excision. Excision of warts (Figure 1C) on the head and neck was performed by sharp scalpel until the blood oozed; then, hemorrhage was controlled. Povidone iodine 10% W/V skin solution (BETADINE® antiseptic solution, El-Nile Co. for pharmaceuticals and chemical industries, Cairo, Egypt) was applied on the skin wounds to avoid secondary bacterial infection. All surgically treated cattle were injected with multivitamins (Elyoser Medicine Trading Co., Cairo, Egypt) by intramuscular injection. Recovery of the animals from clinical manifestation was checked 25 to 86 days post-treatment. Pieces of skin warts were collected after surgical excision. The samples were collected in bottles containing sterile saline for the molecular identification of BPV types 1, 2, 4, 5, and 10 by PCR. Skin samples from two apparently healthy cattle were involved as negative controls.

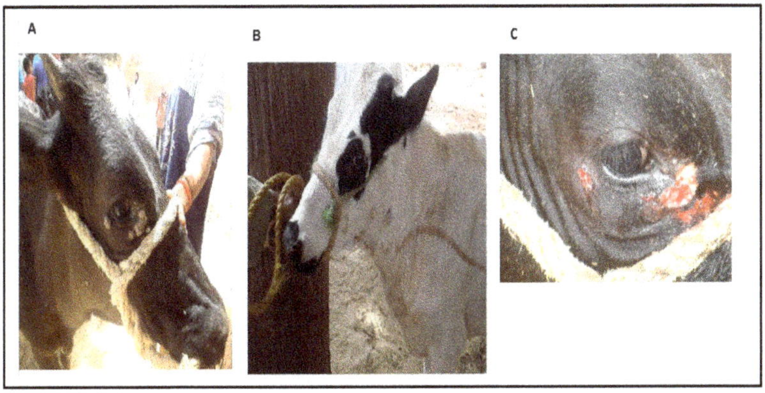

Figure 1. Typical cases of bovine papillomavirus (BPV) infection in cattle with macroscopic cutaneous warts around the eye (**A**), on the neck (**B**), and after surgical removal of cutaneous growths around the eye (**C**).

2.4. Skin Wart Sample Preparations

Samples from cutaneous warts were minced with sterile scissors and homogenized. The samples were then suspended in phosphate-buffered saline (20% w/v PBS) solution and centrifuged at 2000 rpm for 15 min, from which supernatants were stored at −20 °C for PCR tests.

2.5. Polymerase Chain Reaction (PCR)

Molecular identification of BPV-1, -2, -4, -5, and -10 in head and neck skin wart specimens was made with PCR. Oligonucleotide primers were synthesized for the amplification of the L1 gene of BPV-1 and -2, the E7 gene of BPV-4, and the E2 gene for BPV-5 and -10 according to protocols described elsewhere [33,34]. Primers were synthesized by Metabion International AG, Planegg, Germany and used at a 10-μM concentration. DNA extraction was carried out using a QIAamp® MiniElute® Virus Spin Kit (QIAGEN, GmbH, Hilden, Germany) based on the manufacturer's instructions. Negative control skin samples were also involved. PCR amplification was done following a protocol described elsewhere [33], using a Thermo Scientific PCR Master Mix (Thermo Scientific, Waltham, MA, USA). The PCR conditions and time-temperature program was as follows: 95 °C for 10 min for initial melting, 30 cycles of 94 °C for 45 s (melting), 50 °C for 45 s (annealing), and 72 °C for 1 min (extension), followed by 72 °C for 7 min (final extension). Visualization of the PCR products by gel electrophoresis was performed as reported elsewhere [35].

2.6. PCR Product Sequencing and Analysis

Purification of PCR products from agarose gel was done using a QIAquick Gel Extraction kit (Qiagen Inc., Valencia, CA, USA). The ABI Prism BigDye™ Terminator v3.1 Cycle sequencing kit was used for DNA sequencing of the PCR amplicon using an ABI PRISM 3130x1 Genetic Analyzer (Life Technologies, Carlsbad, CA, USA). Analysis of the sequencing data was performed using ClustalW (http://www.ebi.ac.uk/Tools/msa/clustalw2/). The alignment *.aln output file was utilized for the neighbor-joining phylogenetic analysis, as well as divergence, and identity percent calculation was carried out via Mega software v5.2.2 (http://www.megasoftware.net/)

2.7. Developing Recombinase Polymerase Amplification-Nucleic Acid Lateral Flow Immunoassays (RPA-NALF) for Point-of-Need Molecular Identification of BPV

A point-of-need rapid molecular assay comprising an isothermal RPA amplification step with BPV-1-specific primers for the detection of conjugated amplicons with a lateral flow strip was developed to detect BPV-1.

2.7.1. Oligonucleotide Primers for RPA

Primers were designed to amplify a 105-bp fragment based on the sequence of the virus gene (accession sequence MH543316) targeted for RPA amplification. The forward primer (5′CCTGATCCCAATCAATTTGC-3′) was labeled with DIG, and the reverse primer (5′-AGAGGCTGCCCTCTGGAC-3′) was labeled with Biotin. A BLAST search (http://www.ncbi.nlm.nih.gov) indicated no potential cross-hybridization of the primers with other bovine papillomaviruses, capripoxviruses, or bovine herpesvirus 2 (BHV2).

2.7.2. BPV-1 RPA Amplification

The twistAmp™ Basic Kit (TwistDx Ltd., Cambridge, UK) was used for isothermal RPA. Briefly, 4.8 µl of forward and reverse primers (480 nM of each), 29.5-µl rehydration buffer, and 11.2 µl of nuclease-free water were added to RPA tubes provided in the kit and containing lyophilized enzyme and other reagents. Additionally, 2.5 µl of 280-nM/Mg acetate was placed on the inside of the tube lid, which was mixed on tube inversion. Finally, 2 µl of DNA from the sample was added to the tube. The tube was briefly centrifuged and placed in a water bath (38 °C) for 30 min. Nontemplate (no sample DNA) controls were also included. Samples with lumpy skin disease virus (LSDV) and sheep poxvirus (SPV) were used as a check for nonspecific amplification. All reactions were repeated three times.

2.7.3. Visualization with Nucleic Acid Lateral Flow (NALF) Strip

Labeled RPA amplicons were assayed using Abington Health Lt (York, UK) PCRD lateral flow (nitrocellulose) strip immunoassay cassette, which can detect DIG/BIO-conjugated amplicons. Following RPA, 5 µl of RPA product and 70 µl of PCRD buffer were loaded into the PCRD cassette sample well, and the cassette was laid horizontally for at least five minutes. The DIG/Biotin amplicon bonded with colloidal carbon coated with anti-biotin detection antibodies (bonded with the biotin label). The carbon-conjugated amplicon migrated as the buffer wicked down the strip. The first test line on the nitrocellulose strip was striped with anti-DIG to capture carbon particles, which aggregated to darken the test line as a visual positive indicator of the amplicon. A second test line (striped with anti-FAM antibodies) was not used in this test. Further downstream, a control line was involved to capture excess carbon particles (not captured at the test lines) and as an indicator that the assay was working properly.

2.7.4. The Limit of Detection (LOD)

Purified BPV DNA standard with 10^6 viral genome copies/µL in Tris-EDTA buffer was used to estimate the minimum copies number of BPV-1 nucleic acid that can be identified via the RPA-NALF assay [36]. Serial dilutions (ten-fold) of purified BPV DNA were spiked into negative samples to estimate the LOD.

2.7.5. BPV RPA-NALF Immunoassay Detection Performance

Thirteen clinical samples (n = 13) collected from suspected cattle and assayed by PCR, along with negative controls, were tested using the RPA-NALF immunoassay test described above.

3. Results

3.1. PCR Detection and Sequence Analysis

As mentioned above, PCR products from skin wart biopsies were visualized by gel electrophoresis. Out of 13 collected samples, 11 (eight female and three male) were positive for the BPV-1 L1 gene, with an amplicon of 301-bp size. BPV-2, -3, -5, and -10 were not detected, and the controls from healthy animals showed no PCR product. Accordingly, the prevalence of BPV-1 in our study population was 3.6% (11 out of 308). The results showed the infection rate more in females (2.6%) than male ones (1.0%). In accordance with sequence analysis, sequencing of the PCR product partial L1 gene showed 100% identity between our 11 positive specimens.

The sequence was submitted to GeneBank (accession: MH543316) and compared with similar sequences (Table 2) from China, India, Sweden, Morocco, Switzerland, Turkey, USA, Croatia, and Japan. The phylogenetic analysis (Figure 2) showed the Egyptian BPV in the same clade and closely related to Indian BPV from cattle that were identified in 2014 at both the DNA and protein sequences. The virus sequenced in the present work revealed 99.7% identity with the Indian virus (accession number HG918265).

Table 2. Detailed information of L1 gene sequences of bovine papillomavirus (BPV) type-1 used in the present study.

Isolate Number	Country of Isolation	Year of Identification	Host Species	Accession Number
BPV 1	Egypt\New Valley Governorate (This study)	2016	Cattle	MH543316
BPV 2	India	2014	Cattle	HG918265
BPV 3	Sweden	1983	Cattle	J02045
BPV 4	China	2017	Cattle	MF045489
BPV 5	Morocco	2017	Cattle	KY746722
BPV 6	India	2012	Buffalo	KF148690
BPV 7	India	2012	Equine	KF114855
BPV 8	Japan	2011	Cattle	AB626705
BPV 9	Switzerland	2017	Cattle	MF384294
BPV 10	Switzerland	2017	Cattle	MF384293
BPV 11	Switzerland	2017	Cattle	MF384292
BPV 12	Switzerland	2017	Cattle	MF384291
BPV 13	Switzerland	2017	Cattle	MF384290
BPV 14	India	2018	Cattle	MK396096
BPV 15	Japan	2016	Cattle	LC426023
BPV 16	India	2018	Cattle	MK173052
BPV 17	Turkey	2018	Cattle	MH197482
BPV 18	Japan	2014	Cattle	LC333380
BPV 19	USA	2012	Equine	KY886226
BPV 20	China	2018	Cattle	MK347523
BPV 21	China	2017	Cattle	MG263871
BPV 22	China	2016	Cattle	MF435917
BPV 23	China	2016	Cattle	MF435916
BPV 24	China	2016	Cattle	KX907623
BPV 25	Switzerland	2017	Equine	MF384284
BPV 26	Switzerland	2017	Equine	MF384283
BPV 27	Switzerland	2017	Equine	MF384282
BPV 28	Switzerland	2017	Equine	MF384286
BPV 29	Croatia	2010	Cattle	JX046521
BPV 30	India	2017	Cattle	LT837966

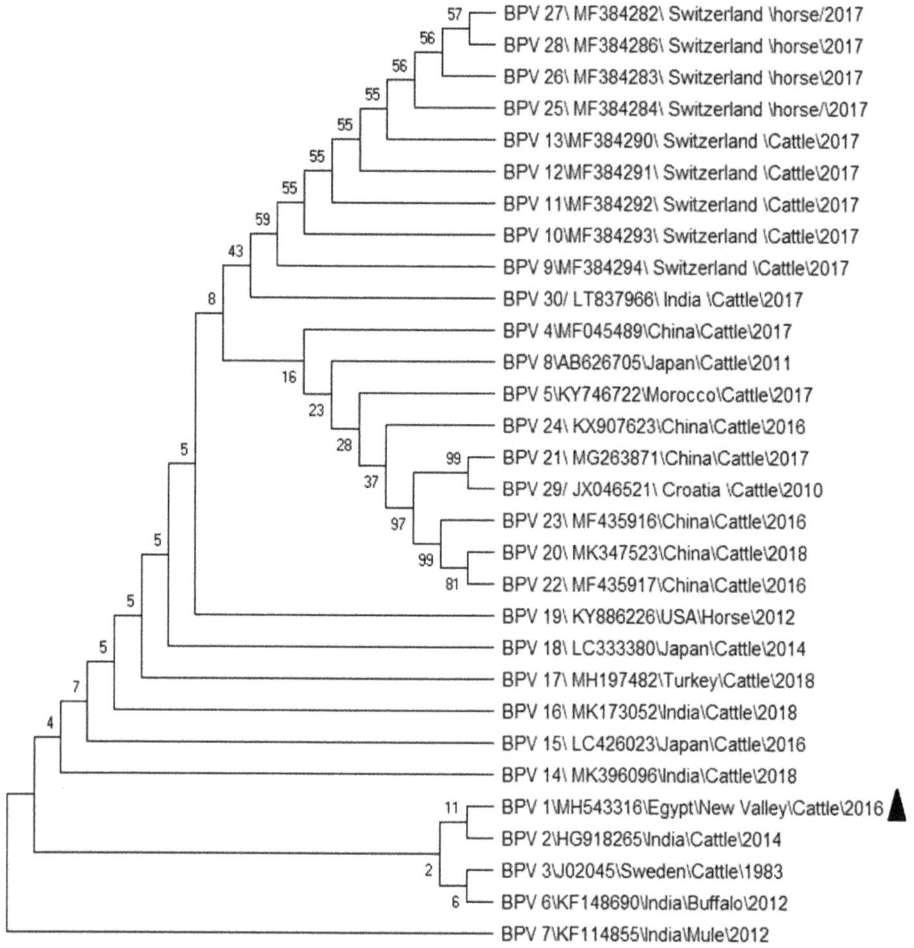

Figure 2. Phylogenetic tree of our bovine papillomavirus type-1 (BPV-1) from cattle with others BPVs that were taken from the GeneBank database based on L1 gene sequences. Numbers at the internal nodes represent the bootstrap probabilities (1000 replicates).

3.2. RPA-NALF Assay Results

As shown in Figure 3, PCRD cassettes were observed after incubation in a horizontal position for 5 min, with dark lines at the control line (C) and test line 1 (L1). Negative controls revealed dark lines only at the control line (C) (Figure 4). The LOD of our assay (based on the previously mentioned serial dilution tests) was approximately 100 viral genome copies per RPA reaction. RPA-NALF immunoassay was used to screen 13 samples for BPV, and it showed a 84.6% positivity rate, which is similar to that obtained by PCR.

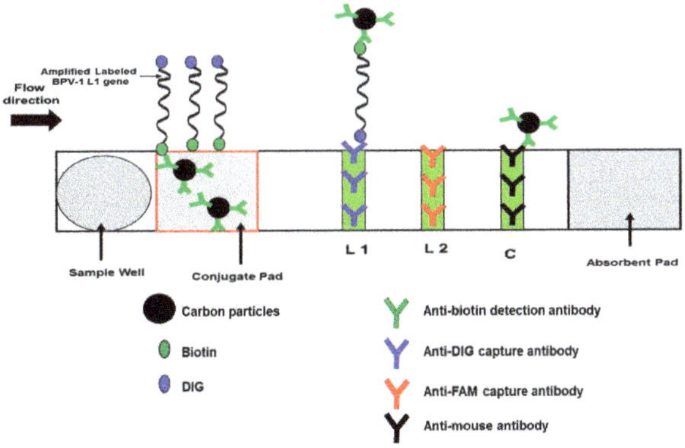

Figure 3. PCRD cassette. The carbon-conjugated biotin antibodies at the conjugate pad bind to biotin of the BPV-1 L1 gene amplicons and flow towards L1 and L2. L1 is lined with anti-DIG monoclonal antibodies to bind the labeled amplicons. L2 is decorated with anti-FAM monoclonal antibodies and will remain free from any carbon particles. C line is the control line that is lined with anti-mouse antibodies and will capture excess carbon-conjugated biotin.

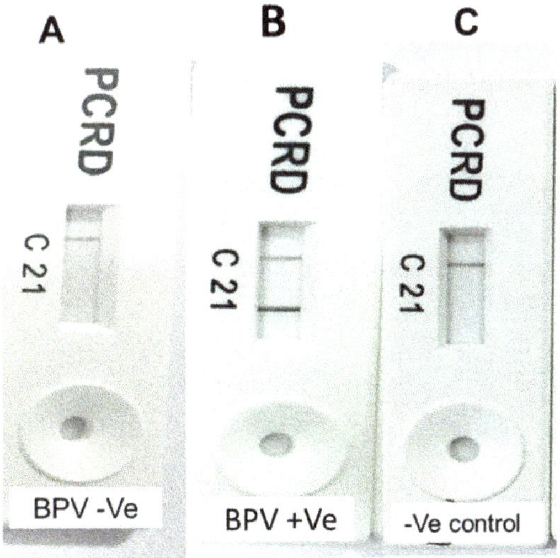

Figure 4. Results of recombinase polymerase amplification (RPA) amplicons identification after 30-min incubation at 38 °C using a PCRD cassette: (**A**) BPV assay revealed a negative reaction, (**B**) BPV assay revealed a positive reaction, and (**C**) negative result of the negative control.

4. Discussion

To the authors' knowledge, BPV is associated with several clinical problems that might result in considerable economic losses in cattle production due to the resulting damage of infected cattle's hides and dairy industries [37–39]. BPV can also affect the udders and teats of lactating cows, which might interfere with the suckling of young calves and milking of infected animals, besides predisposing the animals to secondary bacterial infection, which might result in mastitis [19,40]. Moreover, BPV infection causes gastrointestinal and bladder cancers in cattle, and further, the virus has been confirmed in the peripheral blood [41–44]. Despite the economic impact of BPV, there is insufficient information regarding the types of BPV circulating in Egypt. Interestingly, the present study reports BPV-1 (type 1) infection in cattle less than two years of age in New Valley Province. Furthermore, other BPV types

(BVP-2, -4, -5, and -10) were not detected in wart specimens collected from the symptomatic cattle. Moreover, the phylogenetic analysis revealed that the Egyptian BPV is closely related to strains reported in India. The virus was molecularly identified based on the amplification and sequencing of L1 gene fragments. As shown, a lower prevalence (3.6%) of BPV-1 infection was found in this study than previous studies either at the national or international level [18,19,45,46]. This difference might be attributed to various factors, including differences in cattle management systems, sampling locations, and sample sizes [10,47,48]. In the present work, the higher infection rate of female cattle versus males may be due to the immunosuppression associated with pregnancy and lactation [49]. These observations are consistent with those described elsewhere [50]. In addition, the treatment regime in the current study showed that cattle recovered from 25 to 86 days post-surgical excision. This treatment was similar to that used previously for BP-infected cattle [18]. As depicted in our results, BPV-1 could be only detected in cattle less than two years of age, while examined animals over two years old did not reveal such clinical signs at the time of examination. The history of these older cases revealed that they did not show the external signs of the disease throughout their lives. The lack of infection in older animals may be due to more well-developed immune systems, and the absence of clinical signs in these animals when they were young could be due to their good health status or may be the absence of the source of infection at that time [3,7,10].

In accordance with its diagnosis, several previous studies documented the role played by the molecular methods in the detection and characterization of various strains of BPV [19,51–54]. The present study confirmed the occurrence of BP infection in Egypt and further demonstrated the typing of the causative virus by molecular methods. These methods offer many advantages over the immunological methods that require specific antibodies against strains of BPV that may not be readily available in developing countries such as Egypt [19,51–54]. The two PCR-negative samples of putative BPV specimens may be due to infection by other strains of BPV than those investigated in our study. Sequencing the L1 gene of BPV-1 revealed a close genetic relationship with BPV-1 found in India, suggesting a possible transmission of BPV from India to Egypt. Further studying of the genetic relationships and diversity among BPVs may identify other types of BPV that might circulate in Egypt and provide more information of their places of origin, patterns of spreading, or other causes of cattle warts. Furthermore, investigation of the virus using immunohistochemistry and histopathological methods would be interesting to gain a better understanding of bovine papillomatosis in Egypt

Timely control measures are essential to curtail BPV spread, and therefore, a second aim of the present work was to develop a simple, easy-to-use point-of-need molecular test appropriate for use outside of laboratories, which could provide test results in less than about 30 min. The current work also investigated a test comprising RPA available commercially as a tube-based reaction, with lyophilized reagents in combination with a commercially available NALF strip immunoassay cassette to visually detect amplification products, as demonstrated for the sensitive (LOD: 100 viral genome copies) detection of BPV in samples derived from cattle wart excisions. This test provides a minimally instrumented, simple-to-interpret, fast diagnostic for BPV infection appropriate for a limited-resource setting [55–57]. The development of nucleic acid amplification tests (NAATs) similar to that used in the present study enhances both the sensitivity and specificity of diagnostics of various infectious agents compared to simple immunoassays [58,59]. In addition, the isothermal RPA method obviates the need for an expensive thermal cycler unit as needed for PCR. Further development integrating nucleic acid extraction into simple tests will facilitate their wider use and convenience and improve reliability and performance [60].

5. Conclusions

The present findings concluded that BPV-1 was molecularly confirmed in cattle in Egypt using NAATs. The tests found no incidence of other BPV types (BPV-2, -4, -5, and -10) in cattle wart specimens. Our study revealed the close genetic relatedness of the Egyptian BPV-1 with BPV-1 found in buffalo in India. Taken into account, the control of BPV infection and mitigation of its economic impact can be facilitated by simple point-of-need tests. A simple low-cost combined RPA-NALF test was also developed and validated for the point-of-need molecular diagnostics of cattle suitable for use outside of laboratories. Further studies seem mandatory to investigate the other circulating strains of BPV in Egypt, combined with assessing the risk factors for BP in Egypt being warranted, especially comparing different cattle management systems.

Author Contributions: M.E.-T., M.G.M., Y.F.E., S.M.M., and M.W.E.-S. were involved in the conception of the research idea and methodology design and performed the data analysis and interpretation. A.T., M.S.L., R.B.K., A.A., A.A.S., and E.K.E. participated in the methodology, sampling, the laboratory work and data analysis, and prepared the manuscript for publication. M.E.-T., M.G.M., Y.F.E., S.M.M., M.W.E.-S., and E.K.E., contributed their scientific advice, prepared the manuscript for publication, and did revision. All authors have read and agreed to the published version of the manuscript.

Funding: Mohamed El-Tholoth was the recipient of a scholarship from the Fulbright Visiting Scholar Program.

Conflicts of Interest: The authors declare no conflict of interest.

References

1. Lunardi, M.; Alfieri, A.A.; Otonel, R.A.A.; Alfieri, A.F. Bovine Papillomaviruses—Taxonomy and Genetic. Features. In *Current Issues in Molecular Virology: Viral Genetics and Biotechnological Application*; Intechopen: London, UK, 2013; p. 113.
2. Howley, P.M.; Lowy, D.R. Papillomaviruses. In *Fields' Virology*; Knipe, D.M., Howley, P.M., Eds.; Lippincott Williams and Wilkins: Philadelphia, PA, USA, 2007; pp. 2300–2354.
3. Campo, M. Papillomas and cancer in cattle. *Cancer Surv.* **1987**, *6*, 39–54. [PubMed]
4. Egawa, K. Eccrine-centred distribution of human papillomavirus 63 infection in the epidermis of the plantar skin. *Br. J. Dermatol.* **2005**, *152*, 993–996. [CrossRef] [PubMed]
5. Radostits, O.; Gay, C.; Hinchcliff, K.; Constable, P.; Jacobs, D.; Ikede, B.; McKenzie, R.; Colwell, D.; Osweiler, G.; Bildfell, R. *Veteriary Medicine: A Textbook of the Diseases of Cattle, Sheep, Pigs, Goats and Horses*, 10th ed.; Saunders Ltd.: Philadelphia, PA, USA, 2007.
6. McBride, A.A. Mechanisms and strategies of papillomavirus replication. *Biol. Chem.* **2017**, *398*, 919–927. [CrossRef] [PubMed]
7. Campo, M.S. Papillomavirus and disease in humans and animals. *Vet. Comp. Oncol.* **2003**, *1*, 3–14. [CrossRef] [PubMed]
8. Bernard, H.-U.; Burk, R.D.; Chen, Z.; Van Doorslaer, K.; Zur Hausen, H.; de Villiers, E.-M. Classification of papillomaviruses (PVs) based on 189 PV types and proposal of taxonomic amendments. *Virology* **2010**, *401*, 70–79. [CrossRef] [PubMed]
9. Walker, P.J.; Siddell, S.G.; Lefkowitz, E.J.; Mushegian, A.R.; Dempsey, D.M.; Dutilh, B.E.; Harrach, B.; Harrison, R.L.; Hendrickson, R.C.; Junglen, S.; et al. Changes to virus taxonomy and the International Code of Virus Classification and Nomenclature ratified by the International Committee on Taxonomy of Viruses (2019). *Arch. Virol.* **2019**, *164*, 2417–2429. [CrossRef]
10. Hamad, M.A.; Al-Shammari, A.M.; Odisho, S.M.; Yaseen, N.Y. Molecular epidemiology of bovine papillomatosis and identification of three genotypes in central Iraq. *Intervirology* **2017**, *60*, 156–164. [CrossRef]
11. Borzacchiello, G.; Roperto, F. Bovine papillomaviruses, papillomas and cancer in cattle. *Vet. Res.* **2008**, *39*, 1. [CrossRef]
12. Munday, J.S.; Thomson, N.; Dunowska, M.; Knight, C.G.; Laurie, R.E.; Hills, S. Genomic characterisation of the feline sarcoid-associated papillomavirus and proposed classification as Bos taurus papillomavirus type 14. *Vet. Microbiol.* **2015**, *177*, 289–295. [CrossRef]
13. Daudt, C.; Da Silva, F.; Lunardi, M.; Alves, C.; Weber, M.; Cibulski, S.; Alfieri, A.; Alfieri, A.; Canal, C. Papillomaviruses in ruminants: An update. *Transbound. Emerg. Dis.* **2018**, *65*, 1381–1395. [CrossRef]
14. Corteggio, A.; Altamura, G.; Roperto, F.; Borzacchiello, G. Bovine papillomavirus E5 and E7 oncoproteins in naturally occurring tumors: Are two better than one? *Infect. Agent Cancer* **2013**, *8*, 1. [CrossRef]
15. Lunardi, M.; de Alcântara, B.K.; Otonel, R.A.A.; Rodrigues, W.B.; Alfieri, A.F.; Alfieri, A.A. Bovine papillomavirus type 13 DNA in equine sarcoids. *J. Clin. Microbiol.* **2013**, *51*, 2167–2171. [CrossRef] [PubMed]
16. Bocaneti, F.; Altamura, G.; Corteggio, A.; Velescu, E.; Roperto, F.; Borzacchiello, G. Bovine papillomavirus: New insights into an old disease. *Transbound. Emerg. Dis.* **2016**, *63*, 14–23. [CrossRef] [PubMed]

17. MacLachlan, N.J.; Dubovi, E.J. (Eds.) Chapter 11—*Papillomaviridae* and *Polyomaviridae*. In *Fenner's Veterinary Virology (Fourth Edition)*; Academic Press: San Diego, CA, USA, 2011; pp. 213–223.
18. Salib, F.A.; Farghali, H.A. Clinical, epidemiological and therapeutic studies on Bovine Papillomatosis in Northern Oases, Egypt in 2008. *Vet. World* **2011**, *4*, 53.
19. Ata, E.B.; Mahmoud, M.A.E.; Madboli, A.A. Molecular detection and immunopathological examination of Deltapapillomavirus 4 in skin and udder of Egyptian cattle. *Vet. World* **2018**, *11*, 915–920. [CrossRef]
20. Özsoy, Ş.Y.; Özyıldız, Z.; Güzel, M. Clinical, pathological and immunohistochemical findings of bovine cutaneous papillomatosis. *Ankara Üniv. Vet. Fak. Derg.* **2011**, *58*, 161–165.
21. Silva, M.; Pontes, N.; Da Silva, K.; Guerra, M.; Freitas, A. Detection of bovine papillomavirus type 2 DNA in commercial frozen semen of bulls (Bos taurus). *Anim. Reprod. Sci.* **2011**, *129*, 146–151. [CrossRef] [PubMed]
22. Favre, M.; Breitburd, F.; Croissant, O.; Orth, G. Hemagglutinating activity of bovine papilloma virus. *Virology* **1974**, *60*, 572–578. [CrossRef]
23. Kirnbauer, R.; Chandrachud, L.; O'neil, B.; Wagner, E.; Grindlay, G.; Armstrong, A.; McGarvie, G.; Schiller, J.; Lowy, D.; Campo, M. Virus-like particles of bovine papillomavirus type 4 in prophylactic and therapeutic immunization. *Virology* **1996**, *219*, 37–44. [CrossRef]
24. Pathania, S.; Dhama, K.; Saikumar, G.; Shahi, S.; Somvanshi, R. Detection and quantification of bovine papilloma virus type 2 (BPV-2) by real-time PCR in urine and urinary bladder lesions in enzootic bovine haematuria (EBH)-affected cows. *Transbound. Emerg. Dis.* **2012**, *59*, 79–84. [CrossRef]
25. De Paz, H.; Brotons, P.; Muñoz-Almagro, C. Molecular isothermal techniques for combating infectious diseases: Towards low-cost point-of-care diagnostics. *Expert Rev. Mol. Diagn.* **2014**, *14*, 827–843. [CrossRef] [PubMed]
26. Piepenburg, O.; Williams, C.H.; Stemple, D.L.; Armes, N.A. DNA detection using recombination proteins. *PLoS Biol.* **2006**, *4*, e204. [CrossRef]
27. St John, A.; Price, C.P. Existing and emerging technologies for point-of-care testing. *Clin. Biochem. Rev.* **2014**, *35*, 155. [PubMed]
28. El-Tholoth, M.; Branavan, M.; Naveenathayalan, A.; Balachandran, W. Recombinase polymerase amplification–nucleic acid lateral flow immunoassays for Newcastle disease virus and infectious bronchitis virus detection. *Mol. Biol. Rep.* **2019**, *46*, 6391–6397. [CrossRef] [PubMed]
29. Euler, M.; Wang, Y.; Otto, P.; Tomaso, H.; Escudero, R.; Anda, P.; Hufert, F.T.; Weidmann, M. Recombinase polymerase amplification assay for rapid detection of Francisella tularensis. *J. Clin. Microbiol.* **2012**, *50*, 2234–2238. [CrossRef] [PubMed]
30. Chow, W.H.A.; McCloskey, C.; Tong, Y.; Hu, L.; You, Q.; Kelly, C.P.; Kong, H.; Tang, Y.-W.; Tang, W. Application of isothermal helicase-dependent amplification with a disposable detection device in a simple sensitive stool test for toxigenic Clostridium difficile. *J. Mol. Diagn.* **2008**, *10*, 452–458. [CrossRef]
31. Vincent, M.; Xu, Y.; Kong, H. Helicase-dependent isothermal DNA amplification. *EMBO Rep.* **2004**, *5*, 795–800. [CrossRef] [PubMed]
32. Wang, Z.; Yang, P.P.; Zhang, Y.H.; Tian, K.Y.; Bian, C.Z.; Zhao, J. Development of a reverse transcription recombinase polymerase amplification combined with lateral-flow dipstick assay for avian influenza H9N2 HA gene detection. *Transbound. Emerg. Dis.* **2019**, *66*, 546–551. [CrossRef]
33. Yaguiu, A.; de Carvalho, C.; de Freitas, A.C.; Góes, L.G.B.; Dagli, M.L.Z.; Birgel Jr, E.H.; Beçak, W.; dos Santos, R.d.C.S. Papillomatosis in cattle: In situ detection of bovine papillomavirus DNA sequences in reproductive tissues. *J. Morphol. Sci.* **2017**, *23*, 0-0.
34. Kumar, P.; Nagarajan, N.; Saikumar, G.; Arya, R.; Somvanshi, R. Detection of bovine papilloma viruses in wart-like lesions of upper gastrointestinal tract of cattle and buffaloes. *Transbound. Emerg. Dis.* **2015**, *62*, 264–271. [CrossRef]
35. Viljoen, G.J.; Nel, L.H.; Crowther, J.R. *Molecular Diagnostic PCR Handbook*; Springer Science & Business Media: Berlin, Germany, 2005.
36. Shalaby, M.A.; El-Deeb, A.; El-Tholoth, M.; Hoffmann, D.; Czerny, C.-P.; Hufert, F.T.; Weidmann, M.; Abd El Wahed, A. Recombinase polymerase amplification assay for rapid detection of lumpy skin disease virus. *BMC Vet. Res.* **2016**, *12*, 244. [CrossRef] [PubMed]
37. Carvalho, C.d.; Freitas, A.C.d.; Brunner, O.; Góes, L.G.B.; Cavalcante, A.Y.; Beçak, W.; Santos, R.d.C.S.d. Bovine papillomavirus type 2 in reproductive tract and gametes of slaughtered bovine females. *Braz. J. Microbiol.* **2003**, *34*, 82–84. [CrossRef]

38. Carvalho, R.; Sakata, S.; Giovanni, D.; Mori, E.; Brandão, P.; Richtzenhain, L.; Pozzi, C.; Arcaro, J.; Miranda, M.; Mazzuchelli-de-Souza, J. Bovine papillomavirus in Brazil: Detection of coinfection of unusual types by a PCR-RFLP method. *Biomed. Res. Int.* **2013**, *2013*, 270898. [CrossRef] [PubMed]
39. Catroxo, M.; Martins, A.; Petrella, S.; Souza, F.; Nastari, B. Ultrastructural Study of Bovine Papillomavirus During Outbreaks in Brazil. *Int. J. Morphol.* **2013**, *31*, 777–784. [CrossRef]
40. Campo, M.S. *Bovine Papillomavirus: Old System, New Lessons?* Caister Academic Press: Norfolk, UK, 2006.
41. Dos Santos, R.S.; Lindsey, C.J.; Ferraz, O.P.; Pinto, J.R.; Mirandola, R.S.; Benesi, F.J.; Birgel, E.H.; Pereira, C.; Be, W. Bovine papillomavirus transmission and chromosomal aberrations: An experimental model. *J. Gen. Virol.* **1998**, *79*, 2127–2135. [CrossRef]
42. Freitas, A.C.d.; Carvalho, C.d.; Brunner, O.; Birgel-Junior, E.H.; Dellalibera, A.M.M.P.; Benesi, F.J.; Gregory, L.; Beçak, W.; Santos, R.d.C.S.d. Viral DNA sequences in peripheral blood and vertical transmission of the virus: A discussion about BPV-1. *Braz. J. Microbiol.* **2003**, *34*, 76–78. [CrossRef]
43. Araldi, R.; Melo, T.; Diniz, N.; Mazzuchelli-de-Souza, J.; Carvalho, R.; Beçak, W.; Stocco, R. Bovine papillomavirus clastogenic effect analyzed in comet assay. *Biomed. Res. Int.* **2013**, *2013*, 630683. [CrossRef]
44. Campos, S.; Melo, T.; Assaf, S.; Araldi, R.; Mazzuchelli-de-Souza, J.; Sircili, M.; Carvalho, R.; Roperto, F.; Beçak, W.; Stocco, R. Chromosome aberrations in cells infected with bovine papillomavirus: Comparing cutaneous papilloma, esophagus papilloma, and urinary bladder lesion cells. *ISRN Oncol.* **2013**, *2013*, 910849. [CrossRef]
45. Dagalp, S.B.; Dogan, F.; Farzani, T.A.; Salar, S.; Bastan, A. The genetic diversity of bovine papillomaviruses (BPV) from different papillomatosis cases in dairy cows in Turkey. *Arch. Virol.* **2017**, *162*, 1507–1518. [CrossRef]
46. Rojas-Anaya, E.; Cantu-Covarrubias, A.; Alvarez, J.F.; Loza-Rubio, E. Detection and phylogenetic analysis of bovine papillomavirus in cutaneous warts in cattle in Tamaulipas, Mexico. *Can. J. Vet. Res.* **2016**, *80*, 262–268.
47. Olkeba, W.; Sorba, E.; Belay, A.; Deres; Gebremedhin, E. Prevalence of major skin diseases of cattle and associated risk factors around Ambo town, Ethiopia. *Anim. Health Prod.* **2016**, *64*, 355–365.
48. Araldi, R.; Carvalho, R.; Melo, T.; Pessoa, N.; Sant'Ana, T.; Mazzuchelli-de-Souza, J.; Spadacci-Morena, D.; Beçak, W.; Stocco, R. Bovine papillomavirus in beef cattle: First description of BPV-12 and putative type BAPV8 in Brazil. *Genet. Mol. Res.* **2014**, *13*, 5644–5653. [CrossRef] [PubMed]
49. Goff, J.; Horst, R. Physiological changes at parturition and their relationship to metabolic disorders1, 2. *J. Dairy Sci.* **1997**, *80*, 1260–1268. [CrossRef]
50. Otter, A.; Leonard, D. Fibropapillomatosis outbreak in calves. *Vet. Rec.* **2003**, *153*, 570–571. [PubMed]
51. Reetha, T.; Manickam, R.; Boovalingam, P. Detection of Bovine Papillomavirus in Cutaneous Lesions by Polymerase Chain Reaction (PCR) in Cattle. *Int. J. Curr. Microbiol. Appl. Sci.* **2020**, *9*, 1611–1616. [CrossRef]
52. Fagbohun, O. Molecular Detection Of Bovine Papilloma Viruses Associated With Cutaneous Warts In Some Breeds Of Nigerian Cattle. *Int. J. Biotechnol. Biochem.* **2016**, *12*, 123–130.
53. Han, S.-H.; Park, Y.-S.; Seo, J.-P.; Kang, T.-Y. PCR-based Detection of Bovine Papillomavirus DNA from the Cutaneous Papillomas and Surrounding Environments in the Korean Native Cattle, Hanwoo. *J. Vet. Clin.* **2016**, *33*, 346. [CrossRef]
54. Peng, H.; Wu, C.; Li, J.; Li, C.; Chen, Z.; Pei, Z.; Tao, L.; Gong, Y.; Pan, Y.; Bai, H.; et al. Detection and genomic characterization of Bovine papillomavirus isolated from Chinese native cattle. *Transbound. Emerg. Dis.* **2019**, *66*, 2197–2203. [CrossRef]
55. Mark, D.; Haeberle, S.; Roth, G.; Von Stetten, F.; Zengerle, R. Microfluidic lab-on-a-chip platforms: Requirements, characteristics and applications. In *Microfluidics Based Microsystems*; Springer: New York, NY, USA, 2010; pp. 305–376.
56. Abd El Wahed, A.; Weidmann, M.; Hufert, F.T. Diagnostics-in-a-Suitcase: Development of a portable and rapid assay for the detection of the emerging avian influenza A (H7N9) virus. *J. Clin. Virol.* **2015**, *69*, 16–21. [CrossRef] [PubMed]
57. Faye, O.; Faye, O.; Soropogui, B.; Patel, P.; Abd El Wahed, A.; Loucoubar, C.; Fall, G.; Kiory, D.; Magassouba, N.F.; Keita, S. Development and deployment of a rapid recombinase polymerase amplification Ebola virus detection assay in Guinea in 2015. *Eurosurveillance* **2015**, *20*, 30053. [CrossRef]
58. La Marca, A.; Capuzzo, M.; Paglia, T.; Roli, L.; Trenti, T.; Nelson, S.M. Testing for SARS-CoV-2 (COVID-19): A systematic review and clinical guide to molecular and serological in-vitro diagnostic assays. *Reprod. Biomed. Online* **2020**, *41*, 483–499. [CrossRef] [PubMed]

59. Silva, R.O.S.; Vilela, E.G.; Neves, M.S.; Lobato, F.C.F. Evaluation of three enzyme immunoassays and a nucleic acid amplification test for the diagnosis of Clostridium difficile-associated diarrhea at a university hospital in Brazil. *Rev. Soc. Bras. Med. Trop.* **2014**, *47*, 447–450. [CrossRef] [PubMed]
60. Li, J.; Macdonald, J.; von Stetten, F. A comprehensive summary of a decade development of the recombinase polymerase amplification. *Analyst* **2018**, *144*, 31–67. [CrossRef] [PubMed]

animals

MDPI

Article

Circulation of Indigenous Bovine Respiratory Syncytial Virus Strains in Turkish Cattle: The First Isolation and Molecular Characterization

Zafer Yazici [1,*], Emre Ozan [2], Cuneyt Tamer [1], Bahadir Muftuoglu [2], Gerald Barry [3], Hanne Nur Kurucay [1], Ahmed Eisa Elhag [1,*], Abdurrahman Anil Cagirgan [4], Semra Gumusova [1] and Harun Albayrak [1]

1 Department of Veterinary Virology, Faculty of Veterinary Medicine, Ondokuz Mayis University, 55139 Samsun, Turkey; cuneyt_tamer@hotmail.com (C.T.); kurucayhannenur@gmail.com (H.N.K.); semragumusova@hotmail.com (S.G.); harunalbayrak55@msn.com (H.A.)

2 Department of Veterinary Experimental Animals, Faculty of Veterinary Medicine, Ondokuz Mayis University, 55139 Samsun, Turkey; emre.ozan@omu.edu.tr (E.O.); bahadirmuftuoglu@hotmail.com (B.M.)

3 Veterinary Science Centre, School of Veterinary Medicine, University College of Dublin, Dublin 4, Ireland; gerald.barry@ucd.ie

4 Bornova Veterinary Control Institute, Veterinary Control Institute Directorates, Ministry of Agriculture and Forestry, 35010 Izmir, Turkey; a.anilcagirgan@gmail.com

* Correspondence: zyazici@omu.edu.tr (Z.Y.); ahmedeisa_85@hotmail.com (A.E.E.)

Received: 12 August 2020; Accepted: 18 September 2020; Published: 20 September 2020

check for updates

Simple Summary: Bovine respiratory syncytial virus (BRSV) is an important pathogen of both dairy and beef cattle, and causes huge economic losses annually across the world. This study reports the identification, isolation, and molecular characterization of a new BRSV (subgroup III) strain collected from respiratory distressed cattle in Turkey. The three field isolates obtained showed 100% similarity to each other at the nucleotide (nt) level and were found to be 99.49% and 99.22% identical to another Turkish strain—KY499619—at both (nt) and amino acid (aa) levels, respectively. They were also 97.43% (nt) and 98.44% (aa) similar to the American reference strain KU159366. This important information will inform Turkish BRSV diagnostic and control strategies, as well as highlight the urgent need to better understand the burden that BRSV is placing on the Turkish agricultural sector.

Abstract: Bovine respiratory disease (BRD) is a huge economic burden on the livestock industries of countries worldwide. Bovine respiratory syncytial virus (BRSV) is one of the most important pathogens that contributes to BRD. In this study, we report the identification and first isolation, with molecular characterization, of a new BRSV strain from lung specimens of three beef cows in Turkey that died from respiratory distress. After the screening of lung tissues for BRD-associated viruses using a multiscreen antigen-ELISA, a BRSV antigen was detected. This was then confirmed by real-time RT-PCR specific for BRSV. Following confirmation, virus isolation was conducted in MDBK cell cultures and clear CPE, including syncytia compatible with BRSV, were detected. RT-nested PCR, using F gene-specific primers, was performed on the cultured isolates, and the products were sequenced and deposited to Genbank with accession numbers MT179304, MT024766, and MT0244767. Phylogenetic analysis of these sequences indicated that the cattle were infected with BRSV from subgroup III and were closely related to previously identified American and Turkish strains, but contained some amino acid and nucleotide differences. This research paves the way for further studies on the molecular characteristics of natural BRSV isolates, including full genome analysis and disease pathogenesis, and also contributes to the development of robust national strategies against this virus.

Keywords: BRSV; cattle; isolation; respiratory disorders; sequencing

1. Introduction

Bovine respiratory disease (BRD) is a term used to describe respiratory disease in cattle caused by single or a range of pathogens. It is a complex disease, with multiple viruses, bacteria, and parasites potentially involved [1,2]. BRD can negatively affect production and is therefore considered a major economic burden on the livestock industry worldwide [1,3]. Bovine respiratory syncytial virus (BRSV), also called *Bovine orthopneumovirus*, is an important pathogen of this complex [2,4,5]. BRSV belongs to the genus *Orthopneumovirus* of the family *Pneumoviridae* in the order *Mononegavirales* [6] and has a negative sense, single-stranded RNA genome. The non-segmented virus genome consists of 10 genes that encode 11 proteins: Two non-structural proteins (NS1 and NS2); a nucleocapsid (N) protein; a phosphoprotein (P); a matrix protein (M); glycoproteins SH, G (attachment), and F (fusion); M2-1 and M2-2 (control transcription and RNA replication); and RNA polymerase (L) [7,8].

Phylogenetic analysis based on both F and G proteins has led to a subdivision of BRSV into eight subgroups, denoted I–VIII [7,9–11]. These subgroups tend to separate geographically; subgroup I BRSV strains are typically isolated in the UK and Switzerland, whereas subgroup II normally includes strains from the Netherlands, Denmark, Belgium, France, and Japan [9,12]. The strains from the USA are commonly included in subgroup III, while some strains from the USA and other European countries fall into subgroup IV [7,9]. Finally subgroups V and VI include BRSV strains usually found in Belgium and France [9]. Subgroups VII and VIII are a recent addition and are predominantly seen in Europe, particularly in Italy and Croatia [7,10]. In addition, a putative new BRSV subgroup, tentatively named subgroup IX, has been proposed, in order to classify recent strains isolated from Brazil, which have mutations in the immunodominant region of the G protein [11].

BRSV predominantly infects cattle, although sheep and goats can also be infected [8,12]. The virus is mainly transmitted by direct contact and/or aerosols and both clinical and sub-clinical animals are capable of transmitting [7,13,14]. BRSV outbreaks can occur in all ages of animals, but young calves (particularly those between 2 weeks and 9 months old) are especially vulnerable [12,13].

The clinical manifestations of BRSV infections in cattle can vary from mildly symptomatic to fatal, and the outcome is multifactorial. The breed of cattle; the strain of virus; and the contribution of other viruses, bacteria, and parasites all play a role, alongside other factors, such as management practices and environments [5,14,15]. Although BRSV infection is rarely fatal, it can lead to upper and lower respiratory damage in young calves and is characterized by a fever, cough, decreased feed intake, increased respiratory rate, and nasal discharge [14,15].

There is limited information available about the seroprevalence of BRSV in Turkey and very few BRSV sequences from Turkish isolates have been submitted to GenBank [4,5]. Cases of BRD are plentiful in Turkey and some have been characterized, but major gaps in our understanding remain, thus limiting the ability to control it [3,16]. In this context, the aim of this study was to present both the first isolation of BRSV in Turkey and its molecular characterization, consisting of both sequencing and phylogenetic analysis.

2. Material and Methods

2.1. Samples

Between December 2018 and January 2019, a veterinarian in the Samsun province of Northern Turkey reported three cases of respiratory disease in beef cattle from the same farm. The cattle were unvaccinated against any BRD-associated viruses, including BRSV. The cattle died from severe respiratory disorders, including pneumonia. Lung tissue samples were taken post-mortem and sent to the Virology Department of The Faculty of Veterinary Medicine, Ondokuz Mayis University, for diagnosis. To differentiate the samples, they were labeled 34TR2018, 43TR2018, and 07TR2019, according to the animal they came from.

2.2. Virus Isolation

For cell culture isolation, approximately 1 g of lung tissue was placed in 5 mL of cold Minimal Essential Medium (MEM) containing 2% penicillin/streptomycin (Sigma-Aldrich, St. Louis, MO, USA), and then homogenized on ice for 1 min at 6000 rpm using a tissue homogenizer (Heidolph Ins., Schwabach, Germany). The homogenate was then centrifuged at 1500× g for 15 min and the supernatant was sterile-filtered (0.22 µm) and stored at −20 °C. For PCR, approximately 30 mg of lung tissue was homogenized with a Tissue-Lyser (Qiagen AG, Hilden, Germany) in 1.8 mL of MEM containing 2% penicillin/streptomycin. Obtained homogenates were clarified by centrifugation at 1500× g for 15 min and the supernatant was then sterile-filtered (0.22 µm) and stored at −20 °C.

MDBK cells were used for the virus isolation studies. Briefly, MDBK cells were cultivated at 37 °C with 5% CO_2 in Dulbecco's Modified Eagle's Medium (DMEM, Gibco, Paisley, UK) supplemented with 10% fetal calf serum (FCS, Sigma-Aldrich) and 1% penicillin/streptomycin (Sigma-Aldrich). Virus isolation from suspected samples was conducted by performing blind passages. Supernatants from tissue homogenates were inoculated onto MDBK monolayers at 37 °C for 60 min and then replaced with DMEM containing 2% FCS. Cells were maintained at 37 °C with 5% CO_2, and checked daily for cytopathic effects (CPE).

2.3. Antigen-ELISA for BRD-Associated Viruses

The lung tissues were tested using a commercially available multiscreen antigen-ELISA kit (Bio-X, Rochefort, Belgium, Cat. No: BIO K, 340/5). The kit has been reported to detect Bovine parainfluenza-3 (BPIV-3), Bovine viral diarrhea virus (BVDV), BRSV, and Bovine herpesvirus-1 (BHV-1), and was used according to the manufacturer's instructions.

2.4. Nucleic Acid Extraction and Amplification

We performed RNA extractions from homogenized lung tissue, as well as infected cell culture lysates, using a GeneJET RNA Purification Kit (Thermo Fisher Scientific, Vilnius, Lithuania), according to the manufacturer's instructions. The extracted RNA was eluted in 75 µL of elution buffer and kept at −80 °C.

For the real time RT-PCR analysis, the primers and the TaqMan probe targeted the N gene of BRSV and have been previously described by Boxus et al. [17]. For the RT-nested PCR, F gene-specific primers were used as previously described by Vilcek et al. [18]. For the first round of RT-nested PCR, we used B1 and B2A primers that amplify a 711 bp product. This was followed by B3 and B4A primers that amplify a 481 bp product. The sequence data of the primers and probe are given in Table 1.

Table 1. Information on the primers and probes used in the analysis.

Primers and Probe	Sequences (5′-3′)	Product Size(bp)	Ref.
F primer	GCAATGCTGCAGGACTAGGTATAAT	124	Boxus et al. [17]
R primer	ACACTGTAATTGATGACCCCATTCT		
Probe	FAM-ACCAAGACTTGTATGATGCTGCCAAAGCA-TAMRA		
B1	AATCAACATGCAGTGCAGTTAG	711	Vilcek et al. [18]
B2A	TTTGGTCATTCGTTATAGGCAT		
B3	GTGCAGTTAGTAGAGGTTATCTTAGT	481	
B4A	TAGTTCTTTAGATCAAGTACTTTGCT		

The real time RT-PCR was carried out using an iTaq™ Universal Probes One-Step Kit (Biorad, Hercules, CA, USA, Cat No: 1725140) on a CFX Connect real time PCR machine (Biorad). The real time RT-PCR reactions were carried out in a final volume of 25 µL containing 5 µL of RNA, 12.5 µL of 2X buffer, 320 nM of each primer, 160 nM of probe, 0.5 µL of RT enzyme, and 5 µL of RNAse-free water. The PCR conditions were as follows: 10 min at 50 °C for reverse transcription and 3 min at 95 °C, followed by 45 cycles at 95 °C for 7 s and 59 °C for 10 s.

The RT-nested PCR was carried out using the Qiagen Onestep RT-PCR kit (Qiagen, Cat No:210212). The first round of PCR was performed in a final volume of 50 μL consisting of 5 μL of RNA, 10 μL of 5X buffer, 400 nM of each primer, 1 μL of dNTP, 1 μL of RT enzyme, and 29 μL of RNAse-free water. The PCR conditions were as follows: 30 min at 50 °C for reverse transcription and 15 min at 95 °C, followed by 35 cycles at 95 °C for 45 s, 50 °C for 45 s, 72 °C for 60 s, and finally a cycle at 72 °C for 10 min. The second round of PCR was also carried out in a final volume of 50 μL containing 5 μL of the first round RT-PCR product, 10 μL of 5X buffer, 400 nM of each primer, 1 μL of dNTP, 1 μL of RT enzyme, and 29 μL of RNAse-free water. The cycling conditions employed for the second round of PCR were as follows: 1 min at 95 °C and 45 s at 95 °C, followed by 35 cycles at 50 °C for 45 s, 72 °C for 1 min, and finally a cycle at 72 °C for 10 min. Positive controls for both RT-PCR tests were provided by the virology laboratory of the Samsun Veterinary Control Institute, Turkey. For the nested PCR, all amplicons were visualized on 1% agarose gels.

2.5. Sequencing and Phylogenetic Analysis

PCR products were purified using a QIAquick PCR purification kit (Qiagen), according to the manufacturer's instructions and then Sanger sequenced by RefGen Biotechnology, Ankara, Turkey (http://www.refgen.com). The sequences were aligned using Bioedit, version 7.2.5, followed by BLAST analysis in GenBank databases [19]. For comparison, we selected seventeen representative isolate sequences from GenBank, including BRSV and human respiratory syncytial virus (HRSV) strains. The phylogenetic tree was constructed with the maximum likelihood method under the Tamura-3 parameter model using MEGA X (Molecular Evolutionary Genetics Analysis-MEGA, version 10.0.5) [20], and the bootstrap values were based on F gene nucleotide (nt) sequences. The tree was assessed using 1000 bootstrap replications. The sequences identified from animals 07TR2019, 34TR2018, and 43TR2018 were deposited in GenBank with the accession numbers MT179304, MT024766, and MT0244767, respectively.

3. Results

3.1. The Identification of Lung Tissue Samples Infected with BRSV

The first step of this study was the screening of all lung tissues for BRD-associated viruses using both the multiscreen antigen-ELISA and real time RT-PCR. All tissue samples were BRSV positive by ELISA, and negative for BVDV, BHV-1, and BPIV-3. The samples were also confirmed to be positive for BRSV by real time RT-PCR.

3.2. Virus Isolation

Lung homogenates from each animal, consisting of 43TR2018, 342TR2018, and 07TR2019, were added to MDBK cultures and incubated. Obvious CPE including syncytia were visible between 3- and 4-days post inoculation (Figure 1).

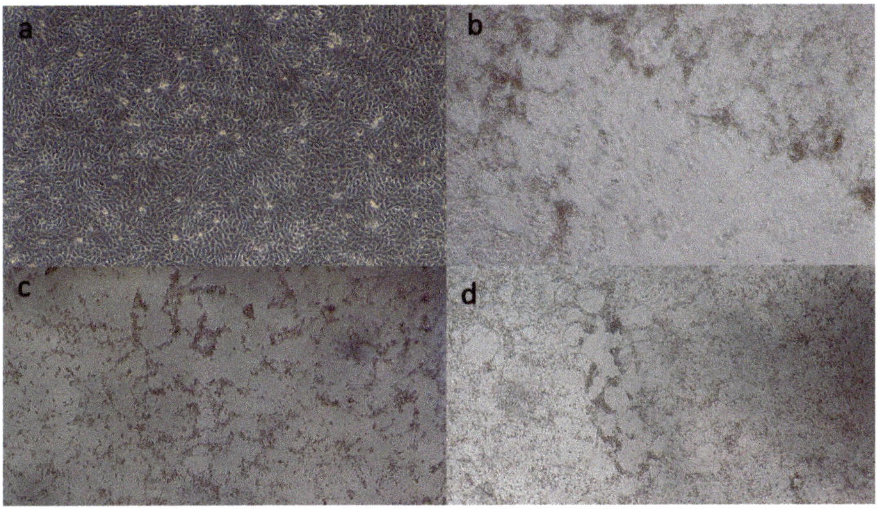

Figure 1. Photos of MDBK cells: (**a**) Cell control; (**b**,**c**) MDBK cells displaying cytopathic effects (CPE) and syncytia formation 72 h post-infection with isolates 43TR2018 and 34TR2018, respectively; (**d**) MDBK cells displaying limited CPE and syncytia foci 72 h post-infection with isolate 07TR2019.

3.3. RT-Nested PCR

Following virus propagation in culture, RNA was extracted from each of the infected MDBK cultures and nested PCR was performed. Based on this, 711 and 481 bp bands corresponding to the F gene were visible for 43TR2018 and 07TR2019, while only a 481 bp band, corresponding to the second round of PCR, was visible for isolate 34TR2018.

3.4. Sequencing and Phylogenetic Analysis

Following the RT-nested PCR, the 481 bp fragments were sequenced. As detailed in Table 2, the sequencing showed that the three isolates—MT179304, MT024766, and MT024767—had a 100% similarity to each other at the nucleotide (nt) level. Furthermore, the three isolates were found to be 99.49% and 99.22% identical to another Turkish strain—KY499619 [3]—at both nt and amino acid (aa) levels, respectively. The three isolates presented here were also 97.43% (nt) and 98.44% (aa) identical to the American reference strain KU159366.

As depicted in Figure 2, the phylogenetic analysis of the F gene revealed that our isolates—MT179304, MT024766, and MT024767—are in the same cluster in subgroup III, together with isolates KY499619 and KU159366, based on the nucleotide sequence.

Interestingly, however, there are some small amino acid differences that exist between these newly presented isolates and KY499619 and KU159366 (Table 3). Unlike the three isolates presented here, in isolate KU159366, a Threonine (T) at position 118 is an Alanine (A) and a Threonine (T) at position 173 is a Serine (S), while a Lysine (K) at position 176 is a Glutamic Acid (E) in isolate KY499619.

Table 2. Percentage of nucleotide and amino acid similarity between the isolates identified in this study (marked with *) and other bovine respiratory syncytial virus (BRSV) strains obtained from Genbank. NA: Not available.

			Amino Acid Similarities (%)												
	GenBank Number	**Strain Name and Country**	**NC038272**	**FJ543091**	**M82816**	**D00953**	**MG947594**	**KU159366**	**KY499619**	**MT179304***	**MT024766***	**MT024767***	**AF092942**	**AF124561**	**MF153477**
Nucleotide Similarities (%)	**NC038272**	ATCC51908 NA		96.05	96.05	97.65	98.44	93.60	92.77	93.60	93.60	93.60	98.44	100.00	95.24
	FJ543091	BRSV-25-BR Brasil	96.14		98.44	95.24	96.05	89.38	88.51	89.38	89.38	89.38	94.42	96.05	91.09
	M82816	NA NA	96.14	99.49		95.24	96.05	90.24	89.38	90.24	90.24	90.24	94.42	96.05	91.93
	D00953	RB 93 NA	98.20	96.40	96.40		97.65	91.93	90.24	91.09	91.09	91.09	96.05	97.65	92.77
	MG947594	Lovsta 2016 Sweden	97.69	95.89	95.89	98.46		91.93	91.09	91.93	91.93	91.93	96.85	98.44	93.60
	KU159366	USII/S1 USA	96.14	93.06	93.57	94.60	94.09		97.65	98.44	98.44	98.44	93.60	93.60	93.60
	KY499619	BRS/TR/Erz/2014 Turkey	95.63	93.06	93.57	94.09	93.57	97.43		99.22	99.22	99.22	92.77	92.77	92.77
	MT179304 *	07TR2019 Turkey	95.63	93.57	94.09	94.09	93.57	97.43	99.49		100.00	100.00	93.60	93.60	93.60
	MT024766 *	34TR2018 Turkey	95.63	93.57	94.09	94.09	93.57	97.43	99.49	100.00		100.00	93.60	93.60	93.60
	MT024767 *	43TR2018 Turkey	95.63	93.57	94.09	94.09	93.57	97.43	99.49	100.00	100.00		93.60	93.60	93.60
	AF092942	ATue51908 Germany	99.49	95.89	95.89	97.94	97.43	96.14	95.63	95.63	95.63	95.63		98.44	95.24
	AF124561	A2Gelfi France	99.49	95.63	95.63	97.69	97.17	95.63	95.12	95.12	95.12	95.12	98.97		95.24
	MF153477	BRSV-UnepJab-1 NA	96.66	93.06	93.06	95.12	94.60	94.86	94.34	94.34	94.34	94.34	96.66	96.14	

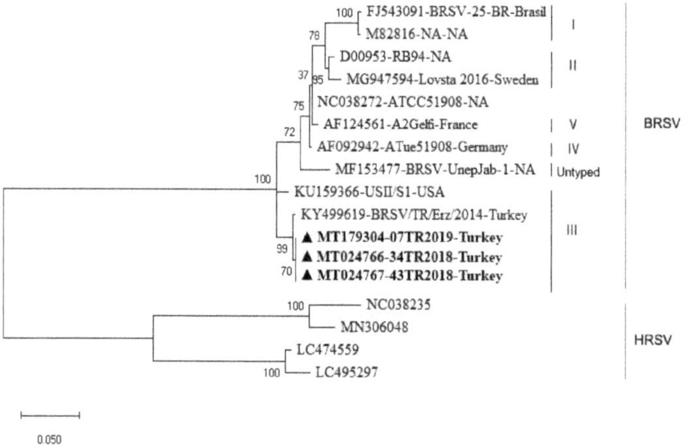

Figure 2. The phylogenetic analysis of the BRSV strains isolated in this study. The tree was constructed from a partial analysis of the BRSV F gene using the maximum likelihood method with MEGA X software. The robustness branching pattern was tested with 1000 bootstrap replications. According to the phylogenetic tree, the current strains were in subgroup III (marked in bold and with a ▲). The BRSV sequences were named using their GenBank accession number, strain name, and geographical origin. NA: Not available.

Table 3. Partial alignment of the F gene from the isolates identified in this study (marked with *), with a selection of strains from the different subgroups. NA: Not available.

Sub-Groups	GenBank Number	Strain Name	Amino Acid Positions of BRSV F Gene Sequence																			
			67	70	71	75	80	91	100	101	102	104	105	113	114	115	118	124	148	168	173	176
I	FJ543091	BRSV-25-BR	N	N	G	K	K	V	E	P	T	S	S	E	S	I	T	K	I	N	S	K
	M82816	NA	.	.	.	.	.	A	.	.	.	.	.	.	.	.	.	.	.	K	.	.
II	D00953	RB 94	.	.	S	N	.	.	.	.	A	.	.	.	L	.	K	.	.	K	.	.
	MG947594	Lovsta 2016	.	.	S	.	.	.	.	L	A	.	.	.	L	.	.	.	.	K	.	.
III	KU159366	USII/S1	D	K	S	.	.	T	V	.	A	F	N	.	L	M	A	R	.	K	.	.
	KY499619	BRS/TR/Erz/2014	D	K	S	.	.	T	V	.	A	F	N	.	L	M	.	R	.	K	T	E
	MT179304 *	07TR2019	D	K	S	.	.	T	V	.	A	F	N	.	L	M	.	R	.	K	T	.
	MT024766 *	34TR2018	D	K	S	.	.	T	V	.	A	F	N	.	L	M	.	R	.	K	T	.
	MT024767 *	43TR2018	D	K	S	.	.	T	V	.	A	F	N	.	L	M	.	R	.	K	T	.
IV	AF092942	ATue51908	.	K	S	.	.	.	.	.	A	F	.	.	L	.	.	.	V	K	.	.
V	AF124561	A2Gelfi	.	.	S	.	.	.	.	.	A	F	.	.	L	.	.	.	.	K	.	.
	NC038272	ATCC51908	.	.	S	.	.	.	.	.	A	F	.	.	L	.	.	.	.	K	.	.
Untyped	MF153477	BRSV-UnepJab-1	.	K	S	.	Q	I	.	.	A	F	.	G	L	T	.	R	.	K	.	.

4. Discussion

BRD is an economically important condition in the worldwide livestock industry that can be caused by a number of different viruses, bacteria, and parasites, individually or in combination [2,21]. The disease is typically caused by early virus infection, followed by bacterial secondary infection that can lead to lung damage and pneumonia-like illnesses [2,21]. Surprisingly, we have recently observed cattle with severe, sometimes fatal, BRD, associated with just single-pathogen infections, such as BRSV, BPIV3, or BHV-1 [3,5,22].

To investigate this and to understand potential changes in the viruses that may be causing an increased virulence, it is vital to be able to isolate and study the viruses in question. Previous studies in Turkey have mainly been diagnostic in nature, with limited phylogenetic analysis [4,5,23,24]. We present here, for the first time, the isolation and growth in culture of BRSV from infected cattle, phylogenetic analysis of the aforementioned isolates, and the identification of differences between them and previous isolates from Turkey and abroad. In this study, lung tissues from diseased animals were collected post-mortem and screened for the most common BRD-associated viruses, including BVDV, BHV-1, BPIV3, and BRSV, using commercially available ELISA kits, and only a BRSV antigen was found to be present [5]. No screening for bovine coronavirus or bacteria in the lung tissue was carried out, so the contribution from these pathogens to the disease state of the animals cannot be ruled out. Following a positive ELISA, lung homogenates were added to the cell culture and observed daily until CPE including syncytia and round apoptotic cells were visible. The isolation of BRSV in culture can be challenging because the virus is relatively labile and can struggle to grow in culture; however, this successful isolation now opens the door to extensive studies that would not have been possible otherwise [25–27].

The F gene of BRSV encodes a major structural protein that is commonly targeted by the adaptive immune response. It is a protein that is central to virus entry into cells, as well as being responsible for the fusion of infected cells with adjacent cells, resulting in the formation of large multinucleated syncytia [28]. Furthermore, the F gene is also a highly conserved region of the BRSV genome compared with the G gene [11]. The results of partial sequencing of the F gene of the current three isolates revealed that they were 100% identical to each other and were closely related to the sequence submitted (KY499619) from Turkey by Timurkan et al. [3]. We determined that the current strains—MT179304, MT024766, and MT024767—had a 99.49% nt and 99.22% aa similarity to the KY499619 strain. When compared to an international strain—KU159366—the isolates had a 97.43% nt and 98.44% aa similarity.

Phylogenetic analysis classified the isolates in subgroup III, similar to isolate KY499619, which was previously identified in Turkey and KU159366 from the USA. Considering the geographical location of Turkey, one could imagine a scenario where European strains would be readily imported into Turkey as globalization and international trade may hold potential risks for the spreading of diseases [29]; however, this does not seem to be the case for the outbreak on the farm in the present study. The amino acid change at position 118 is particularly interesting because that is the −2 position for an N-glycosylation sequence. The −2 position can have an influence on the efficiency of glycosylation of the local Asparagine [30]. Position 118 is also in the middle of the virokinin that is cleaved from the fusion protein of BRSV and is known to increase pulmonary inflammation during infection [31,32]. It is possible that this glycosylation efficiency may impact cleavage at the fusion protein furin cleavage sites, or that the amino acid change may impact the function of the virokinin itself. The second amino acid difference identified in the fusion protein compared to strain KY499619 is in the F2 subunit. Changes in this region could impact antibody recognition and may have consequences for vaccine development. All of these questions are areas for future exploration using the isolates in culture from this study.

Turkey has strong economic links to the USA and live animals are transported to Turkey from this region [33]. This is a possible source of the virus and illustrates the risks associated with globalized trade. Animals are known to harbor BRSV without symptoms, meaning the virus could easily be transported without detection [3], and constant introductions of new strains will increase the diversity of viruses in circulation, thus potentially complicating control efforts.

While the sample number is small in this study and from just one farm, it is a clear warning to the agricultural industry in Turkey that variant strains of BRSV exist in Turkey—variants that may have an increased virulence—and an increased molecular understanding of those variants is needed, along with better, more widespread surveillance and control strategies, in order to reduce the impact of this virus.

5. Conclusions

It is believed that BRSV is endemic in Turkey; however, minimal information is available on the prevalence of the virus, along with an understanding of the strains present. In order to successfully control infection, defining the target is essential. This study reports the identification and isolation of a new strain of BRSV that has not previously been identified in Turkey. It was associated with animals that died from respiratory distress and the strain shows amino acid differences in the Fusion protein (compared to the only other Turkish isolate) that are known to contribute to virulence. Importantly, the virus has been isolated in culture, which will allow further investigations into its virulence and the significance of those amino acid changes.

Author Contributions: Conceptualization, Z.Y., H.A., E.O., and G.B.; methodology, C.T., B.M., H.N.K., and A.E.E.; software, E.O., and B.M.; validation, Z.Y., E.O., and G.B.; formal analysis, E.O. and Z.Y.; investigation, C.T., B.M., H.N.K., and A.E.E.; writing—original draft preparation, Z.Y.; writing—review and editing, G.B., E.O., S.G., A.A.C., and A.E.E.; supervision, Z.Y. All authors have read and agreed to the published version of the manuscript.

Funding: This research received no external funding.

Conflicts of Interest: The authors declare that no conflict of interest.

Ethical Statement: No ethical statement is needed for this study because the samples were collected from necropsied animals due to the virus infection. No culling has been done for the sampling process.

Data Availability: All data are available online. Sequences obtained in this study can be found in the NCBI GenBank database at https://www.ncbi.nlm.nih.gov/nucleotide/.

References

1. Fulton, R.W. Bovine respiratory disease research (1983–2009). *Anim. Health. Res. Rev.* **2009**, *10*, 131–139. [CrossRef] [PubMed]
2. Headley, S.A.; Okano, W.; Balbo, L.C.; Marcasso, R.A.; Oliveira, T.E.; Alfieri, A.F.; NegriFilho, L.C.; Michelazzo, M.Z.; Rodrigues, S.C.; Baptista, A.L.; et al. Molecular survey of infectious agents associated with bovine respiratory disease in a beef cattle feedlot in southern Brazil. *J. Vet. Diagn. Invest.* **2018**, *30*, 249–251. [CrossRef] [PubMed]

3. Albayrak, H.; Yazici, Z.; Ozan, E.; Tamer, C.; Abd El Wahed, A.; Wehner, S.; Ulrich, K.; Weidmann, M. Characterisation of the First Bovine Parainfluenza Virus 3 Isolate Detected in Cattle in Turkey. *Vet. Sci.* **2019**, *6*, 56. [CrossRef] [PubMed]
4. Hacioglu, I.K.; Coskun, N.; Duran, S.; Sevinc, S.; Alkan, F. Phylogenetic Analysis of Bovine Respiratory Syncytial Virus from Calves with Respiratory Disorders. *Kafkas Univ. Vet. Fak. Derg.* **2019**, *25*, 251–256. [CrossRef]
5. Timurkan, M.O.; Aydin, H.; Sait, A. Identification and Molecular Characterisation of Bovine Parainfluenza Virus-3 and Bovine Respiratory Syncytial Virus-First Report from Turkey. *J. Vet. Res.* **2019**, *63*, 167–173. [CrossRef]
6. International Committee on Taxonomy of Viruses. 2019 Release. Available online: https://talk.ictvonline.org/ictv-reports/ictv_online_report/negative-sense-rna-viruses/mononegavirales/w/pneumoviridae/738/genus-orthopneumovirus/ (accessed on 3 September 2020).
7. Bertolotti, L.; Giammarioli, M.; Rosati, S. Genetic characterization of bovine respiratory syncytial virus strains isolated in Italy: Evidence for the circulation of new divergent clades. *J. Vet. Diagn. Invest.* **2018**, *30*, 300–304. [CrossRef]
8. Taylor, G.; Wyld, S.; Valarcher, J.F.; Guzman, E.; Thom, M.; Widdison, S.; Buchholz, U.J. Recombinant bovine respiratory syncytial virus with deletion of the SH gene induces increased apoptosis and pro-inflammatory cytokines in vitro, and is attenuated and induces protective immunity in calves. *J. Gen. Virol.* **2014**, *95*, 1244–1254. [CrossRef]
9. Valarcher, J.F.; Schelcher, H.B.; Bourhy, H. Evolution of Bovine Respiratory Syncytial Virus. *J. Virol.* **2000**, *74*, 10714–10728. [CrossRef]
10. Krešić, N.; Bedeković, T.; Brnić, D.; Šimić, I.; Lojkić, I.; Turk, N. Genetic analysis of bovine respiratory syncytial virus in Croatia. *Comp. Immunol. Microbiol. Infect. Dis.* **2018**, *58*, 52–57. [CrossRef]
11. Leme, R.A.; Agnol, A.M.D.; Balbo, L.C.; Pereria, F.L.; Possatti, F.; Alfieri, A.F.; Alfieri, A.A. Molecular characterization of Brazilian wild-type strains of Bovine respiratory syncytial virus reveals genetic diversity and putative subgroup of the virus. *Vet. Q.* **2020**, *40*, 83–96. [CrossRef]
12. Sarmiento-Silva, R.E.; Nakamura-Lopez, Y.; Vaughan, G. Epidemiology, Molecular Epidemiology and Evolution of Bovine Respiratory Syncytial Virus. *Viruses* **2012**, *4*, 3452–3467. [CrossRef] [PubMed]
13. Hoppe, I.B.A.L.; Medeiros, A.S.R.; Arns, C.W.; Samara, S.I. Bovine respiratory syncytial virus seroprevalence and risk factors in non-vaccinated dairy cattle herds in Brazil. *BMC Vet. Res.* **2018**, *14*, 208. [CrossRef] [PubMed]
14. Urban-Chmiel, R.; Wernicki, A.; Puchalski, A.; Dec, M.; Stęgierska, D.; Grooms, D.L.; Barbu, N.I. Detection of bovine respiratory syncytial virus infections in young dairy and beef cattle in Poland. *Vet. Q.* **2014**, *35*, 33–36. [CrossRef] [PubMed]
15. Baptista, A.L.; Rezende, A.L.; Fonseca, P.D.A.; Massi, R.P.; Nogueira, G.M.; Magalhães, L.Q.; Headley, S.A.; Menezes, G.L.; Alfieri, A.A.; Saut, J.P.E. Bovine respiratory disease complex associated mortality and morbidity rates in feedlot cattle from southeastern Brazil. *J. Infect. Dev. Ctries.* **2017**, *11*, 791–799. [CrossRef]
16. Yazici, Z.; Gumusova, S.; Tamer, C.; Muftuoglu, B.; Ozan, E.; Arslan, S.; Bas, O.; Elhag, A.E.; Albayrak, H. The first serological report for genotype C bovine parainfluenza 3 virus in ruminant species of mid-northern Turkey: Traces from the past. *Trop. Biomed.* **2019**, *36*, 803–809, Scopus EID: 2-s2.0-85073422601.
17. Boxus, M.; Letellier, C.; Kerkhofs, P. Real Time RT-PCR for the detection and quantitation of bovine respiratory syncytial virus. *J. Virol. Methods* **2005**, *125*, 125–130. [CrossRef]
18. Vilcek, S.; Elvander, M.; Ballagi-Pordány, A.; Belák, S. Development of nested PCR assays for detection of bovine respiratory syncytial virus in clinical samples. J. *Clin. Microbiol.* **1994**, *32*, 2225–2231. [CrossRef] [PubMed]
19. Hall, T. BioEdit: A user-friendly biological sequence alignment editor and analysis program for Windows 95/98/NT. *Nucleic Acids Symp. Ser.* **1999**, *41*, 95–98.
20. Kumar, S.; Stecher, G.; Li, M.; Knyaz, C.; Tamura, K. MEGA X: Molecular evolutionary genetics analysis across computing platforms. *Mol. Biol. Evol.* **2018**, *35*, 1547–1549. [CrossRef]
21. Kurcubic, V.; Dokovic, R.; Ilic, Z.; Petrovic, M. Etiopathogenesis and economic significance of bovine respiratory disease complex (BRD). *Acta Agric. Serb.* **2018**, *45*, 85–100. [CrossRef]

22. Albayrak, H.; Tamer, C.; Ozan, E.; Muftuoglu, B.; Kadi, H.; Dogan, F.; Cagirgan, A.A.; Elhag, A.E.; Akman, A.; Kurucay, H.N.; et al. Molecular identification and phylogeny of bovine herpesvirus-1 (BoHV-1) from cattle associated with respiratory disorders and death in Turkey. *Med. Weter.* **2020**, *76*, 358–361. [CrossRef]
23. Alkan, F.; Ozkul, A.; Bilge-Dagalp, S.; Yesilbag, K.; Oguzoglu, C.; Akca, Y.; Burgu, I. Virological and serological studies on the role of PI-3 virus, BRSV, BVDV, and BHV- 1 on respiratory infections of cattle. I. The detection of etiological agents by direct immunofluorescence technique. *DTW. Dtsch. Tierarztl. Wochenschr.* **2000**, *107*, 193–195. [PubMed]
24. Yesilbag, K.; Gungor, B. Seroprevalence of bovine respiratory viruses in North-Western Turkey. *Trop. Anim. Health Prod.* **2008**, *40*, 55–60. [CrossRef] [PubMed]
25. Almeida, R.S.; Domingues, H.G.; Coswig, L.T.; D'Arce, R.C.F.; Carvalho, R.F.; Arns, C.W. Detection of bovive respiratory syncytial virus in experimentally infected balb/c mice. *Vet. Res.* **2004**, *35*, 189–197. [CrossRef] [PubMed]
26. Santangelo, P.; Nitin, N.; LaConte, L.; Woolums, A.; Bao, G. Live-cell characterization and analysis of a clinical isolate of bovine respiratory syncytial virus, using molecular beacons. *J. Virol.* **2006**, *80*, 682–688. [CrossRef] [PubMed]
27. Bortolin Affonso, I.; de Souza, A.; Cavalheiro Martini, M.; Bianchi dos Santos, M.; Rosado Spilki, F.; Weis Arns, C.; Issa Samara, S. Detection of an untyped strain of bovine respiratory syncytial virus in a dairy herd. *Semin. Cienc. Agrar.* **2014**, *35*, 2539–2549. [CrossRef]
28. Valentova, V. The antigenic and genetic variability of bovine respiratory syncytial virus with emphasis on the G protein. *Vet. Med.* **2003**, *48*, 254–266. [CrossRef]
29. Dean, A.S.; Fournié, G.; Kulo, A.E.; Boukaya, G.A.; Schelling, E.; Bonfoh, B. Potential risk of regional disease spread in West Africa through cross-border cattle trade. *PLoS ONE* **2013**, *8*, e75570. [CrossRef]
30. Domingues, H.G.; Spilki, F.R.; Arns, C.W. Molecular detection and phylogenetic analysis of bovine respiratory syncytial virus (BRSV) in swabs and lung tissues of adult cattle. *Pesq. Vet. Bras.* **2011**, *31*, 961–966. [CrossRef]
31. Valarcher, J.F.; Furze, J.; Wyld, S.G.; Cook, R.; Zimmer, G.; Herrler, G.; Taylor, G. Bovine respiratory syncytial virus lacking the virokinin or with a mutation in furin cleavage site RA(R/K)R109 induces less pulmonary inflammation without impeding the induction of protective immunity in calves. *J. Gen. Virol.* **2006**, *87*, 1659–1667. [CrossRef]
32. Zimmer, G.; Rohn, M.; McGregor, G.P.; Schemann, M.; Conzelmann, K.K.; Herrler, G. Virokinin, a bioactive peptide of the tachykinin family, is released from the fusion protein of bovine respiratory syncytial virus. *J. Biol. Chem.* **2003**, *278*, 46854–46861. [CrossRef] [PubMed]
33. Okur-Gumusova, S.; Tamer, C.; Ozan, E.; Cavunt, A.; Kadi, H.; Muftuoglu, B.; Eisa Elhag, A.; Yazici, Z.; Albayrak, H. An investigation of the seroprevalence of crimean-congo hemorrhagic fever and lumpy skin disease in domesticated water buffaloes in Northern Turkey. *Trop. Biomed.* **2020**, *37*, 165–173, Scopus EID: 2-s2.0-85086915081.

animals

MDPI

Brief Report

Molecular Evidence of *Hemolivia mauritanica*, *Ehrlichia* spp. and the Endosymbiont *Candidatus* Midichloria Mitochondrii in *Hyalomma aegyptium* Infesting *Testudo graeca* Tortoises from Doha, Qatar

Patrícia F. Barradas [1,2], Clara Lima [3], Luís Cardoso [4], Irina Amorim [1,5,6], Fátima Gärtner [1,5,6] and João R. Mesquita [1,2,7,*]

1 Institute of Biomedical Sciences Abel Salazar (ICBAS), University of Porto, 4050-313 Porto, Portugal; patriciaferreirabarradas@gmail.com (P.F.B.); iamorim@ipatimup.pt (I.A.); fgartner@ipatimup.pt (F.G.)
2 Epidemiology Research Unit (EPIUnit), Instituto de Saúde Pública da Universidade do Porto, 4050-091 Porto, Portugal
3 Department of Biological Sciences, Microbiology Laboratory, Faculty of Pharmacy, University of Porto, 4050-313 Porto, Portugal; claramlima@gmail.com
4 Department of Veterinary Sciences, and Animal and Veterinary Research Centre (CECAV), University of Trás-os-Montes e Alto Douro, 5000-801 Vila Real, Portugal; lcardoso@utad.pt
5 Institute for Research and Innovation in Health (i3S), University of Porto, 4200-135 Porto, Portugal
6 Institute of Molecular Pathology and Immunology of the University of Porto (IPATIMUP), 4200-135 Porto, Portugal
7 Department of Veterinary Clinics, ICBAS-UP, Rua de Jorge Viterbo Ferreira 228, 4050-313 Porto, Portugal
* Correspondence: jrmesquita@icbas.up.pt

Citation: Barradas, P.F.; Lima, C.; Cardoso, L.; Amorim, I.; Gärtner, F.; Mesquita, J.R. Molecular Evidence of *Hemolivia mauritanica*, *Ehrlichia* spp. and the Endosymbiont *Candidatus* Midichloria Mitochondrii in *Hyalomma aegyptium* Infesting *Testudo graeca* Tortoises from Doha, Qatar. *Animals* **2021**, *11*, 30. https://dx.doi.org/10.3390/ani11010030

Received: 10 December 2020
Accepted: 24 December 2020
Published: 26 December 2020

Simple Summary: Due to the veterinary and medical importance of pathogens transmitted by *Hyalomma aegyptium*, we tested ticks removed from *Testudo graeca* tortoises for the presence of *Anaplasma*, *Ehrlichia*, *Hemolivia*, *Babesia* and *Hepatozoon*. Forty-three percent of the examined adult ticks were infected with at least one agent. The most prevalent agent identified was *Hemolivia mauritanica* (28.6%), followed by *Candidatus* Midichloria mitochondrii (9.5%) and *Ehrlichia* spp. (4.7%). Our study reported for the first time *H. mauritanica*, *Ehrlichia* spp. and *Candidatus* M. mitochondrii in *H. aegyptium* ticks collected from pet spur-thighed tortoises, in Qatar, providing data that adds to the geographical extension of these agents.

Abstract: Tick-borne agents constitute a growing concern for human and animal health worldwide. *Hyalomma aegyptium* is a hard tick with a three-host life cycle, whose main hosts for adults are Palearctic tortoises of genus *Testudo*. Nevertheless, immature ticks can feed on a variety of hosts, representing an important eco-epidemiological issue regarding *H. aegyptium* pathogens circulation. *Hyalomma aegyptium* ticks are vectors and/or reservoirs of various pathogenic agents, such as *Ehrlichia*, *Anaplasma*, *Babesia* and *Hepatozoon/Hemolivia*. *Ehrlichia* and *Anaplasma* are emergent tick-borne bacteria with a worldwide distribution and zoonotic potential, responsible for diseases that cause clinical manifestations that grade from acute febrile illness to a fulminant disease characterized by multi-organ system failure, depending on the species. *Babesia* and *Hepatozoon/Hemolivia* are tick-borne parasites with increasing importance in multiple species. *Testudo graeca* tortoises acquired in a large animal market in Doha, Qatar, were screened for a panel of tick-borne pathogens by conventional PCR followed by bidirectional sequencing. The most prevalent agent identified in ticks was *Hemolivia mauritanica* (28.6%), followed by *Candidatus* Midichloria mitochondrii (9.5%) and *Ehrlichia* spp. (4.7%). All samples were negative for *Babesia* spp. and *Hepatozoon* spp. Overall, 43% of the examined adult ticks were infected with at least one agent. Only 4.7% of the ticks appeared to be simultaneously infected with two agents, i.e., *Ehrlichia* spp. and *H. mauritanica*. This is the first detection of *H. mauritanica*, *Ehrlichia* spp. and *Candidatus* M. mitochondrii in *H. aegyptium* ticks collected from pet spur-thighed tortoises, in Qatar, a fact which adds to the geographical extension of these agents. The international trade of *Testudo* tortoises carrying ticks infected with pathogens of veterinary and medical importance deserves strict control, in order to reduce potential exotic diseases.

Keywords: endosymbionts; *Hemolivia*; surveillance; tortoises; tick-borne pathogens; ticks

1. Introduction

Ticks are known as important vectors of many viral, bacterial and protozoan infectious microorganisms capable of producing disease in both humans and animals [1]. As hematophagous arthropods, while taking a blood meal, they can transmit pathogens to susceptible hosts, supporting the enzootic cycles of many infectious agents in various ecosystems and being regarded as major human and veterinary public health problems [2]. Nevertheless, these arthropods also harbor intracellular bacteria that are apparently not detrimental to humans, animals or even to ticks themselves. Symbionts, such as *Candidatus* Midichloria mitochondrii, are obligately intracellular bacteria, and in some cases are closely associated with the presence of known pathogens, such as *Rickettsia parkeri* [3]. Symbiotic, commensal and pathogenic microorganisms harbored by ticks can positively influence pathogen transmission or interfere with their maintenance in the tick [4]. For example, *Coxiella*-like endosymbionts seem to impair the transmission of *Ehrlichia chaffeensis* by *Amblyomma* ticks [5], whereas the presence of *Francisella* sp. endosymbionts increases the colonization success of pathogenic *Francisella novicida* in *Dermacentor andersoni* ticks [6].

Hyalomma aegyptium is a three-host life cycle hard tick endemic in North Africa, Balkan countries, the Middle East, Caucasus, Central Asia, Afghanistan and Pakistan, whose adult stage main hosts are Palearctic tortoises of the genus *Testudo* [7–9]. However, adult ticks, together with the less host-specific nymphs and larvae, also feed on various vertebrates, such as domestic animals (dogs, cattle, pigs, horses), wild animals (birds, boar, deer, foxes, jackals, hamsters, hares, hedgehogs, mustelids, squirrels) and humans [10–15]. This wide host range yields a variety of pathogen transmission scenarios between the numerous hosts, becoming a concern under an eco-epidemiological point of view.

Various known pathogens have been detected in *H. aegyptium* ticks, such as Rickettsia aeschlimannii and Rickettsia africae [16], *Borrelia burgdorferi* s.l. [17] and Borrelia turcica [18], *Hepatozoon kisrae* [19], *Coxiella burnetii* [20] and *Hemolivia mauritanica* [21]. The last one is the most widely distributed blood parasite of turtles, but its geographical distribution still remains cryptic [22].

Due to the veterinary and medical importance of pathogens transmitted by *H. aegyptium* ticks and their wide host range, ticks from *Testudo graeca* acquired in an animal market in Doha, Qatar, were screened for several pathogens, namely, *Ehrlichia*, *Anaplasma*, *Babesia* and *Hepatozoon/Hemolivia*.

2. Materials and Methods

2.1. Study Area

A country located on the eastern side of the Arabian Peninsula, Qatar has a desert climate with an arid and hot summer characterized by temperatures ranging between 25 °C and 46 °C. Rainfall is scarce (75.6 mm per year), falling with erratic patterns from October to March. Doha is the country's capital and its largest city.

2.2. Specimen Collection and Processing

2.2.1. Ticks

Ticks included in this study were previously collected and screened for the presence of *Rickettsia* spp. in 2019 [16]. Briefly, a total of 21 ticks were removed from two pet tortoises (*T. graeca*), which had been acquired from one of Qatar's largest animal markets just before presentation at Parkview Pet Center Veterinary Clinic for a health check and ectoparasitic control in May 2018, Doha. The animal market had a total of 20 animal stores, four of which sold tortoises (averaging 10–15 tortoises per store). The removed ticks were previously identified to the species level as *Hyalomma aegyptium* [16] using the morphological criteria already described and further confirmed by PCR using mitochondrial genes (12S and 16S rDNA) as molecular targets [23,24].

2.2.2. Detection of *Ehrlichia/Anaplasma*, Babesia and *Hepatozoon/Hemolivia* DNA in Ticks

Tick extracted DNA by the alkaline hydrolysis [25] was tested for the presence of *Ehrlichia*, *Anaplasma*, Babesia and *Hepatozoon/Hemolivia* by conventional PCR in the Pathology and Immunology Department of the Institute of Biomedical Sciences Abel Salazar, Porto University, according to previously described protocols (Table 1). For PCR, the KAPA HiFi HotStart ReadyMix, KAPA Biosystems (Woburn, MA, USA) was used according to the manufacturer's instructions. The amplification was performed in Bio-Rad T100^{TM} Thermal Cycler. Aliquots of each PCR product were electrophoresed on 1.5% agarose gel stained with Xpert Green Safe DNA gel stain (Grisp, Porto, Portugal) and examined for the presence of the specific fragment under UV light. DNA fragment size was compared with a standard molecular weight, 100 bp DNA ladder (Grisp, Porto, Portugal). Distilled water was used as negative control.

Table 1. Primer sequences used for the detection of tick-borne agents.

Target Gene	Primer Sequence	bp	References
16S rRNA	EHR16SD: 5′-GGTACCYACAGAAGAAGTCC-3′ EHR16SR: 5′-TAGCACTCATCGTTTACAGC-3′	345	[26]
18S rRNA	PIRO-A: 5′-AATACCCAATCCTGACACAGGG-3′ PIRO-B: 5′-TTAAATACGAATGCCCCCAAC-3′	408	[27]
18S rRNA	HEP-F: 5′-ATACATGAGCAAAATCTCAAC-3′ HEP-R: 5′-CTTATTATTCCATGCTGCAG-3′	666	[28]

2.2.3. Sequencing and Phylogenetic Analysis

All *Ehrlichia*-positive and *Hemolivia*-positive amplicons obtained were sequenced for genetic characterization. Amplicons were purified with Exo/SAP Go (Grisp, Porto, Portugal), and bidirectional sequencing was performed with the Sanger method at the genomics core facility of the Institute of Molecular Pathology and Immunology of the University of Porto. Sequence editing and multiple alignments were performed with the BioEdit Sequence Alignment Editor v7.1.9 software package, version 2.1 (Ibis Biosciences). The sequences obtained were subjected to the basic local alignment search tool (BLAST) [29–31] using the non-redundant nucleotide database (http://blast.ncbi.nlm.nih.gov/Blast.cgi).

3. Results

From the PCR analysis of *H. aegyptium* (n = 21), three (14.2%) were positive for the *Ehrlichia/Anaplasma* 16S rRNA gene, and six (28.6%) were positive for *Hepatozoon* 18S rRNA gene. Bidirectional sequencing and BLAST analysis of consensus sequences of partial 16S rRNA gene of *H. aegyptium* tested showed that two shares 99.11% identity with *Candidatus* M. mitochondrii sequences from France (GenBank accession no. EU780455), and one of tested *H. aegyptium* presented the highest identity (98.64%) with *Ehrlichia* spp. (GenBank accession no. KX987321) and *E. ewingii* (GenBank accession no. MN148616) sequences from China.

Phylogenetic analysis was performed for 16S rRNA sequences to obtain information about their genetic relatedness with other *Candidatus* M. mitochondrii and *Ehrlichia* species. Clustering with reference sequences confirmed the final classification as *Candidatus* M. mitochondrii (Figure 1) and *Ehrlichia ewingii* (Figure 2).

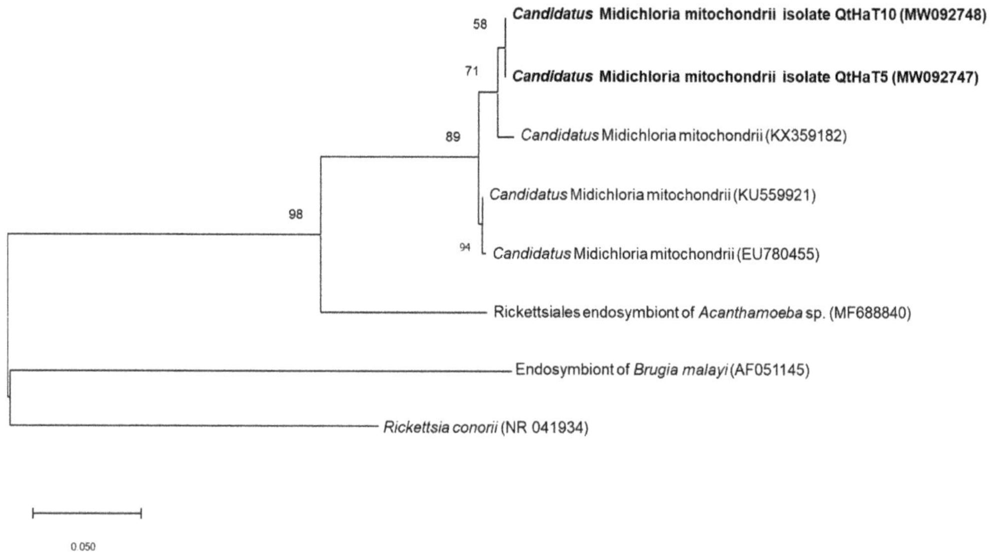

Figure 1. Molecular *Candidatus* M. mitochondrii identification according to phylogenetic analysis using the maximum likelihood method and Tamura-Nei model with the 16S rRNA gene. The analyzed sequences are in bold. The accession numbers for nucleotide sequences from GenBank are presented with species names. The branch numbers mean bootstrap support (1000 replicates). The tree is drawn to scale, with branch lengths measured in the number of substitutions per site.

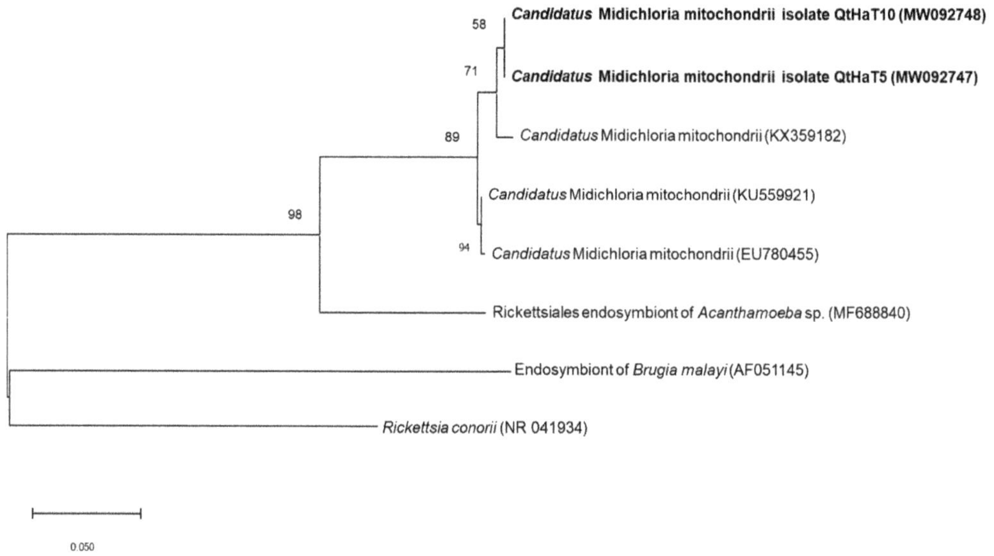

Figure 2. Molecular *Ehrlichia* sp. identification according to phylogenetic analysis using the maximum likelihood method and Hasegawa-Kishino-Yano model with the 16S rRNA gene. The analyzed sequences are in bold. The accession numbers for nucleotide sequences from GenBank are presented with species names. The branch numbers mean bootstrap support (1000 replicates). The tree is drawn to scale, with branch lengths measured in the number of substitutions per site.

When screening the 21 ticks for the 18S rRNA gene, 5 were found positive for *H. mauritanica*. Further characterization of the 18S rRNA sequences showed a nucleotide identity between 99.70% and 99.84% with *H. mauritanica* sequences from the blood of *Tes-*

tudo graeca from Syria (GenBank accession no. KF992707) and Greece (GenBank accession no. KF992710). Phylogenetic analysis was performed for 18S rRNA sequences and confirmed clustering with *H. mauritanica* reference strains (Figure 3).

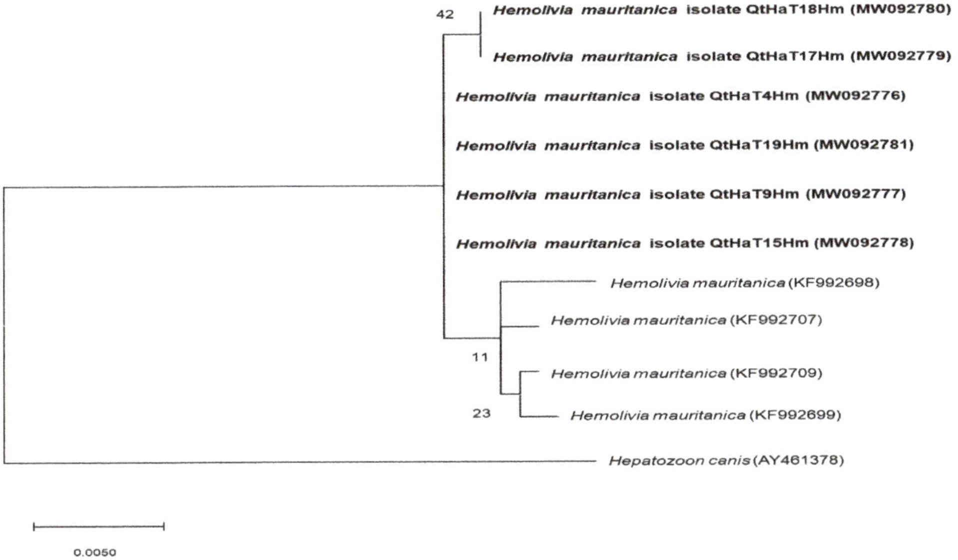

Figure 3. Molecular *Hemolivia mauritanica* identification according to phylogenetic analysis using the maximum likelihood method and Hasegawa-Kishino-Yano model with the 18S rRNA gene. The analyzed sequences are in bold. The accession numbers for nucleotide sequences from GenBank are presented with species names. The branch numbers mean bootstrap support (1000 replicates). The tree is drawn to scale, with branch lengths measured in the number of substitutions per site.

No amplification was obtained for *Babesia* spp. nor *Hepatozoon* spp. One (4.8%) of the ticks was co-infected with *Ehrlichia* spp. and *H. mauritanica*.

The following accession numbers were assigned to the sequences obtained in this work: MW092747 and MW092748 (16S rRNA gene fragment of *Candidatus* M. mitochondrii), MW092750 (16S rRNA gene fragment of *Ehrlichia* spp.) and MW092776 to MW092781 (18S rRNA gene fragment of *H. mauritanica*).

4. Discussion

This report presents the molecular findings for a panel of tick-borne pathogens from a total of 21 *H. aegyptium* ticks previously removed from two *Testudo graeca* tortoises acquired in a large animal market in Doha, Qatar.

In 38% of the 21 *H. aegyptium* collected from *T. graeca* tortoises, tested for *Ehrlichia/Anaplasma*, *Hemolivia/Hepatozoon* and *Babesia* spp., at least one agent was detected. The most commonly detected agent was *H. mauritanica*, with 28.6% of the *H. aegyptum* ticks being positive for it, followed by the endosymbiont *Candidatus* M. mitochondrii, 9.5%, and bacterium *Ehrlichia* spp., 4.8%. *Hemolivia mauritanica* and *Ehrlichia* spp. co-infection was detected in one *H. aegyptium*.

Hemolivia mauritanica is a pathogen of tortoises and has *H. aegyptium* as the definitive host [11]. The results obtained in this study are in accordance with previous prevalence levels from Lebanon (38%), Algeria (30.4%) and Bulgaria (14%), but are much lower when compared with results observed in Turkey (82%), Romania (84%), Syria (82%) and Greece (81%) [32].

The molecular analysis of a 345 bp stretch of the 16S rRNA gene showed that a sequence found in a tick presented the highest identity with *Ehrlichia* spp.

Ehrlichia spp. are maintained in complex zoonotic systems involving vector ticks and reservoir hosts. These agents affect both humans [33] and animals such as dogs, ruminants [34,35] and even deer [36]. Infected humans [33] and dogs [37] may manifest fever, malaise, leucopenia, thrombocytopenia and abnormal liver function. Tick species that are vectors of these pathogens, such as *Amblyomma*, *Dermacentor*, *Rhipicephalus*, *Ixodes*, *Haemaphysalis* and *Hyalomma*, also parasitize humans, thus posing a considerable risk [38]. Our results demonstrate a lower occurrence of *H. aegyptium* infected with *Ehrlichia* spp. (4.7%) when compared with recent work, which has shown an occurrence of 30.2% [38].

Candidatus M. mitochondrii, an α-proteobacterial symbiont first detected in *Ixodes ricinus*, has a unique intramitochondrial lifestyle [39]. It was the first bacterium shown to reside within the mitochondria and the possible role in ticks is yet to be determined [40]. In the present study, *Candidatus* M. mitochondrii was detected in *H. aegyptium* ticks collected on *T. graeca* from Qatar. As far as we know, this is the first report of the detection of this symbiont in *H. aegyptium* ticks.

Our study reports for the first-time detection of *H. mauritanica*, *Ehrlichia* spp. and *Candidatus* M. mitochondrii in *H. aegytium* ticks collected from pet spur-thighed tortoises, in Qatar, a circumstance which contributes to characterizing the geographical distribution of these agents. The current dimension and growth of international wildlife trade is known not only to act as an avenue for the spread of disease [41] but also poses an important risk to global biodiversity, as well as having an impact on social and economic development [42]. Importation of tick-infested tortoise, later found to be carrying zoonotic pathogens, have been reported in the past [16,43].

5. Conclusions

Our study reports for the first-time the detection of *H. mauritanica*, *Ehrlichia* spp. and *Candidatus* M. mitochondrii in *H. aegytium* ticks collected from pet spur-thighed tortoises, in Qatar, a circumstance which contributes to characterizing the geographical distribution of these agents and shows the need of strict surveillance and control to reduce potential non-native diseases while assisting animal conservation.

Author Contributions: P.F.B. and J.R.M. were involved in the conception of the research idea and methodology design and performed the data analysis, interpretation and prepared the manuscript for publication; C.L. was involved in sampling; L.C., C.L., I.A. and F.G. reviewed the manuscript. All authors have read and agreed to the published version of the manuscript.

Funding: This research received no external funding.

Conflicts of Interest: The authors declare no conflict of interest.

References

1. De la Fuente, J.; Antunes, S.; Bonnet, S.; Cabezas-Cruz, A.; Domingos, A.G.; Estrada-Peña, A.; Johnson, N.; Kocan, K.M.; Mansfield, K.L.; Nijhof, A.M.; et al. Tick-Pathogen Interactions and Vector Competence: Identification of Molecular Drivers for Tick-Borne Diseases. *Front. Cell. Infect. Microbiol.* **2017**, *7*, 114. [CrossRef] [PubMed]
2. Wikel, S.K. Ticks and Tick-Borne Infections: Complex Ecology, Agents, and Host Interactions. *Vet. Sci.* **2018**, *5*, 60. [CrossRef] [PubMed]
3. Budachetri, K.; Kumar, D.; Crispell, G.; Beck, C.; Dasch, G.; Karim, S. The tick endosymbiont *Candidatus* Midichloria mitochondrii and selenoproteins are essential for the growth of *Rickettsia parkeri* in the Gulf Coast tick vector. *Microbiome* **2018**, *6*, 141. [CrossRef] [PubMed]
4. Bonnet, S.I.; Binetruy, F.; Hernández-Jarguín, A.M.; Duron, O. The Tick Microbiome: Why Non-pathogenic Microorganisms Matter in Tick Biology and Pathogen Transmission. *Front. Cell. Infect. Microbiol.* **2017**, *7*, 236. [CrossRef] [PubMed]
5. Klyachko, O.; Stein, B.D.; Grindle, N.; Clay, K.; Fuqua, C. Localization and visualization of a coxiella-type symbiont within the lone star tick, *Amblyomma americanum*. *Appl. Environ. Microbiol.* **2007**, *73*, 6584–6594. [CrossRef] [PubMed]
6. Gall, C.A.; Reif, K.E.; Scoles, G.A.; Mason, K.L.; Mousel, M.; Noh, S.M.; Brayton, K.A. The bacterial microbiome of *Dermacentor andersoni* ticks influences pathogen susceptibility. *Int. Soc. Microb. Ecol. J.* **2016**, *10*, 1846–1855. [CrossRef]
7. Agustín Estrada-Peña, A.D.M.; Trevor, N. *Petney Ticks of Europe and North Africa: A Guide to Species Identification*; Springer International Publishing: Manhattan, NY, USA, 2017; Volume 34, pp. 361–363.

8. Estrada-Pena, A.; Pfaffle, M.; Baneth, G.; Kleinerman, G.; Petney, T.N. Ixodoidea of the Western Palaearctic: A review of available literature for identification of species. *Ticks Tick Borne Dis.* **2017**, *8*, 512–525. [CrossRef]
9. El Mouden, E.H.; Laghzaoui, E.-M.; Elbahi, A.; Abbad, A. A case of massive infestation of a female Spur-thighed tortoise *Testudo graeca* by blood-sucking ticks *Hyalomma aegyptium* (Acari: Ixodidae). *Int. J. Acarol.* **2020**, *46*, 63–65. [CrossRef]
10. Apanaskevich, D.A. [Towards a diagnostic view of *Hyalomma* (Hyalomma) *aegyptium* (Acari, Ixodidae)]. *Parazitologiia* **2003**, *37*, 47–59.
11. Široký, P.; Petrželková, K.J.; Kamler, M.; Mihalca, A.D.; Modrý, D. *Hyalomma aegyptium* as dominant tick in tortoises of the genus *Testudo* in Balkan countries, with notes on its host preferences. *Exp. Appl. Acarol.* **2006**, *40*, 279–290. [CrossRef]
12. Vatansever, Z.; Gargili, A.; Aysul, N.S.; Sengoz, G.; Estrada-Pena, A. Ticks biting humans in the urban area of Istanbul. *Parasitol. Res.* **2008**, *102*, 551–553. [CrossRef] [PubMed]
13. Bursali, A.; Tekin, S.; Orhan, M.; Keskin, A.; Ozkan, M. Ixodid ticks (Acari: Ixodidae) infesting humans in Tokat Province of Turkey: Species diversity and seasonal activity. *J. Vector Ecol. J. Soc. Vector Ecol.* **2010**, *35*, 180–186. [CrossRef]
14. Paştiu, A.I.; Matei, I.A.; Mihalca, A.D.; D'Amico, G.; Dumitrache, M.O.; Kalmár, Z.; Sándor, A.D.; Lefkaditis, M.; Gherman, C.M.; Cozma, V. Zoonotic pathogens associated with *Hyalomma aegyptium* in endangered tortoises: Evidence for host-switching behaviour in ticks? *Parasites Vectors* **2012**, *5*, 301. [CrossRef] [PubMed]
15. Girisgin, A.O.; Senlik, B.; Aydin, L.; Cirak, V.Y. Ectoparasites of hedgehogs (*Erinaceus concolor)* from Turkey. *Berl. Munch. Tierarztl. Wochenschr.* **2015**, *128*, 315–318.
16. Barradas, P.F.; Mesquita, J.R.; Lima, C.; Cardoso, L.; Alho, A.M.; Ferreira, P.; Amorim, I.; de Sousa, R.; Gartner, F. Pathogenic *Rickettsia* in ticks of spur-thighed tortoise (*Testudo graeca*) sold in a Qatar live animal market. *Transbound. Emerg. Dis.* **2019**. [CrossRef]
17. Kar, S.; Yılmazer, N.; Midilli, K.; Ergin, S.; Alp, H.; Gargili, A.; Namık; Üniversitesi, K.; Bölümü, B. Presence of the Zoonotic *Borrelia burgdorferi* sl. and *Rickettsia* spp. in the Ticks from Wild Tortoises and Hedgehogs. *MUSBED* **2011**, *11*, 2011–2166.
18. Güner, E.; Watanabe, M.; Hashimoto, N.; Kadosaka, T.; Kawamura, Y.; Ezaki, T.; Kawabata, H.; Imai, Y.; Kaneda, K.; Masuzawa, T. *Borrelia turcica* sp. nov., isolated from the hard tick *Hyalomma aegyptium* in Turkey. *Int. J. Syst. Evol. Microbiol.* **2004**, *54*, 1649–1652. [CrossRef]
19. Paperna, I.; Kremer-Mecabell, T.; Finkelman, S. *Hepatozoon kisrae* n. sp. infecting the lizard *Agama stellio* is transmitted by the tick *Hyalomma* cf. *aegyptium*. *Parasite* **2002**, *9*, 17–27. [CrossRef]
20. Siroky, P.; Kubelova, M.; Modry, D.; Erhart, J.; Literak, I.; Spitalska, E.; Kocianova, E. Tortoise tick *Hyalomma aegyptium* as long term carrier of Q fever agent *Coxiella burnetii*—Evidence from experimental infection. *Parasitol. Res.* **2010**, *107*, 1515–1520. [CrossRef]
21. Široký, P.; Mikulíček, P.; Jandzík, D.; Kami, H.; Mihalca, A.D.; Rouag, R.; Kamler, M.; Schneider, C.; Záruba, M.; Modrý, D. Co-Distribution Pattern of a Haemogregarine *Hemolivia mauritanica* (Apicomplexa: Haemogregarinidae) and Its Vector *Hyalomma aegyptium* (Metastigmata: Ixodidae). *J. Parasitol.* **2009**, *95*, 728–733. [CrossRef]
22. Laghzaoui, E.-M.; Sergiadou, D.; Perera, A.; Harris, D.J.; Abbad, A.; El Mouden, E.H. Absence of *Hemolivia mauritanica* (Apicomplexa: Haemogregarinidae) in natural populations of *Testudo graeca* in Morocco. *Parasitol. Research* **2020**. [CrossRef] [PubMed]
23. Szabó, M.P.; Mangold, A.J.; João, C.F.; Bechara, G.H.; Guglielmone, A.A. Biological and DNA evidence of two dissimilar populations of the *Rhipicephalus sanguineus* tick group (Acari: Ixodidae) in South America. *Vet. Parasitol.* **2005**, *130*. [CrossRef] [PubMed]
24. Black, W.C.T.; Piesman, J. Phylogeny of hard- and soft-tick taxa (Acari: Ixodida) based on mitochondrial 16S rDNA sequences. *Proc. Natl. Acad. Sci. USA* **1994**, *91*, 10034–10038. [CrossRef] [PubMed]
25. Schouls, L.M.; Van De Pol, I.; Rijpkema, S.G.; Schot, C.S. Detection and identification of *Ehrlichia*, *Borrelia burgdorferi* sensu lato, and *Bartonella* species in Dutch *Ixodes ricinus* ticks. *J. Clin. Microbiol.* **1999**, *37*, 2215–2222. [CrossRef]
26. Gal, A.; Loeb, E.; Yisaschar-Mekuzas, Y.; Baneth, G. Detection of *Ehrlichia canis* by PCR in different tissues obtained during necropsy from dogs surveyed for naturally occurring canine monocytic ehrlichiosis. *Vet. J.* **2008**, *175*, 212–217. [CrossRef]
27. Olmeda, A.S.; Armstrong, P.M.; Rosenthal, B.M.; Valladares, B.; del Castillo, A.; de Armas, F.; Miguelez, M.; Gonzalez, A.; Rodriguez Rodriguez, J.A.; Spielman, A.; et al. A subtropical case of human babesiosis. *Acta Trop.* **1997**, *67*, 229–234. [CrossRef]
28. Inokuma, H.; Okuda, M.; Ohno, K.; Shimoda, K.; Onishi, T. Analysis of the 18S rRNA gene sequence of a *Hepatozoon* detected in two Japanese dogs. *Vet. Parasitol.* **2002**, *106*, 265–271. [CrossRef]
29. Altschul, S.F.; Gish, W.; Miller, W.; Myers, E.W.; Lipman, D.J. Basic local alignment search tool. *J. Mol. Biol.* **1990**, *215*, 403–410. [CrossRef]
30. Benson, D.A.; Karsch-Mizrachi, I.; Lipman, D.J.; Ostell, J.; Rapp, B.A.; Wheeler, D.L. GenBank. *Nucleic Acids Res.* **2002**, *30*, 17–20. [CrossRef]
31. Pruitt, K.; Tatusova, T.; Ostell, J. 18. The Reference Sequence (RefSeq) Project. In *The NCBI Handbook*; National Center for Biotechnology Information: Bethesda, MD, USA, 2002.
32. Javanbakht, H.; Široký, P.; Mikulíček, P.; Sharifi, M. Distribution and abundance of *Hemolivia mauritanica* (Apicomplexa: Haemogregarinidae) and its vector *Hyalomma aegyptium* in tortoises of Iran. *Biologia* **2015**, *70*, 229–234. [CrossRef]
33. Ismail, N.; Bloch, K.C.; McBride, J.W. Human ehrlichiosis and anaplasmosis. *Clin. Lab. Med.* **2010**, *30*, 261–292. [CrossRef] [PubMed]
34. Dantas-Torres, F.; da Silva, Y.Y.; de Oliveira Miranda, D.E.; da Silva Sales, K.G.; Figueredo, L.A.; Otranto, D. *Ehrlichia* spp. infection in rural dogs from remote indigenous villages in north-eastern Brazil. *Parasites Vectors* **2018**, *11*, 139. [CrossRef] [PubMed]
35. Zhang, H.; Chang, Z.; Mehmood, K.; Wang, Y.; Rehman, M.U.; Nabi, F.; Sabir, A.J.; Liu, X.; Wu, X.; Tian, X.; et al. First report of *Ehrlichia* infection in goats, China. *Microb. Pathog.* **2017**, *110*, 275–278. [CrossRef] [PubMed]

36. Yabsley, M.J.; Varela, A.S.; Tate, C.M.; Dugan, V.G.; Stallknecht, D.E.; Little, S.E.; Davidson, W.R. *Ehrlichia ewingii* infection in white-tailed deer (*Odocoileus virginianus*). *Emerg. Infect. Dis.* **2002**, *8*, 668–671. [CrossRef]
37. Sainz, Á.; Roura, X.; Miró, G.; Estrada-Peña, A.; Kohn, B.; Harrus, S.; Solano-Gallego, L. Guideline for veterinary practitioners on canine ehrlichiosis and anaplasmosis in Europe. *Parasites Vectors* **2015**, *8*, 75. [CrossRef]
38. Akveran, G.A.; Karasartova, D.; Keskin, A.; Comba, A.; Celebi, B.; Mumcuoglu, K.Y.; Taylan-Ozkan, A. Bacterial and protozoan agents found in *Hyalomma aegyptium* (L., 1758) (Ixodida: Ixodidae) collected from *Testudo graeca* L., 1758 (Reptilia: Testudines) in Corum Province of Turkey. *Ticks Tick Borne Dis.* **2020**, *11*, 101458. [CrossRef]
39. Epis, S.; Mandrioli, M.; Genchi, M.; Montagna, M.; Sacchi, L.; Pistone, D.; Sassera, D. Localization of the bacterial symbiont *Candidatus* Midichloria mitochondrii within the hard tick *Ixodes ricinus* by whole-mount FISH staining. *Ticks Tick Borne Dis.* **2013**, *4*, 39–45. [CrossRef]
40. Stavru, F.; Riemer, J.; Jex, A.; Sassera, D. When bacteria meet mitochondria: The strange case of the tick symbiont *Midichloria mitochondrii*. *Cell. Microbiol.* **2020**, *22*, e13189. [CrossRef]
41. Karesh, W.B.; Cook, R.A.; Bennett, E.L.; Newcomb, J. Wildlife trade and global disease emergence. *Emerg. Infect. Dis.* **2005**, *11*, 1000–1002. [CrossRef]
42. Wilcove, D.S.; Rothstein, D.; Dubow, J.; Phillips, A.; Losos, E. Quantifying Threats to Imperiled Species in the United States. *BioScience* **1998**, *48*, 607–615. [CrossRef]
43. Erster, O.; Roth, A.; Avni, Z.; King, R.; Shkap, V. Molecular detection of *Rickettsia bellii* in *Amblyomma rotundatum* from imported red-footed tortoise (*Chelonoides carbonaria*). *Ticks Tick Borne Dis.* **2015**, *6*, 473–477. [CrossRef] [PubMed]

MDPI
St. Alban-Anlage 66
4052 Basel
Switzerland
Tel. +41 61 683 77 34
Fax +41 61 302 89 18
www.mdpi.com

Animals Editorial Office
E-mail: animals@mdpi.com
www.mdpi.com/journal/animals

www.ingramcontent.com/pod-product-compliance
Lightning Source LLC
LaVergne TN
LVHW070631100526
838202LV00012B/780
* 9 7 8 3 0 3 6 5 1 8 9 7 8 *